Franz Schmid

Cell Therapy
A new dimension of medicine

Cell
Therapy

Franz Schmid

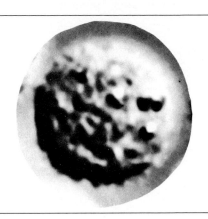

A new
dimension
of medicine

341 illustrations
of which 164 in colour
59 tables

Ott Publishers
Thoune Switzerland

The reproduction of trade marks, brand names
and other registered names or designs in this
book does not give good reason for believing
that, even without special mention, such names
were to be regarded as free within the meaning of
merchandise and trade mark protection
legislation.

Design: Franz Schmid, Aschaffenburg
Printed by
Ott Publishers, Thoune/Switzerland

Contents

CLINIC AND PRACTICE

Preface

Cell Therapy – a new dimension of medicine

The living organism, as a part of the universe, is embedded in the magnitude of the latter's dimensions. Within the wide boundaries of the electron mass of 10^{-31} to the cosmic dimension 10^{17}, life takes up only a small span of 10^{-5} to 10^1, thus only 6 out of 48 dimensions. Life begins at the organizational stage of the single cell and ends in the domain of the multicellular «organism» state. Life is characterized by the capability of the cells to transform the continuous energy and material losses of lifeless nature into new energies and structures. A cellular state deriving from these principles stands in reciprocal harmony with its lifeless environment and is described as healthy. Loss of utilization or deficiency of material of lifeless nature leads to defective functioning of the cellular state, to disease.

The paramount objective of medical treatment should be the restoration of the functional capability of the cells and of their functional associates, the tissues and organs. Medicine today orientates itself towards scientifically registerable symptoms or those deducible by means of technical aids (microscope, electron microscope, biochemical data, electronic recordings). It is thereby neglecting all dimensional areas below and above the so-called objective detection methods and in so doing it defines its limits. Thought levels below the visible correlations with nature, such as in homeopathy, or above them, such as in the embedment of life in earthly and cosmic relations in anthroposophy, lead a reluctant, patient marginal existence in the medical conception of the majority.

It may be that the brilliant idea P. NIEHANS put into practice 50 years ago of making young cells available to diseased or aging organs was erroneous. The idea was, nevertheless, rewarded with practical success. We know today that the implanted cells are decomposed in order of magnitude under microscopic observation, but it is precisely by these easily transportable and incorporable particles that important building substances for the repair of cellular and subcellular defects are supplied to the diseased organism. Moreover, the repair of cellular defects opens the possibility of a new materialization of the elementary functions of life, the utilization of the materials and energies of the environment. Whereupon, not only are symptoms eliminated, but the opportunity exists of producing afresh the fundamental principle of life, and with it health.

The evolution of life embraces a semicircle consisting of maturing, maturity and aging. Disabilities, disorders and diseases increase with the distance from the middle of this semicircle in the direction to the beginning and end of the biological existence. The main field for a therapy aimed at repairing the biological potential therefore lies inevitably in the first and the last decades of life. In the course of practical and clinical experiences the following areas of indications have crystallized:

9

I. Congenital and infantile developmental disturbances
1. Metabolic disorders
2. Chromosome aberrations
3. Insufficiencies and depressions in the blood-forming system
4. Immunologic deficiencies
5. Infantile disturbancies of the central nervous system

II. Degenerative changes caused by old age
6. General devitalization
7. Degenerative manifestations
   a) in the cardiovascular system
   b) in the central nervous system
   c) in the connective tissue
   d) in the digestive tract
   e) in the skin

III. Defective functioning of organs or organ systems arising from constitutional causes or disease
8. Chronic organic diseases of the heart, circulatory system, of the liver, joints
9. Defective functioning of the endocrine system
10. Hereditary degenerative diseases of the central nervous systems

IV. Concomitant tumour therapy
Within this group of indications the documented experimental values in respect of the strength of testimony range between single observations of uncommon diseases and statistical substantiations of up to thousandfold observations.

The implantation treatment with fetal or joung cell suspensions which has taken its place in medical history under the term «Cell Therapy» operates by way of the following therapeutic factors:
1. The rapidly growing intrinsic content of the fetal and young tissues of *biochemical substrates and enzymes.*
2. The fetal tissues' own composition of *minerals and trace elements.*

3. The fetal tissues' own *biological development power* which leads to rapid tissue growth.

Whilst biochemical substances (1) and elements (2) are analyzed in great detail, the biological development power is not measurable with scientific parameters. We know that roots, street pavements and stonework can lift, but we are not a position to interpret and to measure this power. In the therapeutical concept, it plays a big role since it alone makes possible the precondition for the application of the elements and the utilization of enzymes and substrates for new structures.

Away from the indicated connections with microcosm (elements, trace elements, elementary particles) and macrocosm (solar energy, cosmic radiation), cell therapy should always be a wholistic medicine. This means that necessary measures in the conduct of life, nutrition, physiotherapy, psychotherapy and medical treatment must be incorporated insofar as they are required in the individual situation. No form of therapy is a one and only redeeming religion. The «monosymptom – monosubstance» claim of pharmacotherapy is one of the most disastrous dogmatizing efforts of our time.

Cell therapy provides a body, under suitable application, with the opportunity of transforming the elementary function of life, the utilization of environmental energies and materials into new energies and structures. This step in a new dimension in medicine leads, in the longer aspect, from a «medicine for disease» to a «medicine for health», i.e. the therapeutic efforts are not focussed on the elimination of single symptoms of disease but serve in the restoration of the vital elementary functions of an organism.

10

FOUNDATIONS

The cell as a biological elementary unit

From R. HOOKE's discovery (1663) disclosing more than 300 years ago that the bark of the cork-oak consisted of elements similar to honeycombs, all along to modern cell biology a fascinating way leads into ever deeper fields of knowledge. Owing to the «rimmed» cavities seen in the microscopie section, the structures were called «cells». This observation was not introduced into the scientific standard knowledge until the middle of the 19th century. M. SCHLEIDEN (1838) stated that the cell was the basic unit of all plant structures, TH. SCHWANN extended this axiom to animals and plants. With R. VIRCHOW's cell research and his formulation that all life came from cells, cell morphology began to influence and to largely characterize human-medical thinking.

However, nearly another century went by before deeper dimensions were reached from the «little clot protoplasm» or from the «simultaneous existence of nucleus and cellular plasma». The picture of the cell, from historical and modern angles, reflects the technical potentialities of cell research. The structures watched in the light microscope had possessed the mental conceptions for nearly 300 years till the electron microscope opened morphologically new dimensions, till molecular biology and genetics accomplished the step from the mere contemplation of form (structure) to function. This process paralleled the discovery of subcellular structures and elements of organization, which, necessarily, raised the question of their significance (= function within the biological order). Though we believe to have a good conceptual power about the cell, most of the questions of functional interplay within and between the cells are obscure. What we do have, optically, is nothing but a skeleton of structures made visible by chemical influences (colouring) or physical processes (electron-microscopical sections). These methods provide conceptions of structures and space arrangements constituting just the rough brickwork of a house that only allows suppositions about its life and installations. Observations in vivo and cytochemical methods, therefore, help to explain the function of the elementary organization unit of life, namely of the cell.

The *ground plan* of the cell reflects the phylogenetic order. From the most primitive cells, the mycoplasmacateae, the evolution goes via the bacteria, blue algae, the higher plant cells to the complex system of the cells with membrane barriers and complete organelle fitments in multi-cellular and higher organized organisms. The further evolution will probably not continue through variations of the cytoorganelles but will depend on a further differentiation of the interrelations between the cells.

The obligatory building elements of the higher cells include:

1. *Nucleus*
2. *Nucleolus*
3. *Nuclear membrane*
4. *Nucleopores*
5. *Endoplasmatic Reticulum (Ergastoplasm)*
6. *Ribosomes*
7. *Golgi-apparatus*
8. *Vesiculae*
9. *Vacuoles*
10. *Granules of secretion*
11. *Lysosomes*
12. *Mitochondria*
13. *Centriol*
14. *Microtubuli*
15. *Cell membrane (Plasmalemm)*
16. *Desmosomes*
17. *Basic plasma (matrix)*

The form and function of the cell organelles are subject to functionally determined variations of a uniform building principle. The task in the functional unit cell can just be sketched in the scope of this survey.

The *nucleus* consists of chromatin containing DNA, the *nucleolus* constitutes a ball consisting of RNA (ribonucleic acid) in the nucleus. The *nuclear membrane* consists of 2 leaves, the outer

lined with ribosomes and going over into the *endoplasmatic reticulum;* it is interrupted by nucleopores. The so-called *perinuclear space* is between the two membranes.

The *Golgi-apparatus* has various forms, consists of membranes, forms *sacculi, double membranes, vacuoles* and *vesiculae;* it serves for tasks of synthesis and controls and eliminates products of synthesis, which are conveyed on by vesiculae, vacuoles and secretion granules and eventually are eliminated through the cell membrane. The Golgi-apparatus and the endoplasmatic reticulum are connected by the *Gerl complex.*

The protein synthesis takes place on the ribosomes of the *endoplasmatic reticulum.* The density and dimensions of this system (referred to also as *ergastoplasm*) of tubular membranes reflects the synthetizing activity of the cell (see fig. 2).

Mitochondria are elliptic, spheric, rod-shaped and filiform structures $0.3-5\,\mu m$ in length; thanks to their enzymes, they provide the energy for the cell, and therefore are also called energy stations or transformers. According to the activity of metabolism, a cell consequently contains more or fewer mitochondria.

The *microtubuli* and *fibrillary structural elements* are referred to as «metaplasm». Microtubuli have a diameter of $200-300\,\text{Å}$, are of different length and traverse the cytoplasm, but are chiefly oriented in the direction of centriol.

The *centriol* is near the nucleus, mostly in the middle of the cell, at the concave side of the Golgi-apparatus; this area is also called *centrosphere*. Nine groups about $0.5\,\mu$ in length of three mictrotubuli (triplets) form a cylinder of some $0.25\,\mu$ in diameter. The cylinder is surrounded by spherical satellites. The centriol contains extrachromosomal DNA, determines and controls cell division and –

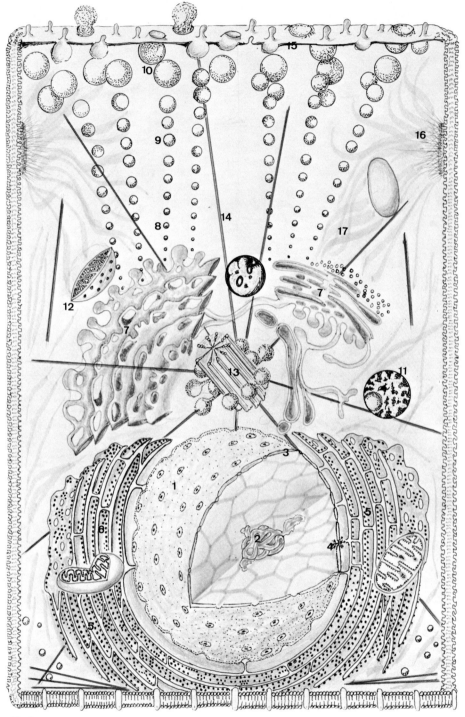

Fig. 1:
Idealized scheme of a *polar cell*

13

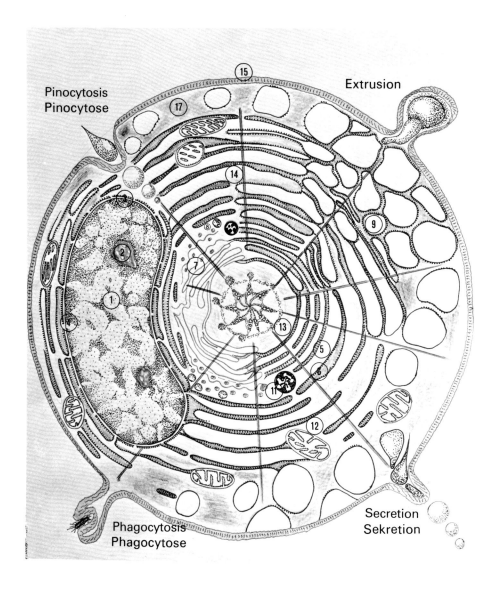

Fig. 2:
Idealized scheme of an *unpolar cell*, immunocyte in the stage of synthesis.

1. *Nucleus*
2. *Nucleolus*
3. *Nuclear membrane*
4. *Nucleopores*
5. *Endoplasmatic reticulum (ergastoplasm)*
6. *Ribosomes*
7. *Golgi-apparatus*
8. *Vesiculae*

9. *Vacuoles*
11. *Lysosomes*
12. *Mitochondria*
13. *Centriol*
14. *Microtubuli*
15. *Cell membrane (Plasmalemm)*
17. *Basic plasma (matrix)*

like the mitochondria – is considered as semi-autonomous in the cell organization.

Lysosomes are spherical to oval, of various density and serve for the intracellular digestion – perhaps also for «autocleaning».

The *cell membrane* (Plasmalemm) consists of 3 layers, has an average thickness of 75–100 Å, and is semipermeable; it regulates the interrelations with the extracellular space and can take up into the cell liquid (pinocytosis) or solid particles (phagocytosis) by advancing and retiring movements (fig. 2). The cell membrane contains enzymes and receptors to recognize foreign substances, hormones and other cells.

Desmosomes are organelles specialized as suctorial discs serving for the cohesion of cells; this clinging function appears from clusters of tonofibrils. Depending on whether the cell moves single in the liquid medium or is bound in the tissue, it is an unpolar (radiary) or polar cell.

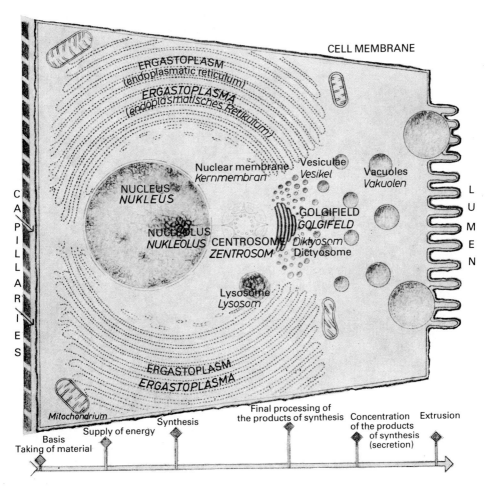

Fig. 3:
Functional scheme of a polar cell (e. g. pancreatic cell)

The *unpolar cell* (fig. 2) has the form of balls or ball-like rotation ellipses and adapts its shape to streaming conditions. The ingestion of material is effected from the surface from various directions, the elimination into various directions determined by laws of structure. The ways of transport are radiary into and out of the cell. Prototypes of these unpolar cells are the blood and exudate cells, specially monocytes, histiocytes and plasma cells. The cells have usually various tasks, are pluripotent and have, partly, kept the omnipotence of embryonal cells.

Cells bound in the tissue are chiefly specialized and polar. As far as they produce secretions (see fig. 3), 3 zones in the course of function must, theoretically, be defined.

1. From a *supply base* via capillaries, biochemical substances are infiltrated into the cells, mostly in connection with fluids.
2. The *zone of synthesis* includes the ergastoplasm, the Golgifeld and the system of vesicles and cisterns.
3. The *products* of synthesis are controlled by the Golgi-apparatus, collected in secretion granules and cisterns, transported towards the apical cell membrane and there, via the cell membrane, deposited either to the nearest cell or into a cavity.

Cells bound in the tissue lose, when specialised, the pluripotence of unpolar cells in the fluid medium and mostly serve for selective tasks of metabolism.

The Nucleus

The core of the cell (nucleus) is an obligatory cell organelle (except for the erythrocytes), usually the most voluminous and most conspicuous formation inside the cell, typically spheric, oval or reniform but very capable of adapting itself to functional requirements. The chromatin built of desoxyribonucleic acid is divided into heterochromatin and euchromatin (interchromatin) with a more active metabolism. The nucleolus (corpuscle of the core) containing ribonucleic acid is embedded in the chromatin substance. The covering of the nucleus separates its «genetic area» from the «economic area» of the cytoplasm. Interruptions of the nuclear covering, the nucleopores, assure an exchange of material between the nucleus and the space of cytoplasm.

Definition

The nucleus is an obligatory cell organelle surrounded by a membrane, which includes the genetic potential in the form of the DNA-containing chromatin and the nucleolus.

Historical data

After the discovery of the cell structure of charcoal and cork by R. HOOKE (1663), it took nearly two centuries till R. BROWN (1837) recognized the nucleus and E. R. v. PURKINJE (1839) postulated that all living creatures consisted of cells (cell theory). At the same time, M. SCHLEIDEN (1838) was the first to describe the nucleolus and recognized the cellular structure of the plants, which recognition was extended to the animal kingdom by TH. SCHWANN in 1839. In his classical work «Microscopic Studies on the Conformity of the Structure and Growth of the Animals and Plants» he defines the cell as a structure of cell mucus, cell wall and nucleus with one or several nuclear corpuscles (cit. H. A. HIENZ, 1971).

The chromosomes were described first by K. W. NÄGELI in 1842. Not until more than 30 years later, E. STRASSBURGER (1875) became aware of their part in mitosis. The name «chromosomes» (chromo = colour–some = body) goes back to H. W. G. v. WALDEYER (1888).

Morphology

The findings resulting from the light microscope became more differentiated by electron-optical information.

The nucleus is spheric, ovoid, reniform, but can adapt itself very well to functional requirements (fig. 7). The contents of the nucleus are formed, in the language of the light-microscopy, by the «nuclear dyestuff» namely the chromatin and the nuclear corpuscle or corpuscles (nucleolus). Electron-optically, two kinds of chromatin can be differentiated: the heterochromatin near the nuclear membrane of the nucleolus consists of osmiophile granules 100–150 Å in diameter and of filaments about 50 Å thick (R. V. KRSTIĆ, 1976). The euchromatin or interchromatin, being less tight to electrons, is between the areas of heterochromatin; in question is probably the chromatin with a more active metabolism (fig. 6, 7).

The chromatin contains the genetic information in its desoxyribonucleic acid structures; the nucleolus includes ribonucleic acid.

Metabolic activity of the nucleus is suggested by deformation and deficiency in chromatin. At the same time, the nucleolus or nucleoli grow, the perinu-

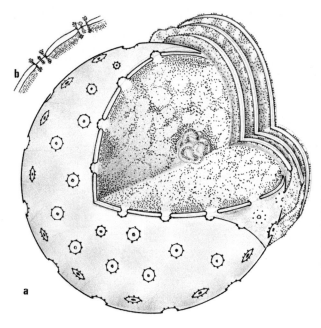

Fig. 4:
Model of nucleus seen from above with segmental section. Nuclear membrane of two layers, with nucleopores, in b) in longitudinal section; heterochromatin and euchromatin and nucleolus. The connections with the endoplasmatic reticulum are lined out on the right.

17

cleolar chromatin increases, a pars amorpha and a nucleolonema can be marked off clearer inside the nucleolus.

The form and structure of the nucleus meet the functional requirements. The nucleus in the head of the sperms e.g. is adapted to the hydrodynamic conditions of sliding and penetrating membranes, as a mediator of the genetic substance comparatively large in proportion to the threadlike cytoplasm. The egg-cell, on the other hand, has a relatively small nucleus and a large space for the cyto-plasm. Nuclei of cylindric epithelia are adapted to the axis of the cylinder, the multi-dimensional osteoblasts have many nuclei.

The nucleus is covered by a mem-brane, or rather, by a system of mem-branes. This covering of the nucleus con-sists of (fig. 4, 5):

a) The Lamina fibrosa nuclei (Zonula nuclei limitans), an optically lighter zone 200–600 Å deep, which sepa-rates the chromatin substance from the (inner) nuclear membrane; it con-sists of microfilaments 20–50 Å thick, and probably represents the nuclear skeleton.

b) The inner layer represents the nuclear membrane proper i.e. the boundary line between the nucleus and the cyt-oplasm.

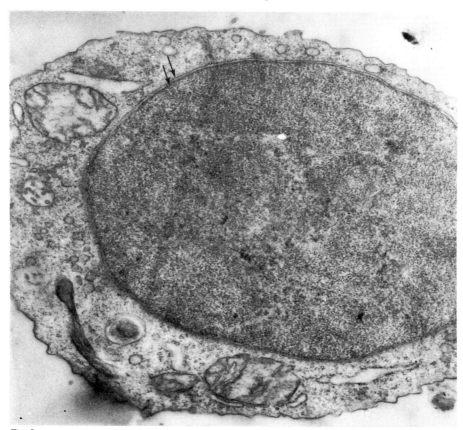

Fig. 5:
Double-layer nuclear membrane (arrows) in a large lymphocyte. Electron-optic final magnif. 1 : 20,000.

c) The outer leaf belongs to the endoplasmatic reticulum and is usually lined with ribosomes.

d) Both leaves are separated from each other by the perinuclear space 200–500 Å deep.

The nuclear covering is interrupted by the nucleopores.

Nucleopores

At the crease of the inner leaf of the nuclear covering adjacent to the outer leaf (fig. 4a, b) a membrane 50–100 Å thick, called diaphragm, spans the gap of the covering structure. Round openings are formed with a mean diameter of about 600 Å – the nucleopores. The centre of a nucleopore includes a consolidation area large about 100 Å, osteophile structures at the edge consolidate to constitute the so-called anulus; these structure elements make the nucleopores look like shooting practice targets when viewed from above.

A hypothetic postulate (FRANKE 1970, KRSTIĆ 1976) maintains that the anulus and the centre of the nucleopores consist of 8 or 1 (for the centre) clusters of thread molecules. These thread molecules span the diaphragm and, partly, project into the nuclear space, with their

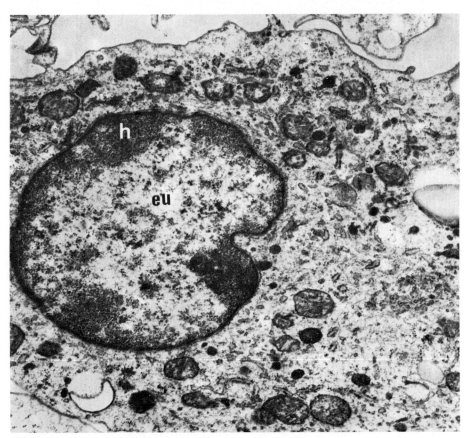

Fig. 6:
Dispersion of *heterochromatin* (h = darker areas in the nucleus) and euchromatin (eu = lighter parts) in a monocyte. Magnif. 1:15,000.

centripetal ends into the cytoplasm (fig. 4b). The areas of nuclear heterochromatin in the zone of the nucleopores are interrupted, which, electron-optically, causes brighter halos within the covering of the nucleus.

Even though it is difficult to make exact assertions about the function of the nucleopores, it can hardly be called in question that they serve for the metabolism between the nucleus and the space of cytoplasm. A quarter of the nuclear surface is occupied by the nucleopores. Through them, elements of the nucleic acids – chiefly aminoacids, purines – get from the cytoplasm into the nucleus. The nucleus for its part infiltrates, via the nucleolus, RNA (ribonucleic acid) through the nucleopores into the space of the cytoplasm.

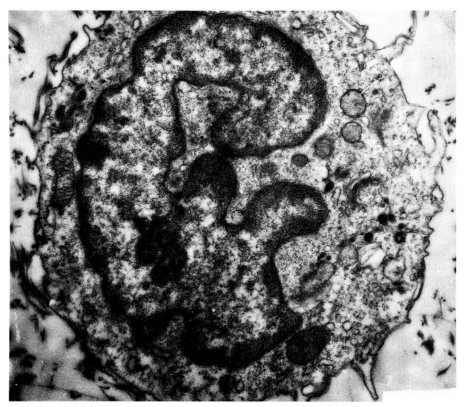

Fig. 7:
Plastic adaptability of the *nuclear form* in a monocyte. Large and optically compact nucleolus. Magnif. 1 : 15,000.

The Nucleolus

constitutes an optically outstanding structure (or 2–3) within the nucleus. A rounded, oval to polymorphous irregular body, the nucleolus (pars granulosa) is closely connected with the lighter areas of the pars fibrosa (amorpha) and the perinucleolar chromatin. The granules of the pars granulosa have a diameter of 150 Å, the filaments of the pars fibrosa about 50 Å (fig. 4, 8).

Whereas the nucleolus, electron-optically, is usually more compact than the neighbouring chromatin substance, it contrasts as a brighter area in the light microscope by panchromatic staining. DNA staining (FEULGEN) leaves the nucleolus invisible in the nucleus, differential staining of nucleic acid (methyl-green pyronin) distinguishes the DNA from the RNA areas of the nucleus.

The nucleolus is integrated into the function of the nucleus and has no membrane. Its purpose is to produce ribonucleic acid (RNA) after the information pattern of the DNA of the nucleus, and to yield it as a mediator of information to the cytoplasm. The M-RNA regulates the synthesis of the ribosomes of the en-

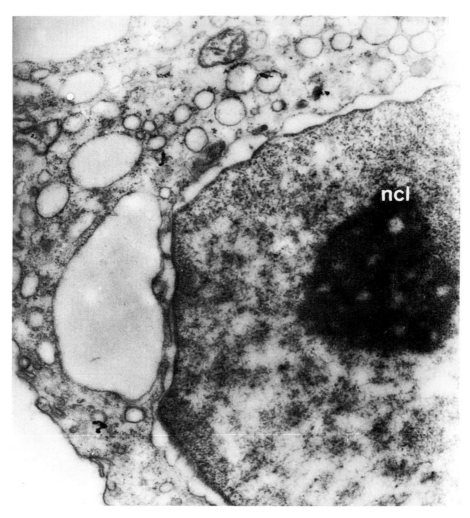

Fig. 8:
Nucleolus (ncl), in which the more compact pars granulosa can be clearly distinguished from the lighter areas of the pars amorpha (fibrosa). Immunocyte in the stage of secretion, final magnif. 1 : 18,000.

doplasmatic reticulum. Metabolic cells therefore contain large or several nucleoli near to or in close contact with the nuclear membrane.

The nucleolus can usually be seen well in the «resting nucleus». During the division of the nucleus it disappears between the prophase and the prometaphase. The RNA synthesis is stopped from the middle of the prophase to the end of the telophase; as soon as the nuclei and the cell membranes of the daughter cells have been retransformed to organelles, the nucleolus reappears.

Function

The biological function of the nucleus is to control the genetic information by means of the nuclear DNA and its morphological aggregates, the chromosomes. The «genetic check point» as an ecological unit inside the cell is separated by a double membrane from the cytoplasm, the «economic space of the cell». The necessary metabolism is effected through the nucleopores. The most active metabolic part of the nucleus is the nucleolus, point of the synthesis and collecting centre of the ribonucleic acid. There are direct relations through the nucleolus and the nucleopores to the space of cytoplasm, here especially to the centriol and the ribosomes of the endoplasmatic reticulum.

Cytomembranes

The *membrane of the cytoplasm* has metabolic functions and protective mechanisms, the solution of which, depending on the biomedium, requires special structures. Membranes, typically, are areas of contact, which separate and mediate. In biology, barriers and mediating surfaces form between morphological and functional units. Membranes fit together without steps and thus include an ecological space. They account for the ingestion, penetration and elimination of substances in this space. The substances can be ingested solid (= phagocytosis) or liquid (= pinocytosis); the penetration is called permeation, and the substances are eliminated in a liquid (= secretion) or solid (= extrusion) form.

The *main function* of the cytomembranes, namely the contact to the environment for the supply of food and protection against harmful influences from outside has antagonistic properties. An increase of the protective function means loss of elasticity, hinders the transport of substances and impairs mobility. Plants reinforce their membranes with cellulose, often by thick layers (bark), animals with scales and spines, or with lime, like the animals in the sea.

The cytomembranes are the *prototype* of the biological membranes inside the organism of the mammals. Their classical description is the *Danielli-Davson model* (Danielli and DAVSON, 1935; DA-NIELLI, 1967). According to it, the membrane of cytoplasm consists of a continuous layer of probably bimolecular lipoids with an insoluble film of proteins on either side (fig. 9). The protein is said to be bound to the layer of lipoids by electrostatic interaction. Moreover, hexagonal phases are supposed to occur inside the watery mixture of phosphorus-lipoids; they can appear especially at higher temperatures ($37°C$) and a low content of water (3%) (STOOKENIUS, 1962). For their arrangement, either linear formation of lipoids (fig. 9) or globular patterns are supposed (LEHNINGER, 1968). HASSELBACH showed recently that both formations are found side by side on the same object. Linear lipoids formations and globular arrangements may, consequently, represent different functional conditions on the same membrane.

The Danielli-Davson model is compatible with the unit-membrane concept (ROBERTSON, 1961, 1966; SJÖSTRAND, 1963; YAMAMOTO, 1963) because the latter includes also three layers. The outer contact layer of the protoplasm represents in the electron microscope a structure unit of three layers having a mean thickness of 70 Å. The detail-dates of structure and function were summarisized by SINGER and NICOLSON (1972) in the «fluid mosaic model». The majority of the proteins are understood as integrated «swimming» elements in a «quasi-fluid» Phospholipid-layer.

Biochemistry

Cytomembranes constitute a formation of lipoid and protein molecules. The inner layer of a cytomembrane consists of a bimolecular lipoid formation, whose hydrophobic poles are turned towards each other. The hydrophilous poles however are pointed at the extracellular and intracellular spaces. The lipoids layer is surrounded by a protein layer «outside» and «inside». The protein molecules constitute unfolded, parallel threads, whose basic direction in the cellular membrane is radial. The protein threads are connected with each other by hydrogen bridges. This pleated-sheet structure explains the elasticity and plasticity of the membrane. Macromolecules can be deposited on the outer and inner sides of the protein layer; this accounts for the high adhesive and binding capability of the membranes.

The differentiated multilayered structure of the cytomembrane provides a several times secured barrier, which is a prerequisite for the bionomy of the enclosed spaces. The organization inside the cell is more differentiated and more complex than the extracellular space. The autonomy of cellular activity and the selective functions of the cell organelles can subsist only while the intracellular complexity continues reciprocally and protected by effective barriers against the extracellular space.

On the other hand, one and the same membrane must regulate selectively the metabolism between the extracellular and intracellular spaces so that sub-stances drawn from the humoral pool for the intracellular metabolic processes can be ingested and superfluous or even harmful substances as well as products of cellular synthesis can be eliminated into the extracellular space. The question whether the cytomembrane has po res is still controversial, but solid and li quid substances can certainly pass, and a gap in the cytomembrane can be made vi sible by lipoid staining. A temporary ga ping in the lipoid layer seems to be the decisive process in the *ingestion* and *extrusion* of larger particles (fig. 29, 176–179).

The lipoid layer is likely to regulate also the *permeation* of dissolved substances through the cytomembrane as well as the *diffusion*. Gaseous substances such as H_2, O_2 and CO_2 permeate readily, electrolytes less so. Neutral lipoids are unsoluable, therefore not permeable, lipoids with acid groups allow to pass the cations, lipoids with alkaline groups the anions (KLIMA, BEUTNER).

Thanks to the different distribution of the ions between the intracellular and extracellular spaces, the cytomembrane

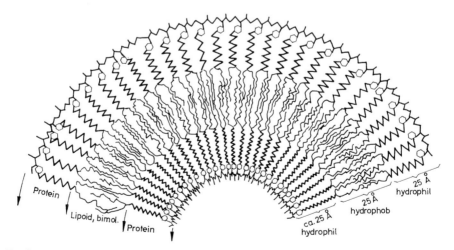

Fig. 9:
Three layers and architectonics of the cytomembrane, which consists, with an average thickness of about 70 Å, of two protein layers and a bimolecular lipoid layer.

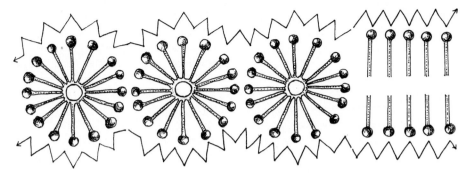

Fig. 10:
Globular arrangement of the membrane layers in a formation favouring the transportation of the membrane.

has an electric potential (= *membrane potential*), which is usually between 50–100 mV, but depends on the functions. This potential compensates the difference of concentrations for K⁺- and Cl-ions. In nerve cells, the resting potential is 50 mV, the action potential (stimulation) is 80–130 mV. The inner side of the membrane is negative when at rest, and positive when excited.

Elementary or alpha-cytomembranes not only serve for cellular boundary barriers but also within the cell divide regions with different functions to form *bionomous units.* A tubular system, the *endoplasmatic reticulum or ergastoplasm,* forms spaces arranged like conveyor belts for cellular synthetic functions (hormones, ferments, antibodies). Cytomembranes enclose *vacuoles,* intracellular cavities containing fluids and substrates, which are better referred to as *vesicles* (small) or *cisterns* (large) because they are not «empty». Finally the nucleus, subject to its own laws, is separated from the cytoplasma space by the nuc-

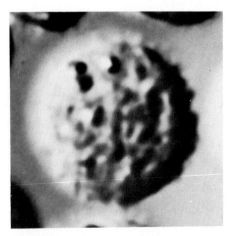

Fig. 11:
Membrane activity of (peritoneal) exudate cells with visible convex and concave areas on the surface.

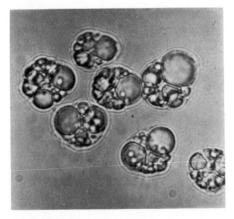

Fig. 12:
Membrane activity of living (peritoneal) exudate cells as seen in the phase-contrast microscope. Several ecological spaces surrounded by membranes within the cells are visible.

lear membrane (fig. 4, 5), same as the energy stations of the cell, the mitochondria (fig. 36–41).

Membranes create and separate more functional spaces where metabolic processes can take place, and whose substrates might endanger or even destroy other parts of cells and cellular organelles unless they were delimited by membranes. Pinocytosis causes in this way vesicles filled with fluid of the extracellular space i.e. having fluids of other quality and concentrations of electrolytes, to be transported through the space of cytoplasm to the Golgifield. Phagocytosis causes solid substances to disintegrate in «digestive vacuoles» (see fig. 176) enclosed by membranes with a pH hardly compatible with the life of the cytoplasmatic space. Here, separated and yet connected with the cytoplasm by permeation and diffusion, the ingested material is broken down into the steps of degradation the cytoplasm can take up without a risk.

Membrane systems separate and connect units of biological functions unbalanced biochemically and physically. The chemico-physical unequality necessary for the performance of differentiated functions can be maintained only by membranes. Membrane systems, consequently, are boundary surfaces regulating selectively the ingestion and extrusion of substances and the exchange of information between the function

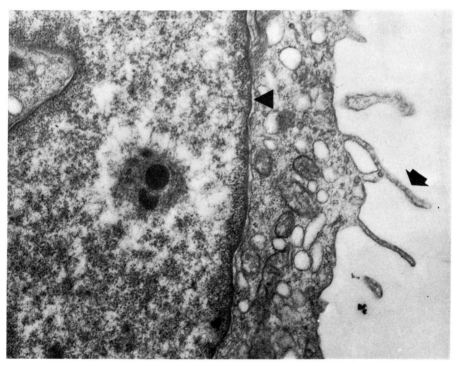

Fig. 13:
Bulges in the cytoplasm-membrane (arrow) of a monocyte. Nuclear membrane (wedge) comparatively thick (1:26,000).

spaces. The development from the monocellular being to the highly differentiated organisms of mammals is inconceivable without systems of membranes. The aging process of living beings is probably accounted for, above all, by an impairment of the functions of cytomembranes.

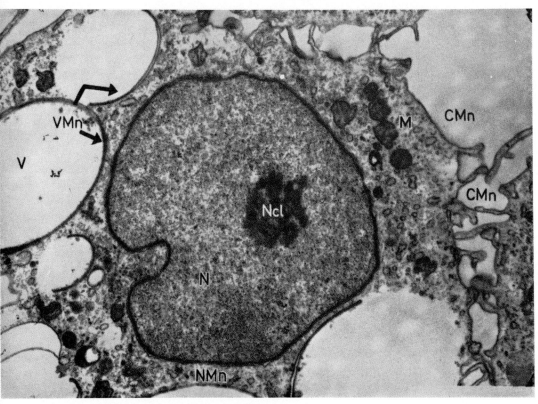

Fig. 14:
Most of the cellular organelles are *ecological spaces* surrounded by membranes such as nucleus, mitochondria, Golgi-apparatus, endoplasmatic reticulum and cytoplasm.

Membrane systems of a monocytary cell.
C Mn = cytoplasm membrane
N Mn = nuclear membrane
V Mn = vacuoles membrane
M = mitochondria, the membrane of which can also be seen

N = nucleus
Ncl = nucleolus
V = vacuole
Electronoptically 1 : 15,000
(SCHMID, WACHSMUTH and WALDECK).

Tab. 1: **Enzymes of the cytoplasm membrane**

Enzyme (synonym) activating ion	Enzyme commiss. No.	Tissue cell-type	Species
acetylecholinesterase	3.1.1.7.	brain synapsis	rat
		erythrocytes	man
alkaline phosphatase	3.1.3.1.	liver	rat
		intestine	rat
		thymocytes	calf
K^+		liver	rat
		kidney	
acid phosphatase	3.1.3.2.	cells	man
		liver	rat
		lymphocytes	pig
		thymocytes-t	calf
phosphatidase-phosphatase	3.1.3.4.	liver	rat
5-nucleotidase	3.1.3.5.	brain: neurons	rabbit
		synaptosomes	rat
		KB-cells	man
		liver	rat
		lymph-nodes, mesent.	pig
		thymocytes	calf
		hela-cells	man
		fat-cells	rat
phosphodiesterase I	3.1.4.1.	liver	rat
		kidney	rat
		hela-cells	man
aminopeptidase (cytosol) intestine	3.4.11.1.	liver	rat
			rat
adenosintriphosphatase ATPase Ca^{2+} and Mg^{2+}	3.6.1.3.		
MG^{2+}		liver	mouse
		liver	mouse
		erythrocytes	man
		thymocytes	calf
		thyroid gland	cat
adenosintriphosphatase MG^{2+}, K^+ and Na^+	3.6.1.3.		
		brain: neuron	rat
		synaptosomes	man
		KB-cells	mouse
		liver	rat
			rat
		heart	man
		erythrocytes	man
		hela-cells	cat
		thyroid gland	rat
		cross-striated muscle	rat
		fat-cells	

Enzyme (synonym) activating ion	Enzyme commiss. No.	Tissue cell-type	Species
nucleotide-pyrophosphatase	3.6.1.9.	liver	guinea-pig rat
adenyl-cyclase F⁻	4.6.1.1.	liver kidney thyroid gland	rat rat cat
entoenzymes on the outside of the plasma-membrane of intact cells			
alkaline phosphatase (p-nitrophenyl phosphatase	3.1.3.1.	polynucl. leukocytes	guinea-pig
5′ nucleotidase (AMPase)	3.1.3.5.	polynucl. leukocytes	guinea-pig
aminopeptidase (cytosol)	3.4.11.1.	hepatocytes	man
adenosintriphosphatase (ATPase)	3.6.1.3.	polynucl. leukocytes	guinea-pig
nucleotide-pyrophosphatase	3.6.1.9.	hepatocytes	man

The Golgi-apparatus

Historical data

In 1898, GOLGI described an «Apparato reticulare interno» in nerve-cells, which was discovered also in other cells of the body in the following years. Lamellary, filamentous structures, granules and vesicles were ascribed to this creation named after him «Golgi-apparatus» (PAPPENHEIMER, 1916). Owing to the variability of the structures depending on the kind of cells and functions, this system as an independent cellular organelle was controversial for decades. PARAT (1928) referred to the netlike structure, represented by impregnation with silver and osmium, as an artifact. HIRSCH (1939) was the first to state that the form depended on the function and mentioned the connection with secretions (pancreas, intestine, salivary glands). In spite of the better morphological differentiation by electron-microscopy opened by DALTON (1952–1956), SIÖSTRAND and HANZON (1954), many controversial interpretations were given later on. However, the independence of this system as cell organelle with synthetic and transporting functions is no longer doubted.

Morphology

The Golgi-apparatus occurs, with few exceptions (erythrocytes, keratinized epidermic cells), in all cells of the vertebrates, and is most conspicuous in se-

29

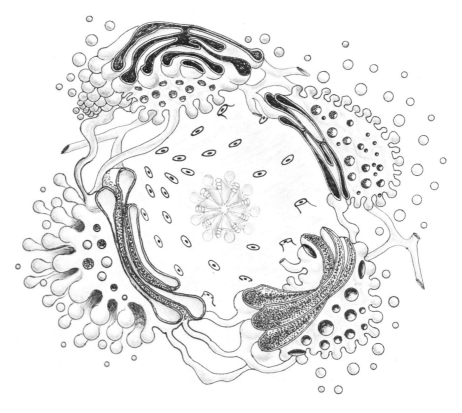

Fig. 15:
Three-dimensional representation of the *Golgi-apparatus* in its structural elements (lamellae and vesiculae) and interrelations to the nucleus and endoplasmatic reticulum.

creting cells i. e. in those which make and eliminate products of synthesis. The Golgi-apparatus, therefore, can be recognized well in cells of the pituitary gland, the Langerhans' islets, the tubular epithelium of the kidneys, the fundic glands of the stomach, adrenal-cortex cells and marrow cells, the neurons of the ganglious cells, the thalamus, the chemoreceptors of Glomus caroticus, the cerebral cortex (MÖLBERT). Several Golgifields connected with each other are found specially in the cells of the thalamus. Less developed are Golgi-apparatuses in skeleton muscles, myocardium, lung, epidermis.

Observations of ovocytes and sper-matocytes, moreover of cells of the oral mucosa have shown how much the morphological formation depends on the functional condition. In the stage of activation e. g. in the stages of incubation and exanthema of viral infectious diseases, the system can clearly be recognized by tubes and granules through cytochemical staining even in the light microscope (fig. 16) whereas these structures cannot be seen in cells at rest and with little metabolic activity.

The Golgi-apparatus consists of the following structural elements: double lamellae called sacculi (fig. 15, 18) for their bilateral club-shaped inflations; cistern-like, rounded, oval or irregular extensions (fig. 18) called vacuoles as they are «optically empty» but actually constitute spaces surrounded by membranes containing fluids and products of synthesis. Further, there are smaller or larger vesicles and granules (fig. 15, 16, 17). As the synthetic functions require high amounts of energy (in our examples synthesis of immunoglobulin) the Golgifield is interspersed with plenty of mitochondria and related intimately to the endoplasmatic reticulum (fig. 18). The orientation round the nucleus is rather conspicuous; if the latter, however, becomes peripherical when a compact, endoplasmatic reticulum is built up (e. g. in immunocytes, plasma cells), the probably more important orientation toward the centrosome (fig. 20) becomes visible (fig. 191).

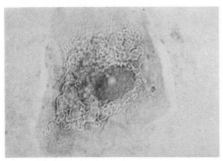

Fig. 16:
Cell of the pharyngeal epithelium in the stage of the measles exanthema, first day. Paranuclear consolidation, surrounded by a close-meshed network of tubes. Best-carmin coloration 1 : 1500.

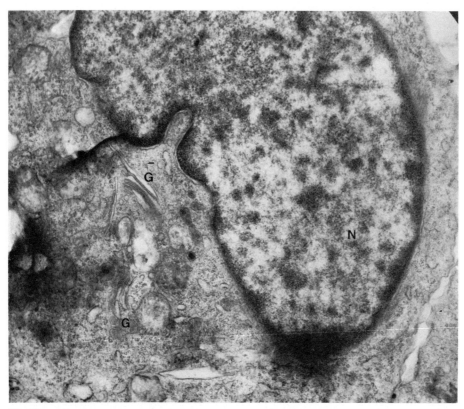

Fig. 17:
Lamellar structures of the Golgi-apparatus (G) in a monocyte-peritoneal exudate guinea-pig, 1 : 20,000. N = nucleus.

are 3–4 (up to 8) smooth double lamellae, which, layered roughly parallel, show a concave and a convex side (fig. 1, 18); these are cytochemically different (KRSTIĆ, 1976). The membranes have a diameter of cytomembranes – 60–80 Å –, the interval of a couple of membranes comes to 50–200 Å (POLLISTER and POLLISTER, 1957); intervals of about 200 Å are more frequent than minor figures. The membrane layers constitute the chromophile part of the Golgi system. The smooth membranes have often terminal club-shaped inflations, which gives the impression of dumbbell-like, parallel layered structures (fig. 15, 17). The membranes are interspersed with pores through which they communicate with the ground substance (fig. 15). The double membranes of the endoplasmatic reticulum (fig. 18) are guided by a flow of the double lamellae; the smooth elements near the Golgifield are referred to as Golgi-bound endoplasmatic reticulum. A connection of the Golgi-apparatus with the nuclear pores (indicated in fig. 15) is probable.

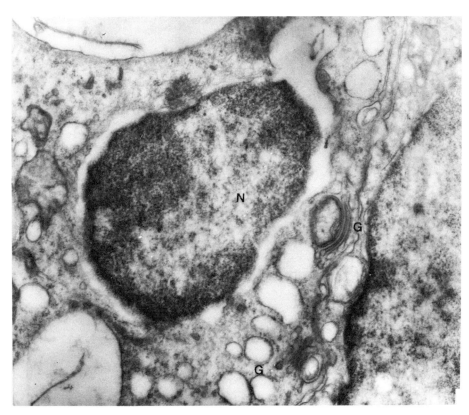

Fig. 18:
Golgi-apparatus (G) with large *vesicles* and *cisterns* in the secretory stage of an immunocyte (plasma cell), 1 : 18,000.

Vesiculae

arise by tying off bulges of membranes after club-shaped or dumb-bell-like extensions of the inner layers (LACY, 1956). POLICARD (1958) demonstrated on human leukocytes that the vesicles and granules split from the chromophobous part of the pairs of membranes so that they are on the convex side turned from the centrosome as shown in the three-dimensional representation of fig. 15; he therefore spoke of a polarity of the Golgifield determined by the centriole. The vesicles serve for the secretion of the products of synthesis as well as for their further chemical processing and their transportation through the cyto-

plasm. The so-called vacuoles are also constituents of this system of ecological spaces in the Golgi-apparatus dependent on the functional circumstances, filled with fluids and surrounded by membranes, somewhat more irregular as to their shape (fig. 18). There are various sizes from these cisterns and vesicles to the granules.

Granules

are found specially in secreting cells (fig. 15, 17). In particular, melanin granules were used to explain the interrelations.

Function

The functional interrelations result from the close relationship between the Golgi-apparatus, the endoplasmatic reticulum and mitochondria. The substances built up in the endoplasmatic reticulum are subject to final processing in the Golgi system before they are transported through the cytoplasm and excretion (secretion, clasmatosis). The products of synthesis «ripened» in the Golgi-membranes are tied off and eliminated through vesicles and granules. A condensation may take place in these ecological substructures surrounded by membranes; but its main function is probably the controlled transportation through the cell. The reduction of the endoplasmatic reticulum in the «starving condition» of the cell is followed by an inhibition of the protein synthesis, a gradual shrinking of the Golgi-membranes while the Golgi-products decrease (MÖLBERT).

Taggings with DL-leucin-4.5-3 H

(CARO and PALADE, 1964) have shown that the contents of cisterns in the endoplasmatic reticulum are tagged already 5 minutes after the injection, and that the Golgifields are tagged after 20 minutes and the zymogen granules show compact concentrations after 1 hour. Zymogen granules, consequently, seem to originate by flowing together and condensating vesicles and cisterns of the Golgi-apparatus. The condensated cisterns, vesicles and granules migrate centrifugally out of the Golgifield.

This principle has been demonstrated in cells of the milk-secreting mamma (BARGMANN and KNOOP, 1959), chondrocytes (SHELDON and KIMBALL, 1962), the Langerhans' islets, follicular cells of the thyroid gland, active cells of the parathyroid gland, hypophysis, neurons and many other secreting cells (survey see MÖLBERT, 1968). The processes were worked out most impressively by the collagenous synthesis (REVEL and HAY,

1963). By means of collagenous pro-phases tagged with radio-elements it has been demonstrated that after the protein synthesis in the ergastoplasm the materi-al is transported to the Golgi-apparatus via separate vesicles. The concentrated protein tagged with 3H-prolin can be identified as fine fibrils in Golgi-cisterns of 0.2–0.5 mi, migrates with the vesicles out of the Golgifield and is found later in the extracellular space as material tagged with radio-elements.

Apart from structural functions, the Golgi-apparatus effects a number of key-processes of the intermediary me-tabolism: the synthesis of the carbohy-drates, specially the glycogen; formation of triglycerides; formation of myelin; formation of pigments. The following enzymes have been identified: alkaline phosphatase in epithelial cells of the small intestine and tubular cells; nucleo-side-diphosphatase in duodenal cells;

acid phosphatases in tubular epithelia and liver cells as well as thyroid cells acti-vated with thyreotropin.

The Golgi-apparatus is extended as a result of great synthetic and secretory ac-tivity of the cells, after application of dia-mox (2-acetyl-amine-1.3.4-thiadiazol-5-sulphonamide), after doses of oestrogen at the epithelium of the uterus of mice, after stimulation with phytohaemagglut-inine in lymphocytes. Intensified trans-portation of fluids receives expression in an increase of large cisterns (MÖLBERT, 1968).

Atrophies or degeneration of Golgi-fields are found in many tumour cells, es-pecially in carcinoma of the bladder (OBERLING, 1959).

The origin of the Golgi membranes has not been explained. Divergent find-ings indicate causalities with the centri-oles, the nuclear membrane and the en-doplasmatic reticulum.

Centrioles

Definition: a centriole or diplosome is a characteristic, semi-autonomous cellu-lar organelle, which, situated between the nucleus and Golgifield, regulates the division of cells by mitosis. If the area round the centriole is included in the function, the unit is called centro-some.

Morphology

The centriole or diplosome (= pair of centrioles of the cell) is situated near the nucleus, in disrounded cells mostly at the concave side – within the Golgifield, here also at the concave side of the bent multilayered Golgi lamellae (see fig. 1, 17, 18). The area round the centri-ole is called *centrosphere;* if the parts of the Golgi apparatus are included in the consideration, *centrosomes* are in ques-tion (fig. 3).

The positions of centrioles form the letter L (KRSTIĆ). Every centriole shows a characteristic formation of the ci-pher 9. Nine groups of microtubuli (trip-lets) about 0.5 mi m long form a cylinder of about 0.25 mi m in diameter (fig. 19). The triplets include angles of about 50°. The diameter of a microtubulus comes to about 200 Å; only the inner microtubu-lus turned to the lumen of the cylinder is circular, the two outer ones have a more crescent-shaped cross-section when viewed from above. Two appendages of an electron-tight material protrude from the inner microtubulus; one of these appendages goes centripetally to the middle of the centriole cylinder and thus forms a ray of a star of 9 rays; the second appendage goes in an obtuse angle to the outer microtubulus of the neighbouring triplet (fig. 21). These branches thus outline more or less the outer wall of the centriole cylinder.

The centriole cylinder is surrounded by a zone of more compact material. Under favourable conditions of representation this zone dissolves to form spherical structures, which a stalk connects with the cylinder. These optically more compact spherical formations are referred to as satellites and are origin and guiding scope for the formation of microtubuli (fig. 21).

In round cells, especially in leukocytes, the centrosome (= centriole + Golgifield) shows a distinct rhythmical oscillation (BESSIS M., 1972). In cell agony these movements of the central cell organelles subside, the cell undergoes some sort of liquefaction, which finally also destroys the centrosome. The centrosome is more resistant than the nucleus. The area of the centrosome is paler in the living cell and free from granules. In the oscillation, the nucleus takes shape round these seemingly more rigid structures. The centriole can just seldom be seen in the optical microscope as the size is close to the limit of dissolubility; under favourable circumstances, it can be recognized as a concentration within radial structures.

The relations between centriole and nuclear membrane are interpreted in different ways. LETTRÉ and LETTRÉ (1958), relying on a voluminous literature, were of the opinion that chromosomes, spindle fibres and centriole constituted a

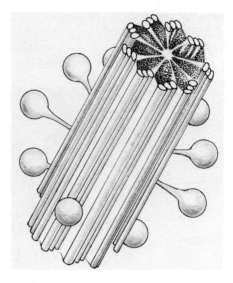

Fig. 19:
Three-dimensional representation of the *centriol.* Cylinder of 27 tubuli in 9 triplets. Radiate satellites.

permanent structural unit, which remained invisible in the interphase of the cell. According to BESSIS and LONQUIN (1950), POLICARD and BESSIS (1953), the nucleus follows the movements of the centriole at a certain interval when the centriole moves away from the nucleus. The classical descriptions of the centriole by DE HARVEN and BERNHARD (1956) as well as STUBBLEFIELD and BRINKLEY (1967) give the following characterization: The centriole consists of 27 tubuli arranged in 9 groups. Three tubuli make a lamella. Every lamella forms an angle of 30° to the surface of the cylinder. Inside the cylinder there is a filamentous structure, with a helix having 8–10 threads to the length of the cylinder. The microtubuli are perpendicular to the axis of the cylinder. In the cells of the haematopoetic apparatus, the satellites are often arranged like spokes

35

round the centriole. The satellites have a diameter of 600–900 Å; they form two pericentriole coronae, from which the microtubuli issue. At the end of cell division the centrioles double by self-reduplication. Polyploid cells – e. g. megacaryocytes – contain up to 30 and even more centrioles.

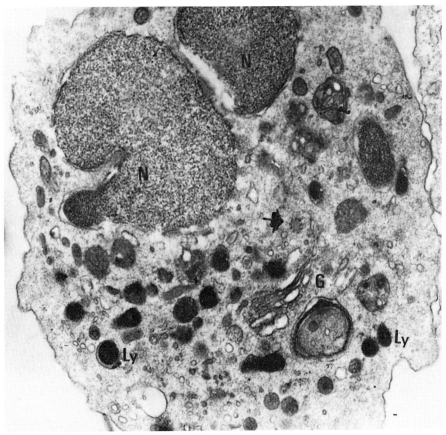

Fig. 20:
Polynuclear peritoneal exudate cell abundant in *lysosomes* (Ly) in the neighbourhood of the Golgi-field (G); N = cut nuclei. The lysosomes are homogenous, compact. Centriol (arrow).

Function

Centrioles have functions in mitosis, in the development of microtubuli as formations of the cell skeleton and for the movement of cells.

In the most important form of cell multiplication – as an expression of the perpetuation of the species of cells – mitosis is controlled by the centriole.

Prophase. In the prophase, chromatin condensations form near the nuclear membrane. The nucleolus is still in good condition, the nuclear membrane intact.

Prometaphase. The next step already shows the function of the pair of centrioles: microtubuli radiate from here and

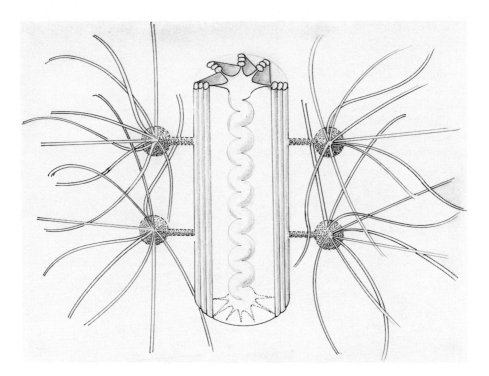

Fig. 21:
Cross-section of a *centriol* with cylinder wall, central helix, satellites and radiating microtubuli.

form the astrosphere when the chromatin masses of the nucleus have moved apart into 2 condensation fields, when the nucleolus has disappeared and the nuclear membrane shows larger or smaller interruptions or duplications. The astrosphere develops in the neighbourhood of the largest dehiscence of the nuclear membrane.

Metaphase. Microtubuli develop from the satellites in the formation of the «metaphasic spindle» (fig. 22) while the centrioles migrate towards the poles. As the chromosomes gather in the equatorial plane of the cell in the form of the so-called «equatorial plate», mitochondria, Golgi-apparatus and endoplasmatic reticulum disperse in equal parts on the halves of the cells. The microtubular apparatus issuing from the centrioles

shows two orienting planes; long bipolar «continuous» microtubuli connect the centrioles of the two cell poles; short «interzonal» microtubuli are between the chromosomes. Thus the metaphasic spindle gets a three-dimensional skeleton, by the long microtubuli in the polar dimension and by the shorter in the Aequatorial plane.

Anaphase. By shortening the chromosomal microtubuli, either half of the chromosomes –the chromatides– is drawn to the corresponding cell pole. By condensation of the chromosomes isolated before, a nuclear fragment develops at either pole and is covered by a nuclear membrane first on the peripheral side.

At the same time, the microtubuli of the equatorial plane shorten and thus cause the constriction in the middle of the cell (fig. 23–26).

Telophase. Through a wider, hourglass-like constriction go compact, nearly parallel, polewise microtubuli surrounded by consolidated substance at the narrowest point. Here, the two halves of the cells are separated later. Nucleus,

nuclear membrane have formed anew in the two halves, and the nucleolus reappears at the end of the telophase.

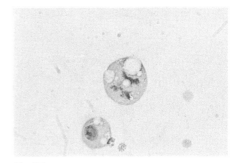

Fig. 24:
Mitosis: the chromosome couples have separated and move towards the cell poles. Monocyte. Alkal. phosphatase colouring.

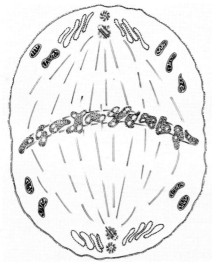

Fig. 22:
Arrangement of the *chromosomes* in the equatorial plane, of the centriols at the opposite cellular poles, of the polar interzonal and equatorial short microtubuli during mitosis.

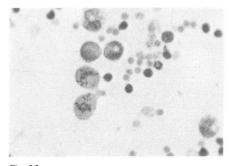

Fig. 25:
Accomplished mitosis with bridge of cytoplasm. Maturing immunocyte, peritoneal exudate, panchromatic.

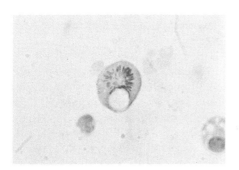

Fig. 23:
Mitosis: dispersion of the chromosomes. Monocyte. Alkal. phosphatase colouring. Peritoneal exudate, guinea-pig.

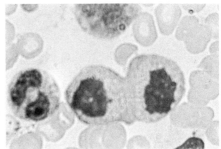

Fig. 26:
The chromosomes have reunited into a nuclear formation at the poles, the cytoplasm is about to contract in the middle. Bone-marrow, panchromatic colouring.

The RNA synthesis stops – as is visible with the nucleolus – from the middle of the prophase toward the end of the telophase. An increase of the lysosomal activity is one of the first signs of the forthcoming mitosis (BECKER and LANE/1965). This indicates a disintegration of structures of the interphase.

Endoplasmatic reticulum

Definition: The endoplasmatic reticulum is a three-dimensional intracytoplasmatic system of membranes, which is found in various forms in every animal cell, except the ripe erythrocytes. The main functions are regulations of transportation and protein synthesis.

Historical data

The knowledge of structure and function is closely connected with the evolution of electron microscopy and with the names of PALADE and PORTER. The most important recognition was won in the years 1953–1960. In 1952/53, PALADE discovered in the electron-optical slide of chicken-embryo cultures a filigrane-like cytoplasmatic ground structure in the form of a «reticulum of filamentous or canalicular structures». The existence of this system was proved by PALADE and PORTER (1954). The membrane system is also called ergastoplasm, but the term «endoplasmatic reticulum» is more common though the membrane system is neither restricted to the «endoplasm» nor is found always in a reticular formation.

The membranes studded with granules (= «Palade granules» = ribosomes) correspond to the basophile regions of the cell; GARNIER (1899) called «ergastoplasm» these regions occurring on secreting glands. The formal distinction of the form studded with ribosomes from the «smooth» form (= smooth-walled membranes) termed «sarcoplasmatic reticulum», «sarcotubular system» or «annulatae lamellae» is probably not justified as here morphological variants of the same principle, dependent on the functional condition, are in question.

Morphology

The endoplasmatic reticulum is a system of membranes originating from the outer nuclear membrane and communicating through nucleopores with the perinuclear space. The framework is constituted by cytomembranes, which, as «unit membranes», are 60–70 Å thick. The inside diameter of these membranes imposing as tubes, varies from 50–300 mμ as long as they run parallel but grows wider in the secreting stage of the synthe sis products to form «little bags» or «cisterns» with larger diameters of round, oval or garland-like shape.

The membranes are «windowed» in the form of rounded or oval openings (fig. 27) probably intended to facilitate changes of space and form. The interior of the endoplasmatic reticulum communicates with the nucleus direct: the outer layer of the nuclear membrane blends into the first lamellae of the membranes of the ergastoplasm. The outer space communicates through the nucleopores direct with the interior of the nucleus and is separated form it only by a «diaphragm» with a central ball of threads.

The outer surface of the lamellae of ergastoplasm is more or less studded with ribosomes: consequently, there is a rough-walled granular form (PALADE, 1955) and a smooth-walled form lacking these granules. Ribosomes can gather in groups and are then called polysomes or polyribosomes (see fig. 31–35).

Function

The formation and compactness of the endoplasmatic reticulum indicate the functional condition. The more intense the rate of protein synthesis, the compacter the ergastoplasm. Compact formations can be found in protein-secreting glands, the «Nissl's bodies» of the neurons correspond to formations of ergastoplasm thickly studded with ribosomes and with free ribosomes. Cells of fatty tissue contain sometimes membranes arranged in concentric layers with granules 250 Å large « phospholipid bodies» (MÖLBERT, 1968). The intensity of these basophilous consolidations has created the term « accessory nucleus».

The changes of form and functions of the ergastoplasm can be observed best when the monocytes turn into immunocytes (plasma cells). A stimulation with antigens provokes first in the perinuclear space a «basophilous» consolidation, which spreads centrifugally in the ripening stage of the immunocytes till the entire cytoplasmatic space is deeply basophilous. These optico-microscopic changes have their electron-microscopic equivalent in a growing compactness of the tubes of ergastoplasm and of the coat of ribosomes. The multiplying structures of ergastoplasm increase the space of cytoplasm, change the relation between the nucleus and cytoplasm at the expense of the nucleus, the nucleus is forced toward the periphery. When the stage of synthesis of the immunocytes changes into the secretory phase, first the spaces between the lamellae extend, the parallel formation of the lamellae is lost, cistern-like extensions to receive the products of synthesis (immunoglobulins) arise. Cytochemical analyses have proved that besides the main function of synthesis and secretion of proteins also the by-products of the metabolic processes are extruded through these systems. After excreting the synthetised proteins, the immunocytes grow poor in lamellae of ergastoplasm and appear dispersed like vacuoles in the optic microscope (fig. 173–192).

Endoplasmatic reticulum without ribosomes is found in the striated muscles (FAWCETT, 1965) and in steroid-producing cells, tubular systems in the striated muscles and myocardium of mammals and in insects (MÖLBERT).

The interior of the endoplasmatic reticulum is, for the most part, homogeneous and less electron-tight than the environment. Homogeneous compact particles up to $350\,m\mu$ in diameter were found in the endoplasmatic reticulum of osteoblasts (ZELANDER, 1959), chondroblasts (PALADE, 1956), exocrine pancreatic cells.

The speed of the metamorphoses described above is considerable. DL-leucin tagged with 3H was identified electron-microscopically in the autoradiogram already after 5 minutes in the ergastoplasm, after 20 minutes in the Golgifield and after 60 minutes in the zymogen granules (CARO and PALADE, 1964). This order is highly significant also in the synthesis of cartilage: 3H prolin – the most important element of the profibrils of tropocollagen – was found first in the endoplasmatic reticulum, then in the Golgifield, later in the extracellular fibrils (REVEL and HAY, 1963).

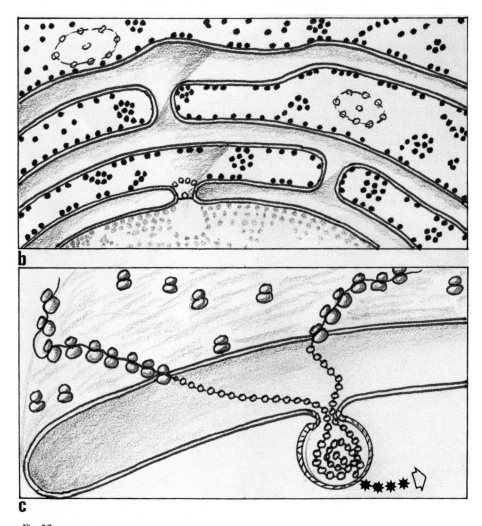

Fig. 27:
Endoplasmatic reticulum in various magnifications.
b) lamellae of ergastoplasm (from an electron-optical picture); membranes of the endoplasmatic reticulum studded with ribosomes and polysomes; below: cut nucleus with nucleopore; c) three-dimensional scheme of an ergastoplasmic lamella studded with polysomes, m-RNA cords between the ribosomes; protein synthesis (chains) and its secretion via cisterns (arrow).

41

The synthetic activity of the cell is characterized by the enlargement and consolidation of the endoplasmatic reticulum. Phases of secretion are distinguished by a dispersion in the form of extensions of the interlamellar spaces and the formation of cistern-like spaces. The lamellae of ergastoplasm disappear when the protein synthesis is terminated or prevented. A decrease to complete depletion was seen in starving animals (BERNHARD et al., 1952). But remainders of ergastoplasm can be traced even under extreme starving conditions (FAWCETT, 1955). The changes are reversible after supplies of substrate. The ribosomes settle on the lamellae first in the neighbourhood of the nuclear membrane and cell membrane. An important function in the activation is attributed to the nucleolus. Hypoxy causes a vacuolation in the liver-cells (MÖLBERT). This mechanism is ascribed to the pathogenesis of myocardial infarction, to the degeneration of the ganglious cells in asphyxia, to the necrosis of striated muscles in ischemia and to the degeneration of tubular epithelium in the case of engorged kidney. The strongest vacuolar degenerations are observed in poisonings (hydrocyanic acid, malonic acid, carbon tetrachloride), similar degenerative processes occur in phosphorous poisonings, overdoses of strophantin and L-tri-iodine-thyroxin.

Besides vacuolation, the following phenomena are regarded as degeneration of the endoplasmatic reticulum:

1. Consolidations into myelin figures – epinuclear formation (e. g. in cirrhosis of the liver, after administration of actinomycin-D).
2. Autophagous vacuoles (LANE and NOVIKOFF, 1965), observed after administrations of thiohydantoin, thioacedamide, aethionin, actinomycin D, aflatoxin B1, carbon tetrachloride, after intense UV-radiation and X-ray therapy, in cases of alcoholism and viral hepatitis.
3. Occurrence of lysosomes and cytosomes; this phenomenon is closely connected with the mitotic activity of the organs.

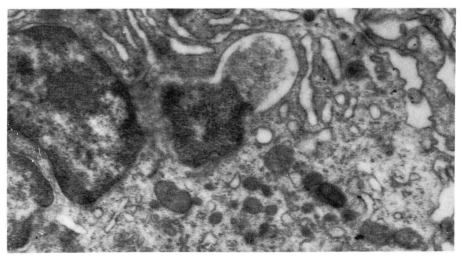

Fig. 28:
Incipient formation of the endoplasmatic reticulum in a maturing immunocyte of the peritoneal exudate in the upper part of the picture. Magn. 1:20,000.

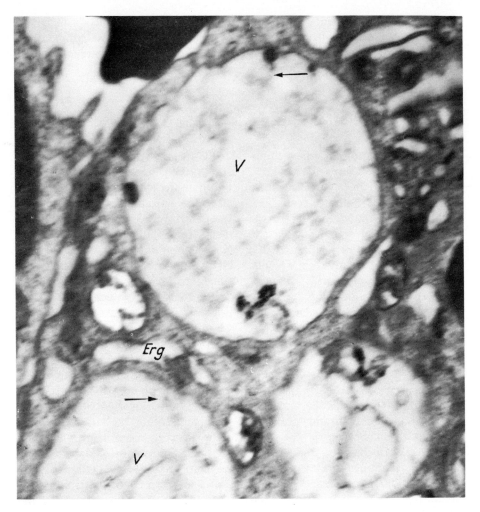

Fig. 29:
Extension of the interlamellar spaces of the endoplasmatic reticulum of an immunocyte in the stage of secretion; secretion of the synthesis products (immunoglobulins) into cistern-like bulges of the interlamellar spaces by pressure filtration. Magn. 1 : 20,000.

Ribosomes

Ribosomes are cellular organelles serving for the protein synthesis. They consist of ribosomal ribonucleic acid (r-RNA) and proteins of cytoplasmatic origin. The subunits consisting of large and small particles are larger in eucaryote cells (80 S) than in procaryotes (70 S).

For the functional ripening, Messenger ribonucleic acid (m-RNA) and transfer-ribonucleic acid (t-RNA) supplied from the nucleolus are necessary. The synthesis products of the ribosomes are polypeptide chains and proteins, which are secreted through vesicles into the interspaces of the endoplasmatic reticulum.

The ribosomes originate probably from the nuclear membrane or from the nucleus, and perform their function either free or at the surface of the endoplasmatic reticulum in the cytoplasm.

Ribosome aggregates are called polysomes.

Historical data

After BRACHET's (1933) first assumptions that the ribonucleic acid (RNA) occurred chiefly in the cytoplasm, cytochemical methods (FEULGEN et al., 1937, BEHRENS, 1938) located the DNA in the nucleus and the RNA in the cytoplasm. Until then, it had been supposed that RNA was the nucleic acid of the plants, DNA that of the animal cells. BRACHET (1940, 1941) demonstrated significantly a correspondence between the protein-synthesis rate and the quantity of RNA in the cell. CLAUDE found by differential centrifugation (1938–1941) that «infectiosity» of the Rous-sarcoma was bound to small particles, which were traceable in the dark-field microscope and contained ribonucleoprotein and lipids. Only the electron-microscopical studies by PALADE (1955) demonstrated significantly the occurrence of these particles large about 200 Å in all tested cells and therewith the existence as real cell organelles. The terms «small granules» and «microsomes» used by CLAUDE were later changed for «ribosomes», probably in consideration of the constituent of 50% RNA (PETERMAN, HAMILTON and MIZEN, 1954).

By tagging with amino-acid, BORSOOK (1950) found the highest concentration in the «microsomes» 30 minutes after the injection. LITTLEFIELD and KELLER furnished by different experiments (between 1955 and 1957) the conclusive proof that amino-acids are actually incorporated first into the ribosomes.

The statistical significance was established for the existence of ribosomes by various studies on bacteria. The ultracentrifuge provided fractions of particles of 40 S, 29 S and 5 S sedimentation coefficients. These spherical particles of the 40 S fraction contained 40% RNA. CHAO (1957) recognized the elementary significance of the Mg^{++} for the stability of the two ribosome elements with a constant of sedimentation of about 80 S. By the middle of the 1950s, definitive statistical significance (A. TISSIERES, 1974) was established for the existence of the spheric particles 200–300 Å in diameter, which consist about half of RNA and half of protein (i. e. of the ribosomes). After a meeting of the Biophysical Society, D. ROBERTS introduced the term «ribosome».

Structure of the ribosomes

The studies conducted on various species have not yet provided a uniform aspect, less so because the dehydrating processes in electron-microscopical preparations make it difficult to assess the circumstances in vivo. According to AMELUNXEN and SPIESS (1971) as well as NOMOMURA (1971), the smallest subunit is about 230 Å × 120 Å × 140 Å (X-ray model 55 Å × 220 Å × 220 Å in E. Coli),

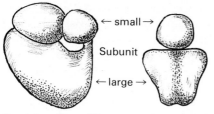

← small →

Subunit

← large →

Frontal profile   Ribosome   Lateral profile

Fig. 30:
Model of *ribosome*

divided into two unequal segments by a notch of 40 Å in diameter. The «large subunit» has a diameter of about 230 Å (see fig. 30).

The best documentations of physico-chemical findings on the structure and function were obtained with ribosomes of E. Coli (K. E. VAN HOLDE and W. E. HILL). Here, the 70 S-ribosomes consist of a 30 S-, a 50 S- subunit and Mg^{++}. The 70 S-particles contain quantities of Messenger RNA (mRNA), polypeptides and protein cofactors varying probably according to the functionary power of the primary cell. The unwashed 30 S subunits have a molecular weight of 1.0×10^6, those washed with NH$_4$CL or units precipitated with (NH$_4$) 2 SO$_4$ a molecular weight of 0.90×10^6. Six proteins seem to be lost by washing (VOYNOW and KURLAND, 1971). The 16 S – RNA constituent (0.53 to 0.64×10^6) is estimated to make 64% in unwashed

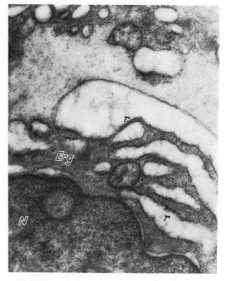

Fig. 31:
Free ribosomes (r) and aggregated to endoplasmatic reticulum. M = mitochondria, N = nucleus. Immunocyte, 1:20,000.

30 S-particles and 71% in washed particles. 16 S-r RNA (= 564.000 daltons) correspond to 1650 nucleotides. 30 S-subunits are asymmetric, with a diameter nearly equal to the 50 S-particle, and highly hydrated.

The high amount of retained water makes it difficult to explain the findings obtained by the electron-microscope because the withdrawal of water causes the ribosome particles to shrink; lyophilisation seems to meet best the natural conditions.

50 S-subunit

The molecular weight of the unwashed 50 S-subunits comes to about 1.7×10^6, to 1.55×10^6 that of washed (NH4CL) or precipitated [(NH4)2 SO$_4$] 50 S-particles; the loss of mass does not reduce the sedimentation coefficient (K. E. VAN HOLDE and W. E. HILL, 1974). The molecular weight of the 23 S-r

RNA was found to range from 1.0×10^6 to 1.1×10^6. The amount of RNA in unwashed 50 S-particles (subunits) is 65%, 71% in the washed; unwashed particles contain about 600.000 daltons of protein, the washed 450,000 daltons.

They seem to be more symmetrical than the 30 S-particles.

45

Small and wide angle X-ray powder diffraction studies of microcrystals of *Escherichia Coli* 70 S ribosomes revealed tetragonal centered macrocells of a = b = 43 nm and c = 52 nm with very strong reflections between 4 nm and 7 nm. This findings were confirmed by electron microscopy. The subcells were found by electron microscopy and X-ray diffraction to have orthogonal axes of a_s = 4.3 nm, b_s = 5.3 nm and c_s = 14.2 nm. (KUCKUK, E. D. 1982).

Ribosomes of eukaryotes have been studied less methodically but are apparently a little larger than those of prokaryotes.

Functionary associations

Ribosomes occur single *(monomeres)*, in groups *(polysomes)* and, obviously under unfavourable biological conditions, in aggregations of crystals (tetrameres, P 422-crystals) (LAKE, SABATINI and NONOMURA, 1974).

Ribosomes seem to be capable of crystallising in various forms. Most of the studies have been conducted on ribosomes of chicken embryos treated with hypothermia (BYERS, 1967). The 166 S-particles in 5-day-old chicken embryos undercooled for 24 hours are ribosomes-tetrameres. Tetrameres are produced from ripe but inactive 80 S-ribosomes. The interribosomal binding seems to depend mainly on the concentration of ions, especially on the Mg^{++}-content of the medium. Tetrameres can deposit into laevorotatory or dextrorotary crystal-lattices of ribosomes. The three-dimensional structure of the monomeres as outlined in a model (fig. 30) from various techniques of investigation shows some criteria of the course of the function as far as they can be reconstructed from the lifeless artificial products of representation. A concise survey is given by fig. 32 (with legend).

In the association of polysomes, the Messenger RNA (m-RNA) cords, in conformity with biochemical findings, can be found among the subunits. The motility (rotation) of the ribosomes seems to be restricted by the connecting RNA cords if the cords traverse several ribosomes in the polysome unit. The diameter of the RNA cords of 15–30 Å suggests that secondary structures of RNA or protein-studded RNA are in question. Laterally, the RNA cord on either side of the ribosome can be followed to where the small and large subunits unite, frontally sometimes to the opaque spot at the boundary of the subunits. Here, probably, the entrance and exit of the ribosome are situated (fig. 30). At least 5 proteins (S4, S7, S8, S15, S20), in case even also S13, can be bound side-specifically to the 16 S-RNA cords of the 30 S-5 subunit of the ribosomes (KURLAND, 1974).

The synthetised polypeptide chains are probably conveyed through small channels in the 50 S subunits of the ribosomes and collected in vesicles (cistern-like bulges) of the endoplasmatic reticulum (fig. 32).

The *enzyme content* of the ribosomes is adapted to the high metabolic efficiency. Earlier enzyme analyses conducted on the «microsome fraction» substantiated the presence of the following enzymes (taking into account any possible impurities of the fraction): ribonuclease, amylase, dipeptidase, trypsin, catalase, cytochrome C, co-enzyme A, ATP-ase, adenylic-acid-phosphatase, alkaline and acid phosphatase, lipase, arginase. The average content of the cytoplasm is exceeded by esterases, cytochrome-c-reductase, glucose-6 phosphate-phosphatase.

Vitamin B_2 and B_6 were identified in the microsome fraction (G. C. HIRSCH, 1955).

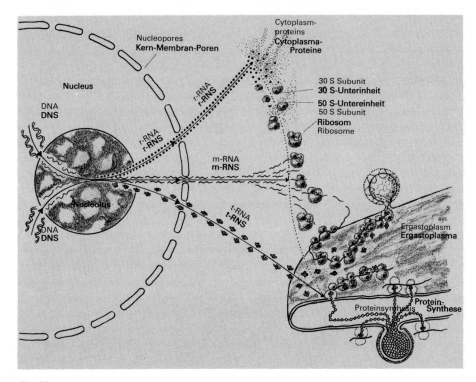

Fig. 32:
Functional cycle of the ribosomes (see text).
The DNA of the nucleus regulates via the intranucleolar DNA three different forms of ribonucleic acids of the nucleolus: r-RNA (ribosomal RNA), m-RNA (Messenger-RNA) and t-RNA (transfer RNA). The ribosomal RNA (r-RNA) gets through the nucleopores into the cytoplasm space and unites with cytoplasm proteins to form the ribosomes.
The Messenger-ribonucleic acid (m-RNA) penetrates through the nucleopores into the cytoplasm where it unites with the ribosomes, which temporarily are enabled to form polypeptide chains of a certain sequence.
The transfer ribonucleic acid (t-RNA) completes the functional unit so caused. The enzymes at the end of the trifoliate t-RNA molecules bind certain amino-acids, the genetic code of the m-RNA molecule is deciphered at the other end of the molecule. This assures the genetically fixed sequence of the amino-acids in the protein synthesis.
Ribosomes occur partly single in the cytoplasm (monomerics), partly – if highly efficient synthesis is necessary – in aggregates on the surface of the endoplasmatic reticulum (so-called polysomes), from where the synthetized proteins are evacuated into the interspaces of the reticulum. Examples of the electron-optical changes of the now following transportation processes are demonstrated in the immunoglobulin synthesis of fig. 31, 33, 34, 186–189.

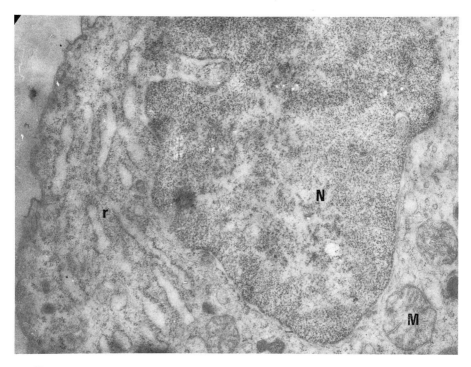

Fig. 33:
Endoplasmatic reticulum thickly studded with ribosomes in a mature immunocyte (peritoneal exudate, guinea-pig after BCG-immunisation). M = mitochondria, N = nucleus. 1 : 20,000.

Reconstruction of the ribosomes

The reconstitution of functional subunits of ribosomes is comparatively easy to conduct experimentally at 37°C within a few minutes (NOMURA and HELD, 1974). 16S-RNA free from proteins (phenol extraction or precipitation of urea-LiCl) is mixed with 30S-ribosome protein. The reconstitution is obtained with 20 mM Mg^{++} ions and with an optimum concentration of ions of 0.37. The 30S-subunits reconstructed with 16S-RNA and purified 30S-ribosome proteins behave physically and functionally like natural ribosomes, only the binding of the S$_1$-protein seems to be weaker. Under these experimental conditions, only 7 of the ribosomal proteins bind primarily to the RNA cord, the rest follow secondarily.

Eukaryotes-ribosomes

Most of the experimental studies of ribosomes were conducted on prokaryotes. Eukaryotes-ribosomes are a little larger than prokaryotes-ribosomes and have about 80 S for the functional ribosome and 60 S or 40 S for the subunits (PETERMANN, 1964); they contain 3 (to 4?) molecules of RNA and somewhat more than 70 proteins. The small subunit consists of an 18 S-RNA cord and about 30 proteins having a total mass of 0.78×10^6 daltons. The RNA constituent comes to 45.5%.

The large subunit consists of a 28 S-, a 5 S-RNA molecule (1.7×10^6) and about 40 proteins $(1.37 \times 10^6$ daltons); the total mass comes to about 3.0×10^6, the RNA constituent to about 59.4%. The growth of the mass of the eukaryotes-ribosomes is caused by the increase of the large subunit whereas the small subunit apparently does not partake of the evolution. Eukaryotes-ribosomes are not uniform and vary from 3.9×10^6 in plants to 4.55×10^6 daltons in mammals. In contrast to the prokaryotes-ribosomes, the reconstruction of eukaryotes-ribosomes from the subunits is difficult, presumably because sufficient quantities of 45S-RNA are not available.

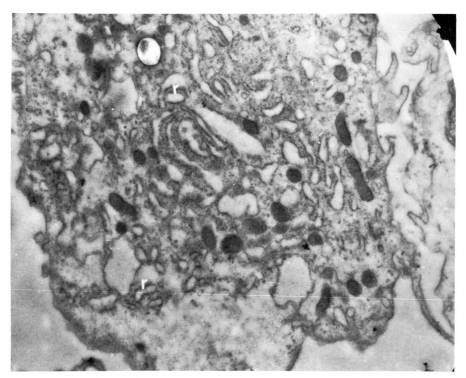

Fig. 34:
Lamellae of endoplasmatic reticulum (r) thickly studded with *ribosomes in mature immunocyte* as the interlamellar interspaces are about to extend (= secretion of the synthetized proteins). 1 : 20,000.

Mitochondria

The term «mitochondria» (thread kernels) goes back to BENDA (1898–1902), who introduced this name for a certain fraction of cell granules inclining to form threads. The function in vesicular breathing was demonstrated first by WARBURG (1913). The statistical significance of their central position in the entire oxydative metabolism was established by the technical possibilities of separating by ultracentrifugation the mitochondria fraction as a large fraction of granules (fig. 36) from the rest of the cellular constituents (SCHNEIDER, 1959; NOVIKOFF, 1961; KLIMA; KRSTIĆ, 1976).

In bacteria, enzymes of the respiratory chain are localised in the peripheral layers of the cytoplasm; higher organisms, however, have special cell organelles for breathing, namely the mitochondria. They are called also «chondriosomes», «chondriochonts» or «plastosomes», «chondriom» in their totality (MEVES, 1907).

Mitochondria are obligatory organelles of all animal cells, with the exception of normocytes. Form and size vary according to the kind of the cells and to their functional activity. The organelles can be made visible, especially by staining with Janus green-B, and can be prepared vitally as greenish-black granules or threads of various sizes. Overdoses of dyestuff produce safranin and a red colour, which causes the degeneration of the mitochondria and immediately the death of the cells. The phase-contrast microscope detects mitochondria during the observation in vivo as moving granules. However, only electron-microscopy (fig. 35–43) has fully disclosed the morphology.

Form and structure

Mitochondria are structures having round, elliptic, filiform, reniform, club-shaped or dumb-bell-shaped cross-sections (fig. 35–43). The diameter of their cross-sections is 0.18 (retina) to 2.0 (myocardium), the length 1.0–5.0 (up to extremely 14.0) mi m; their width varies from 0.2–1.0 mi m (KMENT, KLIMA). In spite of the many different forms, the architectonic structure follows one basic plan: mitochondria have two elementary membranes, an outer one and an inner one, of a total thickness of 100–250 Å. This double-membrane system separates the mitochondria from the rest of the space of cytoplasm. The space between the outer and inner membranes comes to 100–200 Å, and is also referred to as outer phase. The inner membrane forms bulges towards the lumen. These bulges have the function of increasing the surface of the inner membrane; they are also summed up as the inner phase. On the bulges of the inner membrane are ribosome-like particles having a diameter of about 100 Å (fig. 42). According to KRSTIĆ, a liver cell e. g. has about 2500 mitochondria, the surface measures 13 mi m², but the surface of the inner phase some 16 mi m². Depending on the kind of the bulges, several types of mitochondria are distinguished, such as e. g. in transverse bulges:

a) the *Crista type* with Cristae mitochondriales (fig. 38)
b) the *tubulus type* (fig. 39)
c) the *prisma type* (fig. 40)
d) the *sacculus type* (fig. 41).

The elementary particles have a diameter of about 100 Å and are located on a shaft of about 35 Å in diameter. Through this shaft they are connected with the inner mitochondria membrane. There we find structure elements (fig. 42) serving for the enzymatic coupling (b); they contain enzymes of the respiratory

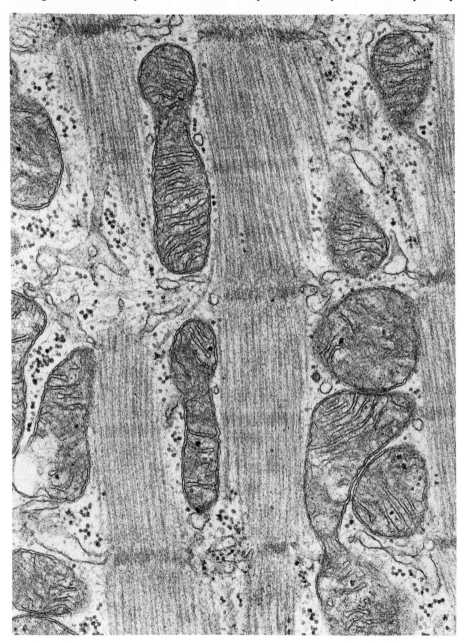

Fig. 35:
Abundance in *mitochondria* in metabolic-active tissues like muscle (H. THEMAN, Münster).

chain (f) and of the cytochrome C (e). In fig. 42, the elementary granules are marked as a, the three-layered inner membranes with b, g and c; b and c mark structural proteins, and g the lipoid layer of the membrane.

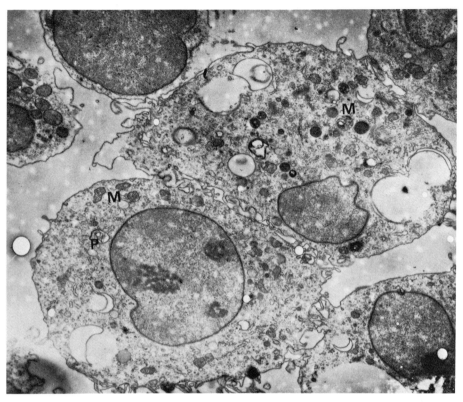

Fig. 36:
«Coarse fraction of granules» = mitochondria in monocytary cells of peritoneal exudate. Guinea-pig. 1:4000.

Outfit of the cell with mitochondria

Number and arrangement of the mitochondria are variable, certain concentrations are found in areas with high metabolic efficiency e.g. in the perinuclear space and in the Golgi-apparatus. The number of the mitochondria, too, depends on the type of the cell and on the metabolism. Embryonic cells contain more mitochondria than cells of adult or aging organisms. Especially liver cells are rich in mitochondria; 1 g of fresh liver is supposed to contain 33×10^{16} mitochondria; glandular cells, renal epithelia, myocardium belong to the organs rich in mitochondria whereas the cells of the thymolymphatic system (thymus, spleen) and the leukocytes are poor in mitochondria.

Related to the *mass of the cell,* a percentage of 15–25% falls to the fraction of mitochondria. Within this fraction of mitochondria, 70% proteins (chiefly enzyme protein), 3% RNA and 27% lipoids can be identified; 60% of this lipoid constituent are phosphatides.

The *membranes* consist of two osmiophile layers each about 70–80 Å thick, between them is a somewhat brighter osmiophobic layer 40–50 Å thick; at least one of the membranes is probably semipermeable. The outer membrane is smooth, the inner membrane shows regular particles with macromolecules.

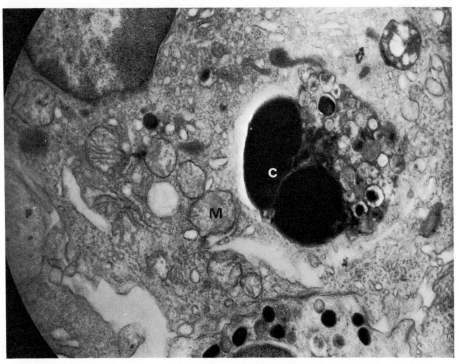

Fig. 37:
Mitochondria (M) with a seemingly empty lumen, in peritoneal macrophages of the guinea-pig, which are about to disintegrate a phagocyted cell (C). Final magnification: 1:20,000.

Function

Mitochondria are carriers of the *energy-metabolism* and of *cellular breathing*. They provide the cell with *oxydative energy* and effect the *release of ATP*. Adenosintriphosphate (ATP) is synthetised from *adenosindiphosphate (ADP)* and *phosphate (P)* in the *elementary particles* of the inner membrane. These elementary corpuscles are therefore called sometimes *ATP-osomes,* not *oxysomes* as formerly (KRSTIĆ). As the ATP is split in connection with the enzymes of the breathing chain, the energy for the cellular activity is released. Of the many functions of the mitochondria in close and changing interrelations to the cytoplasm space, statistical significance has been established for the following:

53

The mitochondria have all enzymes of the Krebs-cycle; tricarbone cycle (fig. 43); respiratory chain coupled with phosphorilation; disintegration of pyru-

tochromoxydase and succino-dehydrogenase (succinic acid-dehydrogenase); the vitamins A and C are required for the function. Aerobians can grow only if the structure and function of the mitochondria are intact.

Still unclear is the question how mitochondria come into existence and multiply, probably they originate from symbionts.

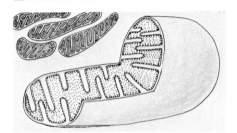

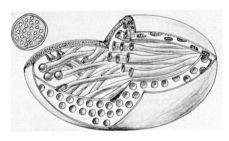

Fig. 38:
Crista-type of the mitochondria

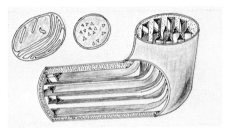

Fig. 40:
Prismatic type of the mitochondria

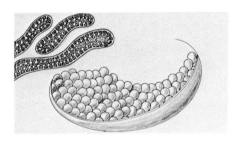

Fig. 39:
Tubulus-type of the mitochondria

Fig. 41:
Sacculus-type of the mitochondria

vic-acid; release of CO_2; transfer of hydrogen on coenzymes and their prosthetic groups; hydrogen is carried through the respiratory chain towards O_2 up to the cytochrome system; participation in the glycerophosphate cycle; formation of energy at 3 sites of the metabolic cycles.

Essential elements are, besides the enzymes mentioned, the key-enzymes cy-

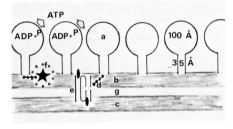

Fig. 42:
Diagram of the inner *surface of mitochondria* (inner phase); see text.

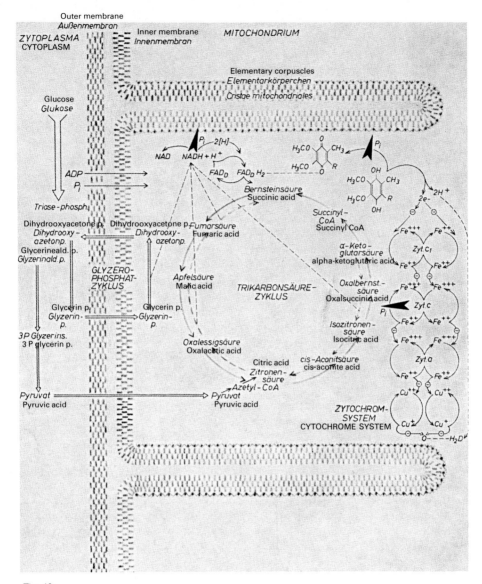

Outer membrane
Außenmembran

Fig. 43:
Metabolic processes in the mitochondria, especially processes for the production of oxydative energy and interrelation to the cytoplasmatic space. Simplified representation after KLIMA.
In the mitochondria, pyruvic acid is disintegrated via the Krebs-cycle by decarboxylation and dehydration; CO_2 ist released and hydrogen transmitted to coenzymes (NAD and FAD). The hydrogen is guided via the respiratory chain towards the O_2 as far as the cytochrome system. At three sites (wedges), energy (Pi) is formed. The formation of the mitrochondria wall and of the Cristae is represented.

55

Microbodies

Peroxysomes and Glyoxysomes

Since the first conference 1969, entitled «The nature and function of Peroxysomes (Microbodies and Glyoxysomes)» has been a tremendous progress in this field, summarized on the second conference 1981 by H. KINDL and P-B. LAZAROW (1982).

The *microbodies* seems to be nothaway a unit. In Trichomonads discovered D. LINDMARK a. M. MÜLLER (1973) microbodies and identified them as «hydrogenosomes». An other type found in Triponosomatids by F. OPPERDOES a. P. BORST (1977) were recognized as «glycosomes». There seems to be no overlap with peroxysomes or glyoxysomes; each of these microbodies has an originally functional system:

Anaerobic transfer of electrons between pyruvate and protons, supporting a substrate-level phosphorylation step for the hydrogenosomes; anaerobic glycolysis from glucose to 3-phosphoglycerate and glycerol, in a manner that is mysteriously selfsupporting ATP, for the glycosomes (DE DUVE 1982). These microbodies are restricted to single groups of protozoa, whereas the peroxy-glyoxysomes are widely distributed throughout the plant and animal kingdom and the microorganisms.

The *evolutionary origin* of the microbodies is not exactly known, since the former hypothesis as derivates of the endoplasmatic reticulum is not generally accepted. DE DUVE proposed, that all different forms of peroxysomes and glyoxysomes in eukaryotic microorganisms, plant an animals are decendants of a common evolutionary ancestor in the role as a primitive respiratory organelle – lacking oxydative Phosphorilation, but capable of oxidizing all major foodstuffs with formation of hydrogen peroxide (H_2O_2). In the superior anaerobic bacteria with the establishment with mitochondria like the eukaryotic cells the function of peroxysomes got lost with the exception of certain functions, especially in gluconeogenesis.

Considerable *biochemical differences* between peroxysomal membranes and the endoplasmatic reticulum were detected by Y. FUJIKI a. o. (1982). It seems, that the peroxysomes are – independent of the endoplasmatic reticulum and the associated membransystem – an enterily isolated population of cell-organelles, similar to the mitochondria.

Following the suggestions of DE DUVE (1982) each type of microbody has some sort of counterpart among the ancient bacteria. Peroxysomes resemble some primitive aerobe, lacking an organized respiratory chain. Hydrogenosomes includes key properties of anaerobic hydrogen-producing bacteria, such as clostridia. The glycosomes could originate from some very primitive anaerobe, because they contain one of the oldest, if not the oldest enzyme system of the biosphere, the glycolysis.

Not unlike this hypothesis the most research-workers believe, that the mitochondria originate from symbionts, loosing with the nucleus the major part of their genetic autonomy.

The *function* is summarized as peroxysmal-β-oxidation. As triglycerols stored fatty acids are the main fuel reserves of animals and readily used by the most tissues with exceptions of a few specialized cells such as nerve cells and erythrocytes (T. HASHIMOTO 1982). The fatty acid degradation goes over the successive oxidation removal of acetyl groups from the carboxyl end of the long chain fatty acids.

Lysosomes

The question whether lysosomes are an independent category of cell organelles has long been a subject of discussion. While studying the intracellular localization of the «acid phosphatase», DE DUVE found this enzyme to be coupled in the ultracentrifugal sedimentation to particles differing from other cellular organelles. Besides the «acid phosphatase», many acid hydrolases were found whereas, in contrast to the mitochondria, the key-enzymes of the citric acid cycle (see fig. 43) do not occur. In homogenates of liver cells still more particles having a sedimentary behaviour differing from that of the lysosomes and containing enzymes not found in lysosomes have been isolated: acid D-amino-oxydase, uricase and catalase.

Lysosomes are nowadays regarded as a special kind of major particles of cytoplasm playing a special part in the intracellular digestion.

Owing to their sedimentary properties, lysosomes are supposed to have a size of 0.4 mi and a density of 1.15 (mitochondria 1.13) on an average. Dyeing in vivo is possible with acridinorange and neutral red; lysosomal enzymes are inhibited by trypan blue. Agents destroying the cytomembranes release also the contents of lysosomes. Proteolytic and lipolytic ferments, mechanical traumata and low pH can release the acid hydrolases. Their transformation (after DE DUVE) is shown in fig. 44. The amount of the lysosomal enzymes is supposed to be large enough to dissolve the entire cellular organisation if a sudden release happens. This postulated lytical property finally led to the name «lysosomes».

Form and function

When phagocyted particles migrate through the cellular membrane, a lysosome appears at the inner limiting surface of the forming digestive cistern even before the outer membrane opening recloses. Constituents of lysosomes flow into the neighbouring tissue (regurgitation). The lysosomes are transported into the periphery of the cells by a regulatory function of the cytoplasmatic microfilaments (see fig. 21) and of the cytoplasmatic microtubuli originating from the centriole region.

The «digestive vacuole» formed after taking up foreign particles contains first no hydrolases and is called «phagosome». After taking up the acid hydrolases, it is sometimes referred to as heterophagous vacuole or phagolysosome. If the lysosomal outfit of enzymes is not capable of disintegrating foreign material, the latter will be stored.

The disintegration of foreign material (heterophagia) seems to proceed otherwise than the intracellular digestion of cellular constituents i.e. autophagia.

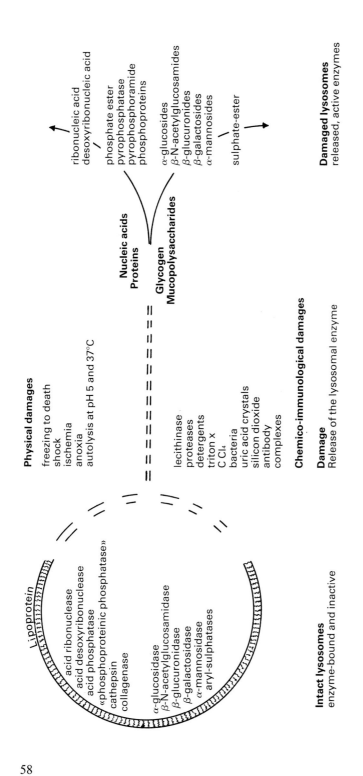

Lipoprotein

acid ribonuclease
acid desoxyribonuclease
acid phosphatase
«phosphoproteinic phosphatase»
cathepsin
collagenase

α-glucosidase
β-N-acetylglucosamidase
β-glucuronidase
β-galactosidase
α-mannosidase
aryl-sulphatases

Intact lysosomes
enzyme-bound and inactive

Physical damages

freezing to death
shock
ischemia
anoxia
autolysis at pH 5 and 37°C

lecithinase
proteases
detergents
triton x
C Cl₄
bacteria
uric acid crystals
silicon dioxide
antibody
complexes

Chemico-immunological damages

Damage
Release of the lysosomal enzyme

**Nucleic acids
Proteins**

**Glycogen
Mucopolysaccharides**

ribonucleic acid
desoxyribonucleic acid

phosphate ester
pyrophosphatase
pyrophosphoramide
phosphoproteins

α-glucosides
β-N-acetylglucosamides
β-glucuronides
β-galactosides
α-mannosides

sulphate-ester

Damaged lysosomes
released, active enzymes

Fig. 44:
Lysosomes
On the left, the circle includes inactive, bound, lysosomal enzymes.
In the middle: physical and chemo-immunological noxious factors, which cause the release of lyso-somal enzymes.
On the right, released, active lysosomal enzymes and their substrate target-substances.

Tab. 2: Lysosomal enzymes[1]

Oxidoreductases act upon hydrogen peroxide	**Hydrolases** acting upon ester compounds	**Hydrolases** acting upon glycosyl compounds	**Hydrolases** acting upon peptide compounds
Peroxidase	arylesterase	lysozyme	glutamate-carboxypeptidase
	triacylglycerol-lipase	neuramidase	carboxypeptidase A
Hydrolases acting upon non-peptide carbo-nitric compounds	cholesterol-esterase	α-glucosidase	(cathepsin A)
	phospholipase A_1	β-glucosidase	carboxypeptidase B
acetylsphingosindeaclase	phospholipase A_2	α-galactosidase	(cathepsin B_2)
aspartylglucosylaminase	acid phosphatase	β-galactosidase	carboxypeptidase C
amino-acid-naphthyl-amidase	phosphatidase-phosphatase	α-mannosidase	lysosom. dipeptidase
benzoylarginin-naphthyl-amidase	phosphoprotein-phosphatase	β-mannosidase	dipeptidylpeptidase I
	phosphodiesterase I	β-N-acetylglucosaminidase	dipeptidylpeptidase II
Hydrolases acting upon acid-anhydrides	desoxyribonuclease II	β-glucuronidase	kininogenin
	ribonuclease II	hyaluron-glucosidase	acrosin
inorganic pyrophosphatase	sphingomyelin-phosphodiesterase	α-N-acetylgalactosaminidase	elastase
	arylsulphatases	α-N-acetylglucosaminidase	cathepsin G
Hydrolases acting upon phosph.-nitrogen-compounds	sulphatase A	α-L-fucosidase	neutral proteinase
	sulphatase B	L-iduronidase	plasminogen activator
phosphoamidase	chondroitin-sulphatase		cathepsin B (B_1)
			cathepsin D
	Hydrolases acting upon sulphurated nitrogen		cathepsin E
			lysosom. collagenase
	heparin-sulphamidase		renin

[1] After data from ALTMANN and KATZ «Cell-Biology» 1976; BARRET A. J. (1972); DEAN R. T. (1975); HERS H. G. and VAN HOFF (1973); ROBINSON D. (1974). Certain enzymes were identified only in lysosomes of certain organs.

The autophagous vacuoles seem to originate from bulges of the endoplasmatic reticulum, which first develop baggy bulges and finally form complete digestive cisterns. Their hydrolytic enzymes originate probably from the vesicles rich in enzymes of the endoplasmatic reticulum or are supplied by connection with lysosomes. Their activity can disintegrate whole endogenic mitochondria.

Form and function – biological magnitudes independent of each other, whose interrelation has always raised fascinating questions in biology – are different:

1. In the granules of the polymorphonuclear granulocytes, probably freshly formed enzymes are stored and then used for intracellular digestion.

2. Endogenic (degenerated, altered) cell constituents are autolysed in the lysosomes, apart from the rest of the cell.

3. As «digestive cisterns» («digestive vacuoles» is misleading because no empty spaces are in question) they disintegrate phagocyted material of extracellular origin.

In granulocytes (microphages) just as well as in monocytes (macrophages), alveolar macrophages and eosinophiles, foreign particles and autogenous substances «estranged from the body» have been disintegrated. Especially when bacteria are phagocyted, lysosomes (fig. 45–47, 20) releasing their contents by autolysis gather round the intracellu-

Tab. 3: **Mechanisms and regulation of the release of lysosomal enzymes from polymorpho-nuclear leukocytes** (Cell biology 1976)

Mechanism	Stimulus for release	Regulation factors

release during phagocytosis	bacteria
	zymosane
	immunocomplexes
	    soluble
	    insoluble
	immunoglobulin-aggregations
	crystals of
	calcium-pyrophosphate	

release without phagocytosis	superficial immunglobulin aggregations superficial immunocomplexes chemotactic factors	contractile proteins microtubuli microfilaments serinesterase energy metabolism cyclic nucleotides calcium
cytotoxic release (destruction after taking particles)	complement components bacteria uric-acid crystals silicon-dioxide crystals	
destruction by membrane-active agents	leukocidin streptolysin O vitamin A antineutrophil antibodies	

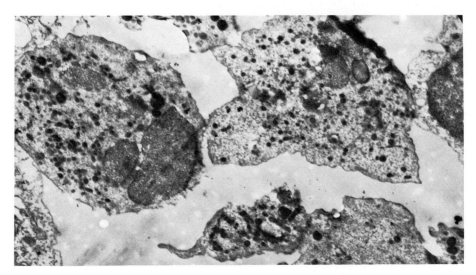

Fig. 45:
Coarse «granulafraction» in polynuclear cells (peritoneal exudate, magnif. 1:5000).

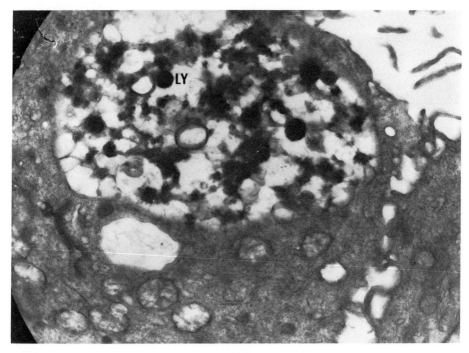

Fig. 46:
Abundance of *lysosomes* in a digestive cistern of a monocyte. Disintegration of a segment nuclear. Lysosomes compact, homogenous, circular (1:40,000).

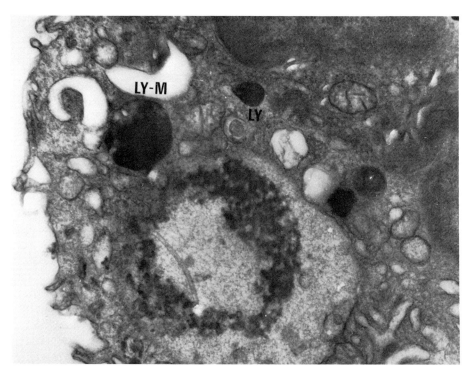

Fig. 47:
Beside the *digestive cistern* of a monocyte, 2 lysosomes and a somewhat larger structure like the «myelin-figures» Ly-M. 1:20,000.

lar digestive cisterns. The hydrolytic enzymes are released (fig. 44) so that the disintegration of the bacteria is quickly effected. The released substance (in question is probably not one but a plurality of substances) has sometimes been called phagocytin (HIRSCH J. G.; MILLER F.).

The ingestion of foreign material is said to involve an increased metabolism of glycolysis, which is believed to account for the acid medium and for the release of the enzymes from the leukocyte granules. The vitamins A, D and K soluble by lipoids reduce the stability of the lysosomes in vitro while hydrocortisone is believed to support this effect.

Heterophagous and autophagous «vacuoles» are sometimes referred to as secondary lysosomes because they form compact residual particles, often in the shape of so-called myelin figures (fig. 47).

Many viewpoints and experimental findings (SCHEIB D.; DEAN R. T.) suggest that the lysosomes play a great biological part in the development and transformation of the rapidly changing tissue formations in the embryonic and foetal life where tissue must be developed and dissolved quickly.

62

Biochemical data

Lysosomal membranes – according to cell biology 1978 – are permeable to

many monovalent salts at $0°C$;
monosaccharides (incl. sedoheptulose);
most of the amino-acids and peptides (mol. weight $< \sim 200$);
neutral forms of weak bases (mol. weight > 500);
3 iodotyrosin (monoiodotyrosin);

impermeable to

many monovalent salts at $37°C$;
disaccharides;
hexitol, hexonic and hexoronic acids;
most of the peptides (mol. weight $> \sim 200$;
various forms of weak bases.

The pH of the lysosomes measured so far in the external medium are about 7.0, those found in the lysosomes range from 4.5 to 6.6.

For the analysis of the non-enzymatic and enzymatic fractions of the lysosomes, the findings rely much on animal material.

The lysosomal enzymes are listed in table 2, their functional relations appear from fig. 44.

Regulatory factors

The effectiveness of lysosomal enzymes and substrates depends on their release. On the one hand, the cell must under resting conditions be protected from the influence of the lysosomal enzymes; on the other hand, endogenic substances foreign to the body or estranged must rely on the disintegration by the lysosomal enzymes. A survey of the known mechanisms of regulating and releasing in the leukocytes having polymorphous nuclei is shown in table 3.

Lysosomal and functional defects are of importance in many so-called storage diseases, especially in mucopolysaccharidosis and sphingolipidosis (see the chapter of lysosomal disorders).

Cytoskeleton

Following the discussions of the last two decades it is now accepted, that the cytoplasm of the most cells is a complex gel, structured by a variety of intracellular filaments, especially *microfilaments, intermediate filaments* and *microtubules* (KOCH, G. L. E., 1981). These units form the socalled *cytoskeleton,* responsible for cell-stability, movements, transport-processes and cell-division (mitosis). In a larger sense also the *Desmosomes* (fig. 1) for the connection between the cells, stability and elasticity of tissues belongs to the cytoskeleton. Whereas the microtubules show a radially orientation with the centriole as centre, the other filaments have a threedimensional architecture.

The present knowledge is limited to certain cell-types of single species. Therefore any categorization is fragmentary (DAVISON, P. F., 1981).

The interrelations between the microtubules-system and the centrioles are considered before (see chapter «Centrioles», pag. 34). In the class of 10 nm intermediate filaments by the antisera-technic are to distinguish the following basic elements:

Vimentin (fibroblast cytoskeletal protein);

Desmin or *Skeletin* (in muscles, skeleton);

Prekeratin (epidermal tonofilaments);

GFAP (glial fibrillary acidic protein).

GFAP (50 kD) of 50,000 Daltons weight, Vimentin (58 kD) and Desmin (56 kD) are homopolymeres, single proteins, which forms their corresponding filaments by association. The tonofilaments of epidermal cells seems to be heteropolymeres, consisting of a mixed population of protomeres (STEINERT, P. H., IDLER, W. W. and WANTZ, M. L., 1980). Components of the *neurofilaments* in vertebrates (fig. 273) are three proteins of 2109,155 and 70 kD, which comigrate with the slowest wave of axoplasmic flow (HOFFMAN, P. N. and LASEK, R. J., 1975).

Experimental fundaments

Apparent progress is the subject of discussions, real progress must be obtained by fighting. This millenial law of science must be stated first if cell therapy is to be understood in the system of modern medicine. A therapy originating from empiricism that claims the capability of regenerating effectively biological structures and of thus influencing ailments defined as uninfluenceable by the modern dogma of medicine, must achieve and prove more than an ordinary chemical substance. Same as in Galilei's times, dogmatists refuse to see what is obvious: medicine is about to cross the threshold between the chemical age and the biological epoch, which depends on the principles of the living substance – and does not rely on the usability of accidental chemical products for the organism. This step from an apparently solid building, often referred to as dogma, is a challenge and arouses hope. Challenged are persons and institutions who identify medicine as a natural science with chemistry and classical physics and, consequently, misunderstand the complexity of life and of its spiritual content. Hopes for the people who «according to the present state of medical knowledge», as the arrogant saying goes, cannot be helped. The fight of dogmatists and institutions aims at the legendary fame of a therapy that helps primarily and for its success was secondarily compelled to furnish proof.

Definition

The name «Cell therapy (originally: cellular therapy)» was derived from the cellular pathology (VIRCHOW). In its most neutral version it means the use of cellular material for therapeutic purposes. In this form, cell therapy belongs to the oldest medical treatments, and includes the following methods:

Transplantations of bone-marrow;
Blood-transfusions;
Implantations of thymus;
Transfusions of thrombocytes;
Concentrates of erythrocytes;
Suspensions of leukocytes.
Transplantation of
  fetal liver cells
  fetal spleen cells
  fetal bone-marrow
  pancreatic cells.

In colloquial usage of the last years, the concept of cell therapy has been identified more with the use of fetal xenogenic tissue. In this restricted formulation, the method can be defined as follows:

Cell therapy is an implantation by injection of (xenogenic) fetal or juvenile suspensions of cells or tissue in physiological solution. The implantation provides the organism of the recipient with a great number of biochemically demonstrable substrates and enzymes found in this concentration and composition only in juvenile tissue.

65

Tab. 4: **Cytochemical identification of enzymes and substrates in fetal tissues**

Enzymes	Substrates
lactatedehydrogenase	desoxyribonucleic acid
non-specific esterases	(FEULGEN; methyl-green pyronin)
alkaline phosphatase	ribonucleic acid (methyl-green pyronin)
dopa-oxydase	nucleotides (toluidin)
adenosin-triphosphatase (ATPase)	alpha-amino groups (ninhydrin)
	SH-groups (after FREDERICH)
	acid and basic substances
	(haematoxylin-eosin; ferric
	haematoxylin)
	lipoids (sudanoblack B)
	lipoid-nuclear coloration (scarlet)
	glycogen (BEST-carmine; PAS; PAS
	after ptyalin)
	polysaccharides

The implantation by injection has essential advantages over the conventional procedures of implantation; they can be outlined as follows:

1. *Implantations by injection bring about a rapid dispersion of the implanted cell material all over the body.*

2. *There are no injuries by implants owing to deficient blood supply during the disintegration of the implant.*

3. *Thanks to the form of suspension, a rapid infiltration into the metabolic processes is possible.*

4. *Organs inaccessible (brain, endocrine glands) or difficult to attain (kidney, liver) by contact transplantation can be reached.*

5. *The fetal tissues with their higher biological potencies are conveyed in the recipient on his own ways of metabolism and used at structurally suited sites. So the organism itself controls and effects a selective incorporation.*

For the implantation by injection, the *intravenous, intraperitoneal, intramuscular* and *subcutaneous* ways of application, theoretically, come into question. The most physiological way, probably, is the intraperitoneal application, which, however, should be used like the intravenous application in exceptional cases only to avoid the risks connected therewith. Most of all, the intramuscular application has been used so far; it constitutes a middle course between the subcutaneous and intraperitoneal ways; its disadvantage: the intramuscular application provokes stretchings and hemorrhages at the sites of injection, which cause secondary processes. The method of choice is the deep subcutaneous, epifascial dispersion of the implantation depot. The injection should be effected completely atraumatically i.e. without resistance, even if large volumes are in question. The injections should preferably be applied to the outer quadrant of the gluteal area and the skin of the abdomen.

Fig. 48–108:
Biochemical substances (substrates and enzymes) contained in lyophilised fetal tissues.

Fig. 48:
Thymus belongs to the tissues *rich in DNA*. Methyl-green (= DNA)-pyronin (= RNA) staining.

Fig. 50:
Identification of *alpha-amino-acid* with ninhydrin.

Fig. 52:
Nucleotides in freshly taken thymus tissue.

Fig. 49:
Fetal cartilage is *abundant in DNA and RNA* (red). Methyl-green-pyronin staining.

Fig. 51:
Identification of *dopa-oxydase*. Laidlaw-Blackberg solution. Concentration of enzymes in the *brain.*

Fig. 53:
Nucleotides in lyophilised thymus tissue. The comparison between fig. 52 and 53 shows in the lyophilisate a higher concentration of substance in proportion to the volume.

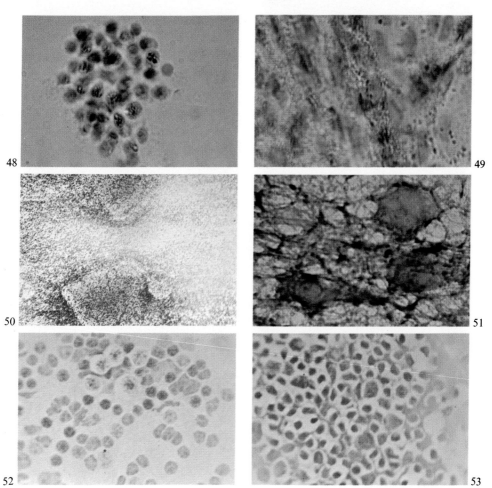

48

49

50

51

52

53

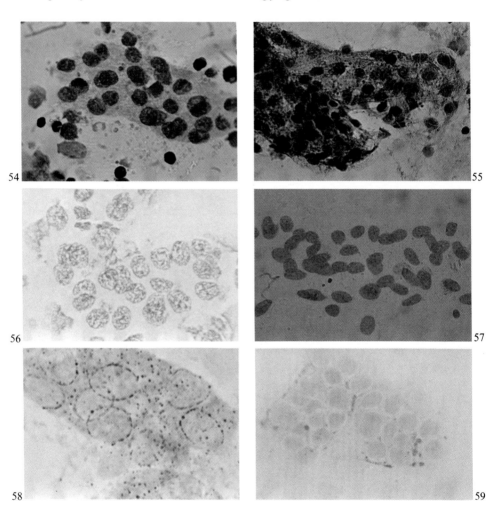

Characteristics

Fetal tissues were chosen first for theoretical considerations, which were later substantiated biochemically and immunologically.

The use of xenogenic (heterologous) suspensions of cells is a necessary consequence of present legislation.

Fetal tissues are used because they contain high concentrations of biochemical substances (substrates and enzymes), concentrations necessary to assure the high demand for material for the growth of fetal structures.

The second reason for the use of fetal cells is the small antigenicity of fetal tissues.

An essential characteristic of cell therapy is the application in the form of implantation by injection. This method is more expedient than the customary procedures of transplantation because the biochemical substrates and enzymes can be used by the body direct, without any secondary degenerative symptoms caused by transplantation changing and rendering them incompatible.

The therapeutic material

The injected suspensions of cells and tissue are taken up by the recipient's organism through phagocytosis and subsequent degradation, and disintegrated into submicroscopic size within two days.

The active substance is constituted by the plurality of the ingested biochemical substrates and enzymes. Of the many biochemical substrates thus made available to the recipient's organism, only part of them have been traced so far in the therapeutic materials of the cellular products (see table 4, fig. 49–108).

The «remedy» is reduced tissue, which is injected by doses of 15 to 55 mg/kg of bodyweight = 2–10 mg/kg of bodyweight of lyophilised substance. An injection of 100 mg of lyophilisate contains 45–75 mg of protein, of which 3–8% of the dry weight (= 6–20% of the whole protein) pass into solution after suspension. The fundamental pharmacological studies were conducted by NEUMANN (1961–1963).

Conclusion:

Tests for pyrogen under DAB 6 did not indicate any pyrogens in doses of 100–150 mg/kg of body weight (rabbit).

Cytochemical comparison between fetal and maternal tissues

Fetus and mother constitute a temporary biological association, separated only by the placenta. They have different functions though in the fetal period the organs are largely differentiated so that there are no fundamental structural differences between the maternal and fetal organs. To find out whether and how far these functional differences within a bio-economic association can be identified cytochemically in the single cell or in the cellular association, was the purpose of this study. Two points are of importance:

1. The preparation of chemical substrates of various cell associations, in qualitative and semiquantitative respect, and the control of the activities in these associations by selective tests on certain substrates and enzymes.

2. On the basis of this cytochemical analysis, the question for differences in the biochemistry of fetal and maternal tissues is studied.

Methods

The starting materials were pregnant sheep, whose fetuses were won by Caesarean section in the twentieth week of gestation. Ten kinds of corresponding tissues of the mothers and fetuses were examined by means of microscopic smears. In question are tissues from the stomach (abomasum), pancreas, brain (cortex), liver, bone-marrow, spleen, muscle, kidney, omentum, lung. These preparations were stained with:

4 nuclear or nucleic-acid preparations

(haemalaun-eosin; ferric haematoxylin; Feulgen; methyl green pyronin); 3 substrates (fat: scarlet red; glycogen: Best's carmine; alpha-amino-acid groups: ninhydrin); 2 enzymes (dopa-oxydase, alkaline phosphatase).

To avoid random results, 4 series of every animal preparation were examined with these nine stainings so that 720 preparations were obtained, of which 800 microphotographic pictures were taken.

Differences between fetal and maternal tissues

Stomach

The conspicuous differences between fetal and adult stomachs is due to the dispersion of nuclear plasma. The cytoplasmatic areas prevail in the fetal preparation, and the nuclear structures are exactly outlined. In the adult preparation, however, the constituents of cytoplasm stand back behind the nuclear structures (fig. 60, 61). The RNA concentration in the adult preparation is correspondingly smaller, with about an equal concentration of DNA. Fat and glycogen are traceable only in minute quantities, partly extracellular, in all stomach preparations (fig. 62, 63). Striking is the high concentration of the alpha-amino-acids, especially in the fetal stomach. The enzymes are more active in the preparation of the adult animal.

Pancreas

All four nuclear stainings depict the nuclei of the fetal tissue stronger than those of the adult preparation (fig. 64, 65). The cytoplasm of the fetal tissue has more structures, which corresponds also to the ample concentration and dispersion of RNA whereas in the pale colour of the cytoplasmatic space of the adult pancreas only a few particles can be traced. Fats can scarcely be identified in the adult preparation though their concentration is quantitatively higher. In the fetal tissues, however, the glycogen staining prevails. Only small quantities of alpha-amino-acids, and no alkaline phosphatase can be found. The rather strong activity of the dopa-oxydase, especially in the fetal preparation, is worth mentioning.

Brain

Characteristic of the cerebral tissues are the strong nuclear structures with their fibrous branches, which probably correspond to dentrite fragments and occur more in the fetal tissue (fig. 66, 67, 68, 69). The DNA is intensely stained, only traces of RNA are found.

Fatty substance and glycogen are contained in all preparations, in the adult tissue if the staining is quantitatively increased (fig. 70, 71). Alpha-amino-acids are amply traceable in both series; the activity of ninhydrin prevails in the fetal

Fig. 60:
Stomach-fetal, ferric hematoxylin-eosin 1:1250. Intense colouration of the cytoplasm.

Fig. 62:
Stomach-fetal, scarlet (1:1250). Good colouration of nucleus, no *fat* traced.

Fig. 64:
Pancreas-fetal, Feulgen (1:1250) High concentration of *DNA,* structures hardly differentiable.

Fig. 61:
Stomach-adult, ferric haematoxylin (1:1250). abvious appearance of the nuclear structures.

Fig. 63:
Stomach-adult, scarlet (1:1250). Good colouration of nucleus, little *fat* traced.

Fig. 65:
Pancreas-adult, Feulgen (1:1250). DNA nuclear colouration less intense than in fig. 64.

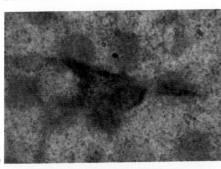

60

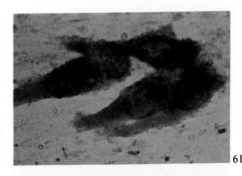

61

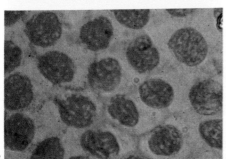

62

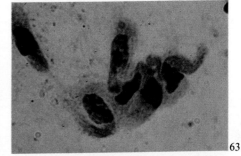

63

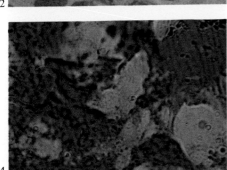

64

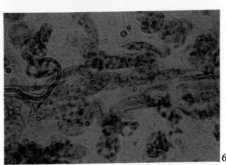

65

preparation. The activity of dopa-oxydase is specially spectacular in the adult preparation where nuclei, membranes and fibre structures are coloured. The alkaline phosphatase is little active in fetal and adult tissues.

71

Fig. 66:
brain-fetal, hemalaun-eosin (1:1250). Little intense cytoplasm colouration, distinct colouration of nucleus.

Fig. 68:
Brain fetal, ferric hematoxylin-eosin (1:30). Many fibriform structures.

Fig. 70:
Brain-fetal, Best-carmine colouration (1:1250). Slight *glycogen* colouration.

Fig. 67:
Brain-adult, hemalaun-eosin (1:1250) Intense cytoplasm colouration of longitudinal structures.

Fig. 69:
Brain-adult, ferric hematoxylin-eosin (1:1250). Intense cytoplasm colouration. Fragment of medullary sheath.

Fig. 71:
Brain-adult, Best-carmine colouration (1:1250). Abundant, island-like concentration of *glycogen.*

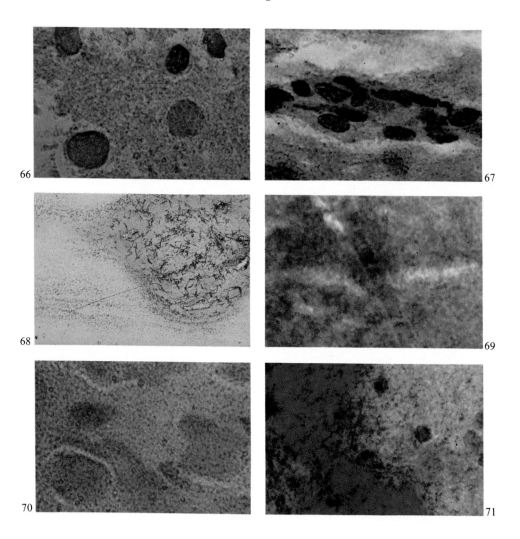

66

67

68

69

70

71

Fig. 72:
Liver-fetal, Feulgen (1:1250).
Nuclei smaller than in the adult preparation.

Fig. 74:
Liver-fetal, ninhydrin (1:30).
Small amount of *alpha-amino-acids*.

Fig. 76:
Bone-marrow-fetal, Feulgen (1:1250). Round
nuclei prevail.

Fig. 73:
Liver-adult, Feulgen (1:1250)
Larger nuclei. Good cytoplasm colouration.

Fig. 75:
Liver-adult, ninhydrin (1:30). Areas abundant in
ninhydrin.

Fig. 77:
Bone-marrow-adult,Feulgen (1:1250).
Fat drops. Reticular structures. Moderate DNA-
colouration within the meshwork.

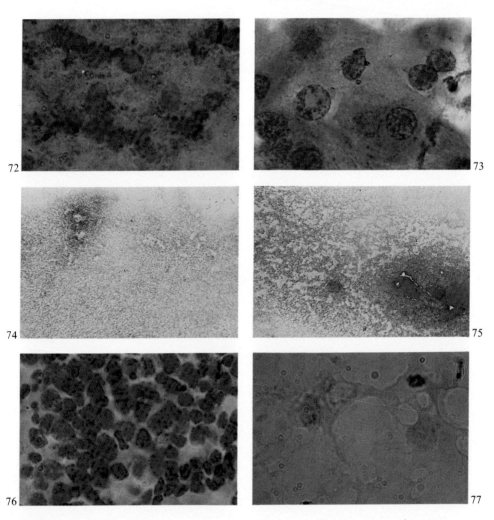

Liver

The nuclear structures of the liver preparations come out well, the small nuclei of the fetal tissues appear more intensely coloured than the very large nuclei of the adult preparations. The cytoplasm takes dye readily but, corresponding to the smaller nuclei, is comparatively better

Fig. 78:
Bone-marrow-fetal, ninhydrin (1:1250). Intense colouration of the cytoplasm.

Fig. 79:
Bone-marrow-adult, ninhydrin (1:1250). Concentration of ninhydrin to trace the alpha-amino-acids in the seams of the meshwork.

Fig. 80:
Spleen-fetal, methyl green-pyronin (1:1250). Intense DNA-colouration of the nuclei. Small amount of RNA as reddish fundamental tone of the ground-substance.

Fig. 81:
Spleen-adult, methyl green-pyronin (1:1250). Fibrous structure and nuclei colourable with methyl green. RNA fundamental tone and particles.

Fig. 82:
Spleen-fetal, scarlet (1:1250). Nuclei clearly structured. Erythrocytes, yellowish. No *fat* traced.

Fig. 83:
Spleen-adult, scarlet (1:1250). Clear nuclear and fibrous structures. More intense colour of erythrocytes. Small amounts of *fat* particles.

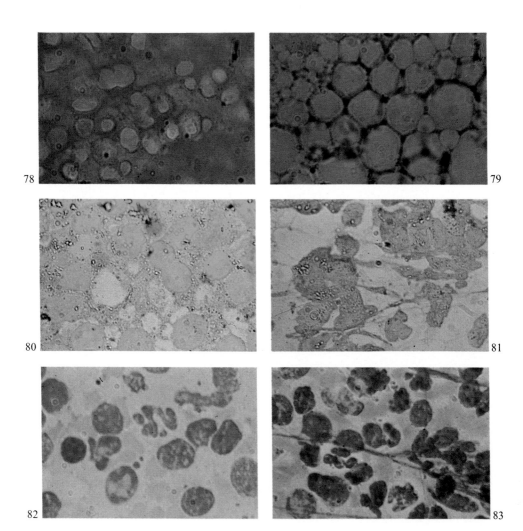

78

79

80

81

82

83

Fig. 84:
Spleen-fetal, dopa-oxydase (1:1250).
Small amount of dopa-oxydase.

Fig. 85:
Spleen-adult, dopa-oxydase (1:1250). Erythrocyte membranes and cytoplasm spaces accentuated.

Fig. 86:
Muscle-fetal, ferric hematoxylin (1:1250).
Reticular structure. Roundish-oval nuclei.

Fig. 87:
Muscle-adult, ferric hematoxylin (1:1250).
Intense striation with oblong, fusiform nuclei.

Fig. 88:
Muscle-fetal, phosphatase (1:1250). Longitudinal striation accentuated by phosphatase colouration.

Fig. 89:
Muscle-adult, phosphatase (1:1250). Transverse striation indicating activity.

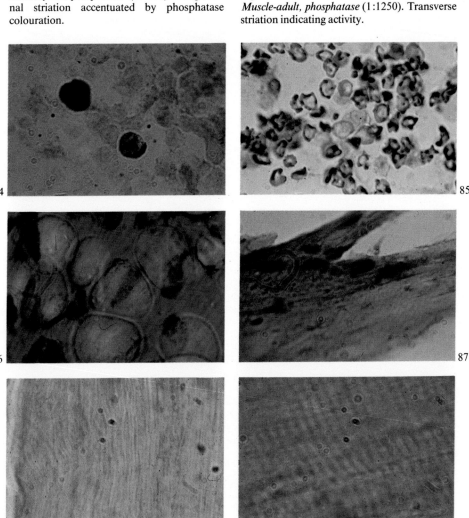

84

85

86

87

88

89

accentuated in the fetal tissue (fig. 72, 73). These findings correspond to the identification of DNA with rela-tively slight RNA activity. Fat can be demonstrated only by traces. The adult, un-like the fetal, animal shows a grest con-

Fig. 90:
Kidney-fetal, hemalaun – eosin (1 :1250). Round, intensely coloured nuclei. Tubular areas.

Fig. 92:
Kidney-fetal, ninhydrin (1 :1250). Small amounts of ninhydrin.

Fig. 94:
Kidney-fetal, phosphatase (1 :1250). Intense colouration. Particles surround the nucleus in the form of crayfish-claws.

Fig. 91:
Kidney-adult, hemalaun – eosin (1 :1250). Less intense colouration of nucleus. Only sporadic deeply coloured cytoplasm.

Fig. 93:
Kidney-adult, ninhydrin (1 :1250). Clear colouration of cytoplasm and nuclear membranes.

Fig. 95:
Kidney-adult, phosphatase (1 :1250). Colouration of the ground substance.

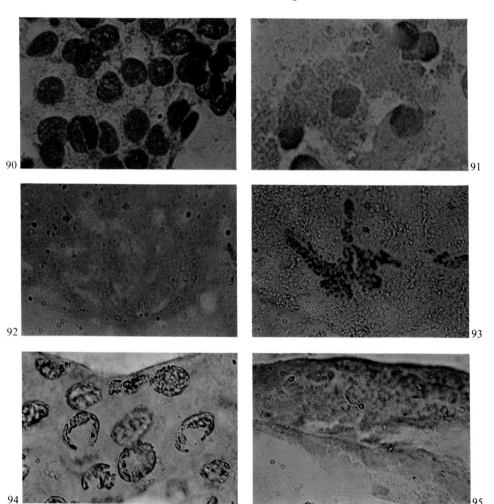

90 91 92 93 94 95

centration of glycogen, which is dispersed into large cells with wide spaces of cytoplasm but attains the most intense colours. Just so, the concentration of alpha-amino-acid is much higher in the adult tissue (fig. 74, 75). The colouring of

76

the adult tissues prevails for both enzymes, and enzymatic activities can clearly be shown in all preparations.

Bone-marrow

The structures of the bone-marrow preparations alone are very different. Whereas in the fetal preparation many round cells prevail and thus the cytoplasm and ground substance are of less importance, fibres and reticular structures with few incorporated cells and much fat predominate in the adult preparation (fig. 76, 77). Consequently, the concentration of DNA in the fetal tissues is high. The colouring of RNA in the adult tissue is very pale but somewhat more concentrated than in the fetal tissue. A higher fat-content can be found in the tissues of the adult animals, in contrast to the fetal tissue. The fetal preparation contains very large amounts of glycogen and alpha-amino-acids (fig. 78, 79). The activity of the alkaline phosphatase can be called strikingly low. The dopa-oxydase is very active and brings about a remarkably intense colouring of the fetal tissues.

Spleen

The fetal tissue is distinguished for its roundish nuclei whereas the adult preparation has much more ground substance, which is transversed by fibriform branches of the nuclei. As the fibres, same as the nuclei, contain much DNA, the preparation of the maternal animal appears richer in nuclei acids. Also the amount of RNA in the adult tissue exceeds that of the fetal preparation (fig. 80, 81). In contrast to the adult splenic tissue slightly interspersed in the nuclei and fibres, no fatty substances can be detected in the fetal tissue (fig. 82, 83). The concentration of alpha-amino-acid

of the spleen corresponds in the mother and fetus; this substance is bound mainly to the reticular ground substances. The rather strong activity of dopa-oxydase concentrates in the cytoplasm space in the adult splenic tissue, and it must be taken into consideration that the intensely coloured erythrocytes of the non-specific dopa-oxydase reaction may easily give a false impression. The fetal preparation contains very little dopa-oxydase (fig. 84, 85). A mean phosphatase activity is in the cells and ground substance of both tissues.

Muscle

Muscle preparations of the mother and fetus differ by the structure alone. Whereas in the fetus longitudinal structures with roundish-oval nuclei possess the picture, the preparations of the adult animal show an intense transverse striation with oblong, fusiform nuclei. The cytoplasm is less coloured in the fetal tissue than in the adult (fig. 86, 87). All nuclei contain much DNA; the concentration in the large nuclei of the adult tissue is lower. Altogether, the intensity of pyronin is high, which is reflected especially by the transverse striation of the adult muscles. Only small quantities of fat can be found in the spaces between the muscle-fibres of the adult preparation. Glycogen occurs in the cytoplasm and ground substance of the fetal and adult muscular tissue. The concentration of alpha-amino-acid is very high in either preparation and is bound to the above-mentioned longitudinal structures in the fetal tissues and to the transverse structures in the adult tissues. The dopa-oxydase stains very intensely in both, the fetal and the adult tissues. The mean activity of phosphatase receives expression very clearly in the longitudinal and transverse structures (fig. 88, 89).

Fig. 96:
Omentum – fetal, hemalaun – eosin (1:1250). Syncitial structure. Dense colouration of nucleus. Obvious eosin colouration of the cytoplasm.

Fig. 98:
Omentum – fetal, scarlet (1:30). Different amounts of fat in arteries and veins.

Fig. 100:
Omentum – fetal, methyl green – pyronin (1:1250). Distinct majority of the pyronin-colouration, which proves the presence of RNA. Island-like formation.

Fig. 97:
Omentum – adult, hemalaun – eosin (1:1250). Fusiform nuclei in longitudinal formations.

Fig. 99:
Omentum – adult, scarlet (1:30). Distinct proof of fat.

Fig. 101:
Omentum – adult, methyl green – pyronin (1:1250). DNA colouration of the nuclei at the connective points of the reticular structure.

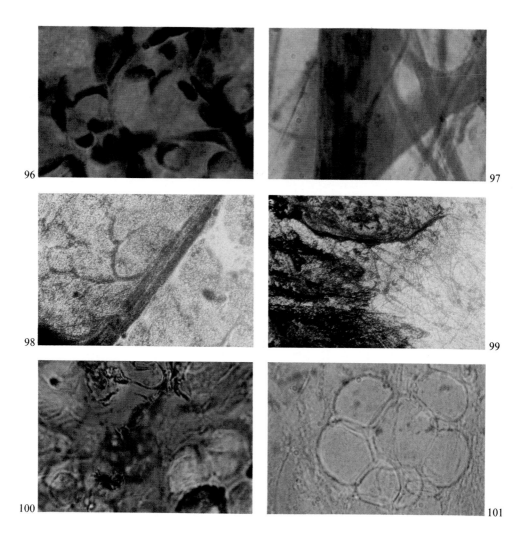

96   97   98   99   100   101

Fig. 102:
Omentum – fetal, dopa-oxydase (1:1250). Intense activity of dopa-oxydase.

Fig. 103:
Omentum – adult, dopa-oxydase (1:1250). Distinct fibrous structure with less intense colouration.

Fig. 104:
Lung – fetal, methyl green – pyronin (1:1250). Strong *RNA* concentration in the cytoplasm.

Fig. 105:
Lung – adult, methyl green – pyronin (1:1250). Good nuclear colouration. Relatively homogenous *RNA* superposition (reddish tone).

Fig. 106:
Lung – fetal, Best-carmine colouration (1:1250). Small amount of *glycogen*.

Fig. 107:
Lung – adult, Best-carmine staining (1:1250). Only traces of *glycogen*.

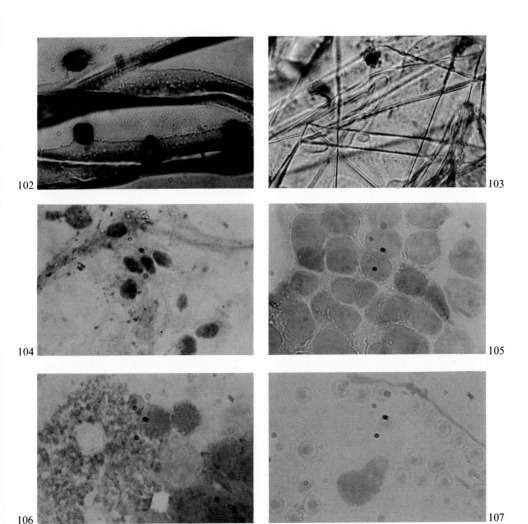

102

103

104

105

106

107

Kidney

The roundish to roundish-oval nuclei of the renal tissue have a compact structure and can be stained deeply with DNA according to their consistency; depending on the quantity of nuclei, the fetal tissue shows a deeper colouring (fig. 90, 91). Traces of RNA can be identified in the adult preparation alone. Fat and glycogen have been found only by traces both in the fetal and in the adult tissues. Quite different is the concentration of the alpha-amino-acids, found highly intense in the adult tissue, chiefly in the cytoplasm, ground substance and nuclear membranes (fig. 92, 93). The dopa-oxydase stains deeply the fetal and adult tissues, without taking into account the effect of the non-specific dopa-oxydase staining of the erythrocytes. The activity of phosphatase is considerably high in both categories of the renal tissue, especially in the space of cytoplasm of the fetal kidney (fig. 94, 95).

Omentum

The fetal omentum preparation is distinguished for alveolar, syncitial, pentagonal to hexagonal structures. The roundish to oval nuclei are localized in the intersections of the syncitium. In contrast thereto, the adult tissue has a fibrous, net-like structure in which oblong, fusiform nuclei prevail (fig. 96, 97). Both tissues, especially the fetal, are interwoven with nets of vessels, veins and arteries mostly running parallel side by side (fig. 98). DNA and RNA, forming islet-like groups, can be seen in both tissues (fig. 100, 101). A high concentration of fat is in the adult tissue (fig. 98, 99). In the fetal tissue, just one of the parallel vessels attracts attention by more intensely stained fat. Glycogen is stained mainly in the fetal tissue. The concentration of the alpha-amino-acids prevails in

the fetal preparation and is massive in the area of the vascular network and islet-like regions, which are rich in ground substance whereas the adult preparation shows the deepest staining on the membranes of the fibre systems. The dopa-oxydase disperses uniformly on the islet-like complexes in the fetal and adult smears (fig. 102, 103). The activity of phosphatase prevails in the fetal tissue but is rather high in both.

Lung

The nuclei of the fetal lung are roundish to oval, poor in structures, very compact and intensely enough stained with DNA whereas the about three times larger, more loosely but more differently structured nuclei of the adult lung show correspondingly smaller concentrations of DNA. The cytoplasm is well stained. The fetal lung contains much RNA in branches of cytoplasm and reticular structures. In the mothers, however, only low concentrations of RNA are found outside the cell nuclei (fig. 104, 105). Fat did not occur in either tissue. Traces of glycogen were identified in a few storage cells, above all in fetal tissue (fig. 106, 107). Alpha-amino-acids are found in both tissues, but the adult tissue has more. High concentrartions of dopa-oxydase are there in both cases. A low activity of phosphatase bound to the membrane systems can be marked for the fetal animal.

The descriptions of the organs have given just a concise survey of the points to be answered. Results can be seen from the summarizing synoptic fig. 108.

Morphologically and cytochemically, there are more differences between fetal and maternal tissues than could be anticipated in any bio-economic association. The morphological structures of the fetal and adult tissues are largely similar, with the following exceptions:

80

1. The fetal tissues have more and smaller nuclei, which appear round to roundish-oval and much more concentrated, more distinct and thus stronger than the voluminous, often oblong-fusiform, loosely structured nuclei of the adult tissues.

Fig. 108:
Synopsis of the cytochemical comparison between fetal (F) and maternal (E) tissues.

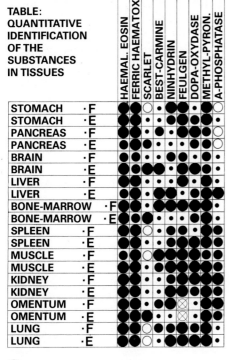

TABLE: QUANTITATIVE IDENTIFICATION OF THE SUBSTANCES IN TISSUES

Columns: HAEMAL. EOSIN, FERRIC HAEMATOX., SCARLET, BEST-CARMINE, NINHYDRIN, FEULGEN, DOPA-OXYDASE, METHYL-PYRON., A-PHOSPHATASE

Rows: STOMACH ·F, STOMACH ·E, PANCREAS ·F, PANCREAS ·E, BRAIN ·F, BRAIN ·E, LIVER ·F, LIVER ·E, BONE-MARROW ·F, BONE-MARROW ·E, SPLEEN ·F, SPLEEN ·E, MUSCLE ·F, MUSCLE ·E, KIDNEY ·F, KIDNEY ·E, OMENTUM ·F, OMENTUM ·E, LUNG ·F, LUNG ·E

● identified in large quantities
● identified in medium quantities
· identified in small quantities
○ no identification possible
⊗ technical impossibility of preparing the product

2. The cytoplasm of the fetal tissues is more uniform and homogeneous. The extranuclear areas of the adult preparations are veined with a network of fibrous, reticular structures so that even in preparations, in which the cytoplasm prevails in proportion to the nucleus: plasma relation in the fetal tissue (e. g. spleen), the compactness of the ground substance appears lower than in the fetal tissues.

3. A syncitial-alveolate formation prevails in fetal omentum and bone-marrow, and a reticular-fibrous formation in the corresponding preparations of the adult animal.

4. The fetal muscle preparations show a longitudinal structure, the adult muscle preparations a distinct transverse striation.

As regards the cytochemical composition, the following is worth mentioning:

a) Fat occurs always in higher concentration in the adult tissue.

b) The proportion of the alpha-amino-acids: glycogen in the fetal and adult tissues depends on the tissue and cannot be generalized.

c) The concentration of nucleic acid, especially the nuclear DNA, is higher in the fetal tissues (exception: spleen) than in the mothers.

d) A uniform tendency of the cytochemically traceable enzymatic activities in the fetal and adult tissues has not been found as the enzymes apparently depend more on the organs than on the age.

Minerals, trace-elements and toxic metals in lyophilized tissues

In an almost biased manner the analysis of biological preparations made in the last decade has focused on the detection of organic compounds. The active substances or compounds sought in biochemical substrates and enzymes were proteins, lipids, carbohydrates, poly- and oligopeptides. In clinical terms, quantities that can be measured or weighed have priority over qualitative estimations. Here, the amount of substances found is sometimes relevant to their biological significance.

The fact that there cannot be any complex functioning compound without an inorganic nucleus is being slowly realized. There can be no hemoglobin without a Fe atom and no chlorophyll without an Mg atom. The red coloured material in the blood of mammals is dependent upon the presence and level of the iron atom, in the same way that the green colouring matter in plants depends upon magnesium. The bivalent ions particularly, magnesium, zinc and copper – represent an indispensable ingredient for the functioning of most enzymes. This significance of the trace elements in the functioning of biological systems encourages you to examine a number of the lyophilizates used in cell therapy with regard to their inorganic content.

Material and method

Minerals were analyzed from 19 different tissues of lyophilized commercial preparations of the «Siccacell-Series». In order to eliminate coincidences, such as seasonal and nutritional factors, each 400 mg of lyophilizate consisted of 4 different batches. Samples of the lyophilizates were numerically numbered and the laboratory conducting the analysis did not know the origin of the tissues.

The analyses were done at the Anamol Laboratories, 105 Scarsdale Road, Don Mills, ON, M3B 2R5. This laboratory, under the management of Dr. Tamari, has long years of experience in the analysis of elements, trace elements and toxic metals – in particular hair analysis. Results and their evaluation are computerized the same way as the results from nutritional analysis.

Results

Results of the analysis have been compiled in 3 tables –
Table 5 – elemental composition of the examined tissues
Table 6 – differences in element distribution in the tissues
Table 7 – differences in mineral or trace element content of female and male tissues – endocrine tissues primarily examined.

On the whole, at first sight the big differences in mineral content of fetal and juvenile tissue lyophilizates are striking. The second finding worth pointing out is the fact that individual elements are only present in specific tissues and missing in others. A third and remarkable finding was the unexpectedly great difference in mineral content between tissues of male and female origin.

Tab. 5: **Content of 21 elements, trace-elements and toxic metals in fetal and juvenile tissues. Values in ppm (pars per mille)**

	Ca	Cr	Co	Cu	Fe	Li	Mg	Mn	Mo	Ni	P	K	Se	Na	V	Zn	Al	As	Cd	Pb	Hg
Cerebrum	502	0,99	0	12,9	124	1,0	694	1,66	0,05	1,42	12330	17890	2,75	12990	0,01	51,9	20,9	5,30	0,46	1,4	12,3
Cerebellum	496	3,12	0,01	35,6	216,8	1,05	1007	2,76	0,16	0,76	13250	21970	0,77	13240	0,20	79,1	67,4	0,53	0,08	0	1,34
Diencephalon	445	2,31	0	25,4	161	0,80	888,8	2,08	0,15	1,10	14030	21010	0,29	12040	0,11	59,2	23,5	0	0,09	0,50	0
Lung	872	1,99	0	23,9	415	1,43	1062	1,77	0,22	0,65	14040	23880	0,14	28280	0,11	96,7	317,4	0,72	0,16	0	1,53
Liver	437	1,34	0	155,1	5293	1,02	954,2	16,11	1,35	1,22	11860	16590	0	8051	0,78	603,3	98,6	0	0,16	0,41	0,76
Spleen	527	1,93	0	24,6	1339	1,20	944,5	1,32	0,18	2,10	12830	18430	0	5892	0,38	70,1	139,1	0	0,17	1,07	0,18
Thymus	597,9	1,99	0	26,6	173,4	0,79	1163	1,97	0,18	0,75	13290	28400	0,22	7895	0,12	83,3	60,2	0,08	0,10	0	1,26
Adrenals ♂	613	1,10	0	13,4	301,9	0,51	587,1	2,94	0,07	0,56	10000	11970	0,20	5289	0	40,1	39,1	0	0,21	0	0
Adrenals ♀	658	17,8	0	19,2	537	0,99	833,9	4,67	0,86	9,27	12910	13830	0,88	5452	0,16	65,9	59,3	0,09	0,60	0	0
Placenta ♂	1150	1,30	0	16,9	651,1	0,88	979,6	1,89	0,17	0,65	13040	16170	0,67	13390	0,15	85,9	36,0	0	0,14	0	0,65
Placenta ♀	770,1	1,40	0	101,9	527,8	0,85	972,9	2,23	0,26	0,60	12230	14490	0,51	14510	0,13	115,1	24,4	0	0,60	0,11	0,35
Testis	919,8	1,59	0	15,7	288,9	0,86	1121	2,90	0,28	1,76	13890	32440	2,20	11700	0,14	131,5	74,7	0	0,21	0	0
Ovary	1077	6,11	0	21,4	345,1	0,84	755,1	2,66	0,33	5,42	11890	18920	1,41	28520	0,04	54,7	616,9	0,63	0,11	0	2,20
Thyreoidgland	851	5,08	0	28,1	281,4	1,31	1027	5,98	0,20	1,35	5653	10420	0,69	11730	0	73,8	111,0	0,50	0,11	0	2,17
Pankreas	3006	12,1	0	102,0	510,6	0,98	1290	5,90	0,63	1,42	13310	18630	0	13430	0,18	198,1	573,7	0,18	0,05	0	0,11
Connective Tissue	3238	5,34	0	41,8	295,3	2,22	1114	2,79	0,22	2,27	6395	9897	0,20	18830	0,15	72,3	74,0	0,20	0,26	0	1,42
Cartilage	13960	3,1	0	11,8	90,1	1,8	2458	2,1	0,1	2,4	13240	5593	0	20350	0,2	93,3	26,6	0	0,1	0	0

The following organs (tissues) were analyzed:

Cerebrum	Hypophysis, male	Thyroid	Lung
Cerebellum	Hyophysis, female	Pancreas	Liver
Diencephalon	Suprarenal gland, male	Thymus	Spleen
	Suprarenal gland,		Connective
	female		tissue
	Testis		Cartilage
	Ovaries		
	Placenta, male fetus		
	Placente, female fetus		

Comment on the various elements

As shown in Tables 5 and 6, the concentration gradient of elements indicated in parts per mille is surprisingly great, as we are concerned here with a purely quantitative evaluation.

Calcium (Ca) – The tissues examined which are richest in calcium are cartilage, connective tissues and pancreas. The tissues with the least amount of calcium are the cerebellum, diencephalon and liver (cartilage 13.960 ppm – liver 437 ppm).

Chromium (Cr) – High concentrations of chromium are found in the female suprarenal glands (17.8), pancreas and ovaries, with the lowest values in the liver, male suprarenal and the cerebrum (0.99). It is worth noting the tremendous difference between the female and male suprarenal glands, i.e. 17.8 vs. 1.10, a ratio also reflected between the ovaries and testes at 6.11 to 1.59.

Cobalt (Co) – Not found in fetal tissues, with the exception of a trace in the cerebellum (0.01).

Copper (Cu) – Also shows a marked difference between the copper-rich organs, liver (155.1), pancreas (102), female placenta (101.9) and the tissues poor in copper, namely male suprarenal glands (13.4), cerebrum (12.9) and cartilage (11.8).

Iron (Fe) – The highest concentration is in the liver (5.293), spleen and male placenta and the lowest concentration in the diencephalon, cerebrum and cartilage (90.1).

Lithium (Li) – Found in connective tissue (2.22), cartilage and lung at relatively high concentrations. Levels are relatively low in the diencephalon, thymus and male suprarenal glands (0.51). Here the ratio is small because of the low initial values.

Magnesium (Mg) – Cartilage (2.458), pancreas and thymus show the highest levels, and the ovaries, cerebrum and male suprarenal glands (587.1) the lowest values.

Manganese (Mn) – Liver (16.11), thyroid and pancreas are at the top, whereas lung, cerebrum and spleen (1.32) are at the low end of the scale.

Molybdenum (Mo) – is found mainly in the liver (1.35), female suprarenal

Tab. 6: **Content- and Conzentrationgraduation of 21 elements, trace-elements and toxic metals in 17 fetal or juvenile tissues. Values in ppm (pars per mille).**

	1	2	3	4	5	6	7	8	9	10	11	12	13	14	15	16	17
Ca	Cartilage 13960	Conn. tiss. 3238	Pankreas 3006	Placenta ♂ 1150	Ovary 1077	Testis 919,8	Lung 872	Thyreoid 851	Placenta ♀ 770,1	Adrenal ♀ 658	Adrenal ♂ 613	Thymus 597,9	Spleen 527	Cerebrum 502	Cerebellum 496	Dienceph. 445	Liver 437
Cr	Adrenal ♀ 17,8	Pankreas 12,1	Ovary 6,11	Conn. tiss. 5,34	Thyreoid 5,08	Cerebellum 3,12	Cartilage 3,1	Dienceph. 2,31	Thymus 1,99	Lung 1,99	Spleen 1,93	Testis 1,59	Placenta ♂ 1,40	Liver 1,34	Placenta ♀ 1,30	Adrenal ♂ 1,10	Cerebrum 0,99
Co	Cerebellum 0,01																
Cu	Liver 155,1	Pankreas 102,0	Placenta 101,9	Conn. tiss. 41,8	Cerebellum 35,6	Thyreoid 28,1	Thymus 26,6	Dienceph. 25,4	Spleen 24,4	Lung 23,9	Ovary 21,4	Adrenal ♀ 19,2	Placent. ♂ 16,9	Testis 15,7	Adrenal ♂ 13,4	Cerebrum 12,9	Cartilage 11,8
Fe	Liver 5293	Spleen 1339	Placenta ♂ 651	Thyreoid. 537	Spleen 527,8	Cerebellum 510,6	Lung 415	Cerebrum 345,1	Pankreas 301,9	Conn. tiss. 295,3	Placenta ♂ 288,5	Thyreoid. 281,4	Spleen 216,8	Ovary 173,4	Adrenals ♀ 161	Cerebrum 124	Adrenals ♂ 90,1
Li	Conn. tiss. 2,22	Cartilage 1,8	Lung 1,43	Cartilage 1,31	Spleen 1,20	Liver 1,02	Thyreoid. 1,05	Cerebellum 1,0	Testis 1,0	Liver 0,98	Placenta ♂ 0,99	Ovary 0,86	Dienceph. 0,85	Ovary 0,84	Thymus 0,80	Thymus 0,79	Spleen 0,51
Mg	Cartilage 2458	Pankreas 1290	Thymus 1163	Testis 1121	Conn. tiss. 1114	Lung 1062	Thyreoid. 1027	Cerebellum 1007	Placenta ♀ 979,6	Liver 954,2	Placenta ♂ 944,5	Dienceph. 888,8	Spleen 833,9	Ovary 795	Cerebrum 694	Cerebrum 587,1	
Mn	Liver 16,11	Adrenals ♀ 5,98	Pankreas 5,90	Adrenals ♀ 4,67	Testis 2,94	Placenta ♀ 2,90	Lung 2,79	Testis 2,76	Placenta ♀ 2,66	Spleen 2,23	Cartilage 2,1	Dienceph. 2,08	Thymus 1,97	Dienceph. 1,89	Lung 1,77	Cerebrum 1,66	Spleen 1,32
Mo	Liver 1,35	Pankreas 0,63	Cartilage 0,63	Ovary 0,33	Testis 0,28	Lung 0,26	Lung 0,22	Conn. tiss. 0,22	Thyreoid. 0,20	Spleen 0,18	Dienceph. 0,18	Thymus 0,17	Cerebellum 0,16	Dienceph. 0,15	Cartilage 0,1	Adrenals ♀ 0,07	Adrenals ♂ 0,05
Ni	Adrenals ♀ 9,27	Cartilage 5,42	Cartilage 2,4	Conn. tiss. 2,27	Spleen 2,1	Testis 1,76	Pankreas 1,42	Cerebrum 1,42	Placenta ♂ 1,35	Liver 1,22	Dienceph. 1,10	Cerebellum 0,76	Thymus 0,75	Liver 0,65	Placenta ♂ 0,65	Conn. tiss. 0,60	Adrenals ♂ 0,56
P	Lung 14040	Dienceph. 14030	Testis 13890	Pankreas 13310	Thymus 13290	Cerebellum 13250	Pankreas 13240	Placenta ♂ 13040	Cerebrum 12910	Spleen 12830	Cerebrum 12330	Placenta ♀ 12230	Ovary 11890	Liver 11860	Thyreoid. 10000	Conn. tiss. 6395	Thyreoid. 5653
K	Testis 32440	Thymus 28400	Lung 23880	Cerebellum 21970	Dienceph. 21010	Ovary 18920	Pankreas 18630	Spleen 18630	Cerebrum 17890	Liver 16590	Placenta ♂ 16170	Adrenals ♀ 14490	Adrenals ♀ 13830	Adrenals ♀ 11970	Thyreoid. 10420	Conn. tiss 9897	Cartilage 5593
Se	Cerebrum 2,75	Testis 2,20	Ovary 1,41	Adrenals ♀ 0,88	Cerebellum 0,77	Placenta ♂ 0,69	Dienceph. 0,67	Placenta ♀ 0,51	Dienceph. 0,29	Conn. tiss. 0,22	Adrenals ♂ 0,20	Conn. tiss. 0,20	Lung 0,14	Liver 0,14	Spleen 0,14	Cartilage 0	Pankreas 0
Na	Ovary 28520	Lung 28280	Cartilage 20350	Conn. tiss. 18830	Pankreas 14510	Testis 13430	Placenta ♂ 13390	Cerebrum 13240	Cerebrum 12990	Placenta ♀ 12040	Thyreoid. 11730	Lung 11700	Dienceph. 12040	Ovary 8051	Dienceph. 5892	Adrenals ♀ 5452	Adrenals ♂ 5289
V	Liver 0,38	Spleen 0,38	Cartilage 0,2	Cerebellum 0,2	Pankreas 0,18	Placenta ♀ 0,16	Placenta ♂ 0,15	Thyreoid. 0	Placenta ♀ 0,14	Placenta ♀ 0,13	Thymus 0,12	Lung 0,11	Dienceph. 0,11	Ovary 0,04	Cerebrum 0,01	Adrenals ♂ 0	Thyreoid. 0
Zn	Liver 603,3	Pankreas 198,1	Testis 131,5	Placenta 115,1	Lung 96,7	Testis 93,3	Liver 85,9	Thymus 83,3	Cerebellum 79,1	Thyreoid. 73,8	Adrenals ♂ 72,3	Spleen 70,1	Ovary 65,9	Dienceph. 59,2	Ovary 54,7	Dienceph. 51,9	Adrenals ♂ 40,1
Al	Ovary 616,9	Pankreas 573,7	Lung 317,4	Spleen 139,1	Thyreoid. 111,0	Liver 98,6	Testis 74,7	Cerebellum 74,0	Cerebellum 67,4	Placenta ♂ 60,2	Adrenals ♀ 59,3	Thymus 39,1	Cartilage 26,6	Cartilage 24,4	Cartilage 23,5	Dienceph. 23,5	Cerebrum 20,9
As	Cerebrum 5,30	Ovary 0,72	Ovary 0,63	Cerebellum 0,53	Thyreoid. 0,50	Conn. tiss. 0,20	Pankreas 0,18	Adrenals ♀ 0,09	Adrenals ♀ 0	Dienceph. 0	Placenta ♂ 0	Spleen 0	Placenta ♀ 0	Placenta ♀ 0	Testis 0	Cerebellum 0,08	Cartilage 0
Cd	Adrenals ♀ 0,60	Cerebrum 0,46	Cerebrum 0,46	Pankreas 0,26	Placenta ♀ 0,21	Testis 0,21	Lung 0,17	Liver 0,16	Cerebellum 0,14	Adrenals ♀ 0,14	Adrenals ♂ 0,11	Thymus 0,11	Cartilage 0,1	Cartilage 0,1	Dienceph. 0,09	Conn. tiss. 0,08	Cartilage 0,05
Pb	Cerebrum 1,4	Spleen 1,07	Dienceph. 0,50	Liver 0,41	Ovary 0,1	Cerebellum 0	Lung 0	Thymus 0	Adrenals ♂ 0	Adrenals ♀ 0	Placenta ♂ 0	Testis 0	Ovary 0	Thyreoid 0	Pankreas 0	Conn. tiss. 0	Cartilage 0
Hg	Cerebrum 12,3	Ovary 2,20	Thyreoid 2,17	Lung 1,53	Conn. tiss. 1,42	Cerebellum 1,34	Thymus 1,26	Liver 0,76	Placenta ♂ 0,65	Placenta ♀ 0,35	Spleen 0,18	Pankreas 0,11	Dienceph. 0	Adrenals ♀ 0	Testis 0	Testis 0	Cartilage 0

85

glands and the pancreas. Only traces are found in the diencephalon, male suprarenal glands and the cerebrum (0.05).

Nickel (Ni) – The most surprising distribution pattern of all elements. The highest concentrations are in the generating tissues of the female fetus, female suprarenal glands (9.27) and ovaries (5.92). These are paralleled by 10 times lower levels in the lung and placenta (0.60). A certain similarity can be identified with chromium.

Phosphorus. Highest phosphorus concentrations (P) are found in the loung (14.040), diencephalon and testes, with the lowest in the male suprarenal glands, connective tissue and thyroid (5.653).

Potassium (K) – Shows a steep gradient between the tissues rich in potassium, such as testes (32.440), thymus and lung, and the tissues with very little potassium, namely thyroid, connective tissue and cartilage (5.593).

Selenium (Se) – Tissues rich in selenium are the cerebrum (2.75), testes and ovaries; tissues low in selenium or free from selenium are cartilage, spleen, liver and placenta, with a 0-value.

Sodium (Na) – Represents the second largest quantitative share of the intracellular elements after potassium. The high values in the ovaries (28.520), lung and cartilage are paralleled by low values in the spleen and the suprarenal glands (5.289).

Vanadium (V) – Does not reach the 1.0 ppm in any tissue, with liver (0.78),

spleen and cartilage showing the highest values. Thyroid and male suprarenal glands do not contain any vanadium.

Zinc (Zn) – Found in large quantities in the liver (603.3), pancreas and testes. The concentration is lowest in the ovaries, cerebrum and the male suprarenal glands (40.1). There is also an interesting ratio between the testes (131.5) and ovaries (54.7).

Aluminium (Al) – Shows the highest concentrations in the ovaries (616.9), pancreas and lung, and the lowest concentrations in the cerebrum, female placenta, fetus and diencephalon (23.5).

Arsenic (As) – The cerebral hemispheres are alone at the top with 5.30, followed by the lung (0.72) and the ovary (0.63). Most fetal organs do not contain arsenic.

Cadmium (Cd) – Found in the female suprarenal glands and female placenta at 0.60 ppm and in the brain at 0.46 in measurable ranges. In most tissues its values are around or below 0.1 ppm.

Lead (Pb) – Found in the cerebrum (1.4), spleen (1.07) and diencephalon (0.50). Most fetal and juvenile tissues do not contain any lead.

Mercury (Hg) – Found, as for most heavy metals, in the cerebral hemispheres (12.3) but in lower concentrations in the ovaries (2.20) and the thyroid (2.17). Five organs, among them surprisingly the diencephalon, do not contain any trace of lead.

Tab. 7: **Differences in the content on minerals, trace-elements and toxic metals in hormonproducing tissues of males and female origin. Noticable are the following differences: In pituary gland: Calcium, Chromium, Copper, Iron, Lithium. In testis and ovary: Magnesium, Chromium, Nickel, Sodium, Potassium. In adrenals: Chromium, Iron, Molybden, Nickel, Selenium. In placenta: Calcium, Copper, Zinc, Aluminium, Cadmium.**

	Ca	Cr	Co	Cu	Fe	Li	Mg	Mn	Mo	Ni	P	K	Se	Na	V	Zn	Al	As	Cd	Pb	Hg
Adrenals ♂	613	1,10	0	13,4	301,9	0,51	587,1	2,94	0,07	0,56	10000	11970	0,20	5289	0	40,1	39,1	0	0,21	0	0
Adrenals ♀	658	17,80	0	19,2	537	0,99	833,9	4,67	0,86	9,27	12910	13830	0,88	5452	0,16	65,9	59,3	0,09	0,60	0	0
Placenta ♂	1150	1,30	0	16,9	651,1	0,88	979,6	1,89	0,17	0,65	13040	16170	0,67	13390	0,15	85,9	36,0	0	0,14	0	0,65
Placenta ♀	770,1	1,40	0	101,9	527,8	0,85	972,9	2,23	0,26	0,60	12230	14490	0,51	14510	0,13	115,1	24,4	0	0,60	0,11	0,35
Testis	919,8	1,59	0	15,7	288,9	0,86	1121	2,90	0,28	1,76	13890	32440	2,20	11700	0,14	131,5	74,7	0	0,21	0	0
Ovary	1077	6,11	0	21,7	345,1	0,84	755,1	2,66	0,33	5,42	11890	18920	1,41	28520	0,04	54,7	616,9	0,63	0,11	0	2,20
Pituary ♂	972	0,53	0	21	17	0,28	57	2,15	0,27	4,9	6398	9701	0,11	7317	0,34	49	21,6	0	0,25	1,24	0
Pituary ♀	1304	0,71	0	70	20	0,11	63	2,49	0,22	3,5	6409	11240	0,04	8146	0,14	74	17,9	0	0,24	5,14	0

87

Test for toxicity

Acute toxicity (Dosis letalis acuta)

Maximum applicable quantities of 4–5 g/kg of bodyweight of liver, heart, placenta were tolerated by BLH mice without deaths so that a DL 50 (or DL 5) could not be determined. Rats tolerated 350–1750 fold therapeutic doses of placenta without any lethal effect.

Subacute toxicity

Wistar rats treated with a 50fold therapeutic dose did not show any symptoms of subacute toxicity (NEUMANN, 1961). The lyophilisates of liver, heart and placenta were controlled and the death rates, bodyweight, weights of organs, macroscopic and microscopic findings were ascertained.

Subchronic and chronic toxicity

A 50fold therapeutic dose (750 mg) of liver lyophilisate gave just a small difference in weight increase in dogs whereas all other parameters such as temperature, blood-pressure, frequency of the pulse and breathing and leukocyte count showed no measurable differences so that there were no indications for a subchronic toxicity.

Standardization

Reasons of practical therapy require the use of qualitatively and quantitatively constant preparations. While the application of fresh tissues may absolutely be effective and acceptable in the hands of an experienced worker, inadequate safety and the lacking determination of quality and quantity dissuade from using fresh tissue in general medicine. The preparations used must meet the requirements of asepsis. Customary ways, however, such as irradiation or the addition of antibiotics, are not practicable as they would change the native composition of the biological tissues. So lyophilization has after all become the method of choice. The biochemical disintegration of the tissues is stopped at once by rapid freezing and simultaneous removal of fluids so that the freeze-dried substances keep the content of native substance and thus are even superior to so-called fresh tissues. A further advantage of the method is the fact that the preparations can be measured by clear quantities and be analysed by controllable qualities.

Incorporation and distribution of injected foreign tissues

Actually, an organism has three possibilities of coping with foreign tissues:

1. Use (enzymes) or incorporation (substrates) in the own tissues.
2. Disintegration with selective utilization and selective elimination.
3. Elimination in toto.

What becomes of a tissue in a foreign organism depends on the phylogenetic and ontogenetic affinity. The less differentiated the tissues and organisms, the better the mutual tolerance. It is therefore much easier to obtain an incorporation in lower species of animals than in man. Good chances for an effective incorporation in the human organism are offered chiefly by endogenic (transplantations of skin and bones) and homogeneous tissues (transplantations and implantations of bones, bone-marrow, vessel and cornea). Blood transfusions provide at least a functional incorporation. The incorporation of foreign tissues is seldom obtained. But even this is possible with juvenile tissues and good conditions of contact. An effective incorporation will always depend on an intimate contact between corresponding tissues.

If a direct contact between corresponding tissues is not feasible (as in most of the parenterally supplied suspensions of cells and tissues) the chances for a direct incorporation will dwindle. Generally, the other two ways namely disintegration with selective utilization and total elimination will have to be taken. A classical example is the implantation of calf hypophysis; the implant is disintegrated in foreign tissue (skin of the abdomen) and can develop a selective effect or is eliminated as foreign matter in the form of a sterile abscess.

The following tests are to show the principles of dispersing injected tissues. Studied were homogeneous fresh tissues and foreign dry tissues (lyophilisates).

Material and methods

To follow the interrelations between the donor and recipient tissues:
1. single cells ought to be estimable,
2. longitudinal studies must be conducted, without
3. disturbing the physiological regulations of recipient's whole organism.

The studies on the contents of irritable blisters conducted first could not be continued because the hairy animals selected for the test do not develop sufficiently provoked blisters. Consequently, cells of abdominal exudates from white rats and guinea pigs were used as standard objects. The exudates were concentrated by intraperitoneal applications of $5–10cm^3$ of paraffin oil (equal quantities in each series). Suspensions of heterogeneous cells were brought into this exudate rich in cells also by intraperitoneal injection, namely in the

1st test series organspecific, homologeous foreign «fresh cells», in the

2nd test series organdifferent, heterogeneous dry tissues.

To distinguish the cells of the recipient animals from the donor cells or tissues, vital stainings were effected with congo-red, janus-green or trypan blue; dry tissues histologically well differentiable remained unstained. The staining with janus-green had soon to be given up as the mitochondria were injured.

The distribution of the donor and recipient cells in the abdominal exudate was registered by regular punctures within 4–6 days. The cells showing a colour of neither the donors nor recipients were recorded by auramin counter-staining. By this vital labelling, the quotient of distribution was found at any time in the cells obtained by puncture. In addition, tampons of spleen, liver, thymus as well as net-mesenterium preparations from selected animals were made.

The intraperitoneal technique ranges between the intramuscular and intravenous applications, and can therefore be regarded as a model of the administrations customary for man.

Tested were 61 albino rats weighing 180 g on an average. The tests were conducted together with P. ROHRBACH and FLÖRSCHINGER.

Results

1. Homologeous, organspecific cells

Although by rinsing the entire abdominal cavity of a donor animal all cells were transmitted so that, theoretically, equal quantities of donor and own cells must be in the abdominal cavity of the recipient, the first punctures made after 10 to 30 minutes showed many more own cells than donor cells. The relation of vitally stained own cells to vitally stained donor cells was about 3:1 to 6:1, but also proportions of 11:1 were registered. The percentage of donor cells came to 1–14% of all cells in the first puncture (including those not stored). These different capacities of storing cells indicate that practically every animal must be valued individually; still, the following rules can be deduced:

1. Removal of the heterogeneous cells from the site of injection sets in at once;
2. heterogeneous cells diminish in an exponentially declining curve (fig. 110);
3. even after 4–6 days, sporadic cells with the heterogeneous vital substance can be traced.

The foreign, homologeous organoid cells begin to diminish at once and dwindle rapidly, though not in a constantly declining curve.

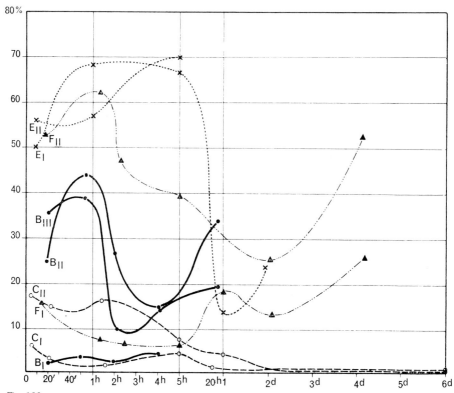

Fig. 109:
Decrease of the own cells marked by vital storage in the peritoneal exudate (guinea-pig).

In contrast thereto, the vitally stained own cells diminish much slower and stay considerably longer in the organism (fig. 109, 112).

The tests did not disclose anything about a fermentative disintegration. It can hardly be supposed that an extracellular fermentative disintegration occurs in the short time during which virtually the donor cells disappear.

2. Heterogeneous (xenogenic) organdifferent cells

The tests described above related to homologous, organspecific cells. Of practical interest were the studies on the situation when tissues of other organs from other bodies were injected under the same conditions. For this purpose, unstained tissues easily identifiable by their morphological properties (siccacell preparations) such as cartilaginous, renal and placenta tissues were used. The tissues were suspended in Ringer solution and injected intraperitoneally in a volume of 2.5 cc (50 mg of dry substance).

Heterogeneous cells disappear very quickly from the site of application. This may occur theoretically
1. by *dissolution*
2. by *phagocytosis*
3. by *transportation-removal*.

The reparations provided safe criteria for a phagocytosis (fig. 114, 119–128) of the heterogeneous cells and certain criteria for an increasing dissolution (fig. 117). Both processes seem to coincide because accumulations of phagocytes around fragments of cells and stain particles of donor cells were largely detected in the autogenous cells. These

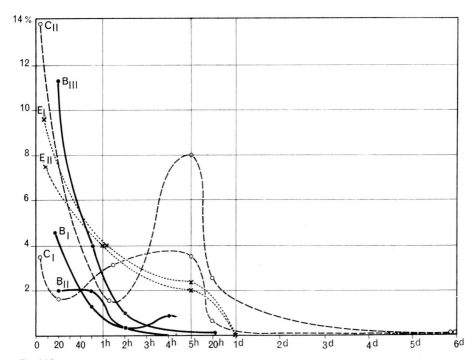

Fig. 110:
Decrease of the homologous donor cells marked by vital storages in the peritoneal exudate. Most of the foreign cells disappear within the first hour after injection.

«mixed colour» cells with much autogenous stain and little heterogeneous stain were found chiefly during the first five hours by 2%–4%, max. 6%.

The disappearance of these cell complexes from the injection area seems to be subject to the same laws as found for the autogenous cells. As complexes of fetal tissue are in question, the disintegration seems to take longer. Many individual pictures indicated that the autogenous cells gather round the heterogeneous tissues (fig. 114, 121–128, 160–189), push branches of protoplasma (fig. 119) to or into the heterogeneous tissue and «eat» the tissue complexes from the periphery. In coping with heterogeneous tissues, the body seems to rely mainly on the dissolution, the parenteral disintegration and the removal by autogenous phagocytes. It has been observed repeatedly that autogenous macrophages can take up in toto and disintegrate other cells (fig. 121, 125, 126).

The lyophilised fetal dry tissues have apparently a less «heterogeneous» effect in the recipient organism as they hardly provoke any changes of cell pictures worth mentioning. The antigenic stimulus is small, the formation of large basophile cells (plasma cells) does not take place or remains abortive. Several days (proved up to 6 days post injectionem) tissue complexes can stay at the site of injection where they are slowly destroyed by phagocytosis.

The removal

Vital labelling has revealed the whereabouts of the autogenous and heterogeneous cells. The rapid disappearance of heterogeneous cells and the longer stay of the autogenous cells charged with stain raise the question of where the cells go. Examinations of organs have shown that the cells are incorporated in the reticulum, mesenterium, in the spleen (fig. 111), liver, bone-marrow, thymus, muscle fasciae, articular coats as well as in the collagenous tissues of the snout, feet and tail i.e. the organs of the loose and reticular connective tissue.

As to this, it is worth mentioning that both the stored autogenous and heterogeneous cells are removed; apparently, therefore, also the autogenous cells are treated as «foreign to the body» from the time of storing.

Nearly equal temporal and topical results were obtained from studies on the distribution of implanted cells with organhomogenates labeled radioactively with L-histidin-2,5-tritium and L-lysin-4,5-tritium (KMENT, ZABAKAS, BINDER, HOFECKER, NIEDERMÜLLER and DREIER, 1968, 1969, 1973).

Summary

The outcome of the test series can be summarized as follows:

1. Injected cells or particles of tissue disappear rapidly from the site of injection, generally within 1 hour, no matter whether homogeneous cells of identical organs or heterogeneous cells of heterogenic, foreign organs are in question; the speed of disappearance is different.

2. Many criteria indicate that the disappearance from the site of injection by disintegration and removal is effected by macrophages. Time seems too short for a fermentative decomposition; but this question cannot be answered by tests.

3. The vitally stained cells are incorporated in the reticular (spleen, bone-marrow, thymus, liver) and loose connective tissue (collagen areas, articu-

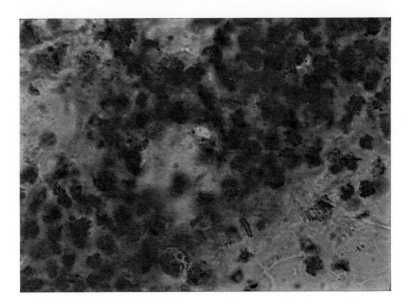

Fig. 111:
Storage of Congo red in the cells of the omentum.

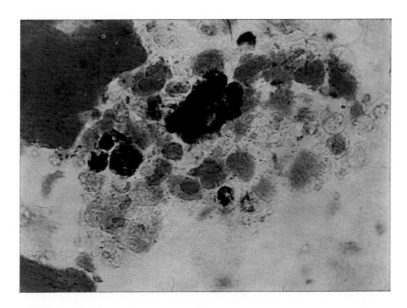

Fig. 112:
Pattern showing the own cells (storage of Congo red) and homologous heterogeneous cells (storage of trypan blue) 30 minutes after injection of the heterogeneous cells. Auramin countercolouration for the identification of the cells without storage.

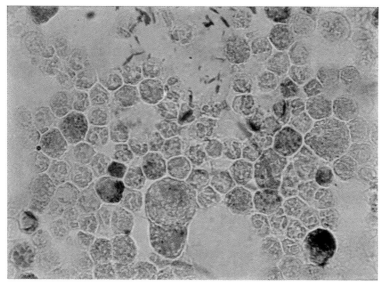

Fig. 113:
Pattern showing vital-stored own cells (Congo red) and homologous foreign cells (trypan blue) 5 hours after the latter's injection.

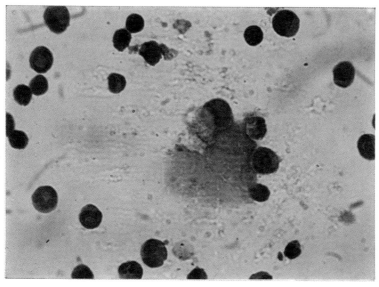

Fig. 114:
Body-produced cells with basophil plasma have «corroded» the remaining tissue of a fetal renal particle.

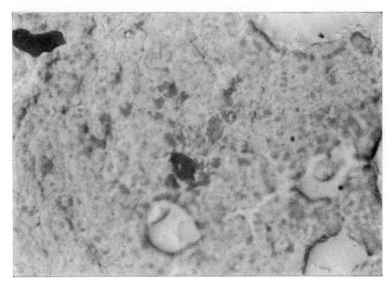

Fig. 115:
Storage of cells carrying vital dyestuffs in the thymus.

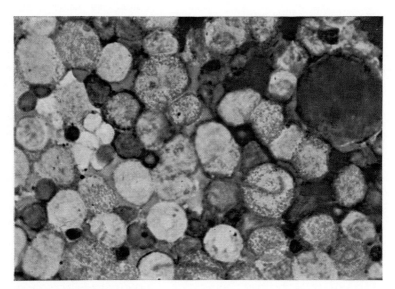

Fig. 116:
Dispersion of own and foreign cells in the spleen. Blue: homogeneous storage with trypan blue, red: heterogeneous cells stored with Congo red.

lar coats, muscle fasciae, peritoneum, mesenterium, omentum). From these tests, however, it can only be concluded that the cells are incorporated in related tissues. As the intraperitoneal application has an intermediate position between the intravenous and intramuscular administrations, the foregoing statement must be restricted. In the intramuscular application, fermentative disintegration may play an important part, but on principle the same mechanisms of disintegration and distribution must be supposed.

4. All partial results indicate that the heterogeneous cells cannot act in toto but as building elements in the size of oligopeptides, enzymes and substructures of biochemical substrates serve as material for the reconstruction of defective cell structures.

Transport-routes and effects

A basic requirement for the application of a medicament or a combination of active agents – as found in biological preparations – is the clarification of the principles governing the absorption and distribution of a remedy in the body. Since cell implants are of a size that can be detected under the microscope, the passage route from the stage of absorption to that of decomposition in submicroscopic particles is much better clarified than is possible and actually the case with many other medicaments.

This has been substantiated by the following tests:

a) Radioactive tagging of the injected tissular suspensions with P^{32} and measuring the radioactive concentration in the organs of the recipient (LETTRÉ, 1955; HARBERS, 1955).

b) Studies on the distribution of implanted cells by radioactive tagging of the organhomogenates with L-histidin-2,5-tritium and L-lysin-4,5-tritium (KMENT, ZABAKAS, BINDER, HOFECKER, NIEDERMÜLLER, DREIER).

c) Longitudinal studies on cellular suspensions tagged with vital stains (congo red, trypan blue, janus green, auramin) in guinea-pigs treated intraperitoneally (SCHMID, 1963).

d) Intravital studies on phagocytosis in guinea-pigs treated with intraperitoneal injections (SCHMID).

These basic experimental tests give the following uniform picture of the conditions of absorption and the fate of the implanted cell lyophilisates:

The heterological fetal tissue particles are loosened up immediately after the injection in net-like fashion, the chromosomes are «despiralized». This process is achieved virtually after 20 minutes. During that time, microphages move into the loosened cell structures and attach – microscopically clearly visible– particles of the implanted cells to their cytomembranes. The process is completed after about two hours to the extent that the entire heterological cell material degrades into small particles and is absorbed by the macrophages i. e. on their cell surface (fig. 117–124).

The second phase of the incorporation of the implanted cell material starts with the phagocytosis of the microphages (loaded with foreign material), which is effected by large mononuclear macrophages. The microphages proper, which are loaded with foreign tissue particles (polynuclear), are evidently felt by the body as being «foreign» and phagocytised by monocytary macrophages.

After 48 hours, this process has continued to an extent that under an optical microscope no implanted fetal cell material is left to be identified (fig. 112–126).

The extent to which the decomposition of the implanted cell material continues, is probably controlled by the recipient organism. On the one hand, there is evidence that the decomposition may take place up to the short-chain peptides (KMENT); on the other hand, there is substantiated proof that the recipient organism incorporates proteins of high molecular weight in specific functions. Cellresident immunoglobines M of a molecular weight of $5 \times 160,000$ are taken over in specific functions; the recipient shows a positive tuberculin reaction three days after the cell transfer and ob tains the transferred property of the life term of the implanted immunoglobines for 3–4 months, without developing tu berculosis. It is irrelevant here whether the donor material is homologous (after exchange transfusions from animal to animal) or heterologic (fluid cells of humans on guinea-pigs, pleura cells, lymphocyte concentrates, spleen-pulp); (M. CHASE, 1945, STAVITSKY, 1948; SCHMID F., 1949–1952; LAWRENCE, 1952; SCHLANGE, H.).

Principles of distribution

Whereas the absorption of implanted cell material, up to the stage of magnitudes identifiable by optical and electronic miscroscopy, has been clarified almost completely, the principles of distribution have been ascertained only in an incomplete manner.

The «Hallstedt principle» advanced by some representatives, according to which planted cells migrate to the «place of need», is difficult to prove or refute by way of experiment. The following stud ies on this partial question are available:

a) Increased growth of corresponding organs (ANDRES, 1953, 1959; MURPHY, 1916; DANCHAKOFF, 1916);

b) Specific effect of cell inoculates in the embryonic and growing organism (ANDRES, 1963); fig. 135a–c.

c) Induction of the growth of organs by implantation of homologous tissues (NEUMANN, 1963).

d) Principles of distribution of injected foreign tissues (SCHMID, 1963).

e) Measuring of radioactive concentration in the organs after application of radioactive tissues (LETTRÉ, HEM-PRICH and SPIRIG, 1953; LETTRÉ, 1954, 1955).

f) Rates of absorption of tagged tissues after splenectomy and experimental renal lesion (HARBERS, 1954).

g) The specific effect of implanted endometrium of rabbits on the uterus of castrated rabbits (BERNHARD and KRAMPITZ, 1960).

h) Studies on the distribution of implanted cells by tritiating organhomogenates (L-histidin-2,5-tritium; L-lysin-4,5-tritium; KMENT, ZABAKAS, BINDER, HOFECKER, NIEDERMÜLLER, DREIER, 1966–1973).

These experimental data can answer satisfactorily two important questions:

1. The injected (implanted) suspended cells and their stages of decomposition are rapidly distributed over the body in an exponentially declining curve, with the main activity taking place within the first hour after application; after five hours, the greater part of the distribution process has been completed. The taggings with

97

radioactive substances and vital staining widely agree in terms of the principle of distribution and in terms of time.

2. The degraded implantation material is removed authentically by microphages (polynuclear) and macrophages (monocytes, histiocytes); it has not been clarified but is probable that submicroscopic fragments are carried along with the flow of fluids.

Regardless of the type of tagging used, high concentrations of the implanted materials can be identified in various organs of the body already one hour after implantation. The tagged cells and their components are mainly, but not exclusively, identifiable in the implanted tissues of corresponding organs.

A few experiments suggest that besides the tissue relationship the «need» of an organ in the recipient organism plays a part. HARBERS (1954) found the rate of absorption of injected liver cells to rise from ordinarily 5–7% a day to 15–20% a day if the liver of the recipient animal was damaged by CCl_4-injections before testing; among these predamaged animals, the nucleic acid fraction in the liver was about double that in healthy animals. LETTRÉ (1955) did not find any specific concentration in the corresponding organs after injection of heart, liver and kidney cells tagged with P^{32}, but after injection of tagged brain cells the increase in activity in the brain of the recipient animal was double the level expected for uniform distribution.

The distribution studies by KMENT et al. (1968–1972) undoubtedly have an indicative value in biostatistics; they show that the highest concentrations of the implanted material are obtained in the corresponding organ. However, this can also be established for other organs and systems.

Increase in growth and action of corresponding organs of the recipient were repeatedly proved statistically (MURPHY, 1916; DANCHAKOFF, 1916; ANDRES, 1953, 1959, 1963; NEUMANN, 1963).

Fig. 117–124:
Fate of the implanted tissues in the recipient's organism.

Fig. 117:
Hypothalamic tissue immediately after implantation in the peritoneal cavity of the guinea-pig.

Fig. 119:
Already in the first hour, endogenic microphages penetrate into the loosened fetal foreign tissues. Microphage: dark colour.

Fig. 121:
After 2 hours, fetal heterogeneous tissues in the peritoneal cavity of the guinea-pig have been attached nearly completely to the membranes of the microphages.

Fig. 123:
Contact of a microphage marked with alkaline phosphatase (dark brick-red), with a monocytary macrophage.

Fig. 118:
Thymic tissue is loosened net-like 20–40 min. after the implantation (DNA disspiralled).

Fig. 120:
The degraded heterogeneous tissue is attached to the membranes of the endogenic microphages (dark colour) within 2 hours; here: cerebral tissue.

Fig. 122:
Within the following 48 hours, the complexes of microphages plus foreign particles are taken for heterogeneous and phagocyted by body-produced macrophages. «Battle of microphages».

Fig. 124:
Destruction of the segment-nuclear microphage (phosphatase colouration = dark red) by a monocyte at the site of injection (peritoneal cavity).

The donor material is degraded in the first hours after the injection of autogenous microphages and, later, macrophages to such an extent that it can no longer be traced optically and is dispersed all over the body. The material is incorporated specifically where the structures are of use and where they are needed. Whereas the cellular contents can rather quickly be disintegrated,

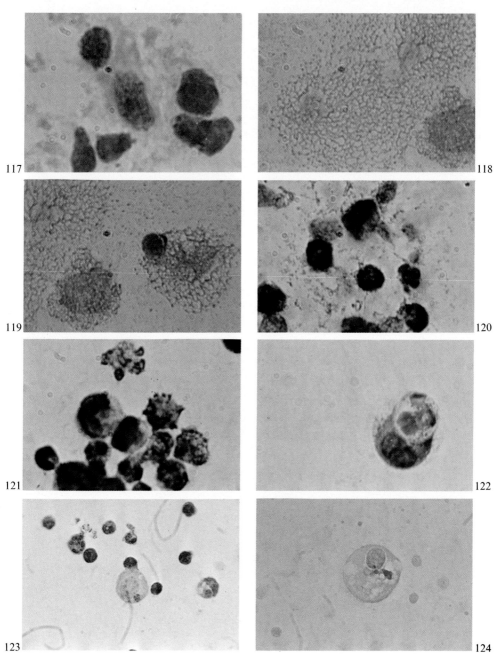

Fig. 125–128:
Disintegration of the microphages in the phagocyting macrophages in electron-optical dimensions. The process takes place in the peritoneal cavity, 2–48 hours after the injection.

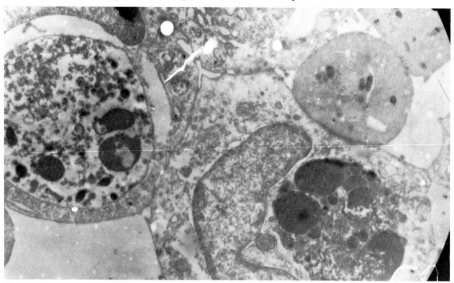

Fig. 125:
2 segment-nuclear microphages in various phases of disintegration (dark) within the cytoplasm of macrophages (1:11,000).

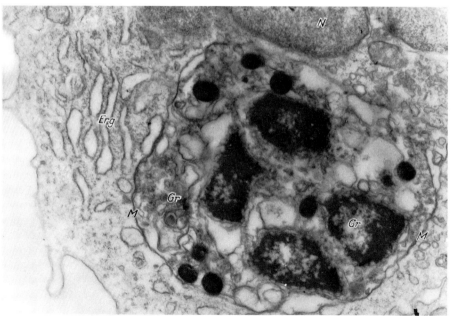

Fig. 126:
Whilst the cytoplasm of the granulocyte (Gr) has much been disintegrated, the nuclear fragments and the membrane (M) are still clearly perceptible. N = nucleus of the macrophage; Erg = ergastoplasm of the macrophage (1:30,000).

transported and incorporated by the recipient organism, the degradation of the membranes charged with heterogeneous particles of the autogenous microphages offers greater difficulties and may provoke immunizing processes.

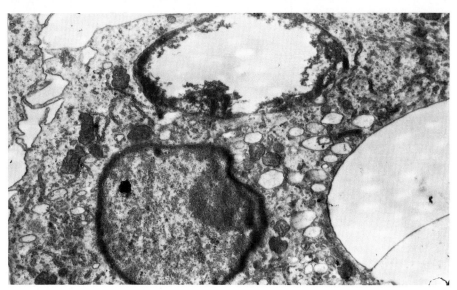

Fig. 127:
The structure of the granulocyte is no longer perceptible, thickened cellular membrane and nuclear particles form a digestive cistern (1:15,000).

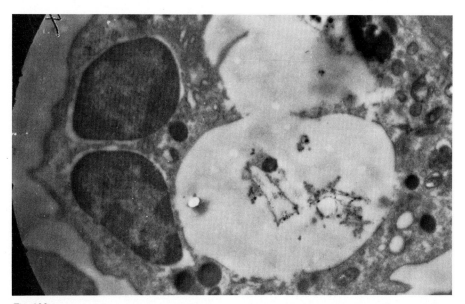

Fig. 128:
The last optical traces in the digestive cisterns of the macrophages are remainders of the granulocyte membrane with particles of heterogeneous tissue and nuclei (1:15,000).

Principle of self-distribution

Under a principle of self-distribution, the macromolecular structures transported in the cells of the organism are incorporated where they are structurally of use. A prerequisite for the therapeutic efficiency of implantations of cells, therefore, is a structural defect of the afflicted tissues i. e. an ecological space for the incorporation of structures.

The metabolic autonomy of the cells assures that

substances that are needed can be built in where their molecular structure permits so;

substances that cannot be disintegrated or infiltrated are wrapped up by antibodies and thus neutralized biologically.

Latency period

A latency period results from the regularities of disintegration and infiltration of the implanted tissues into the paths of autogenous metabolism and structures of the body, between the im-

Fig. 129–132:

In tissular cultures, growth can be stimulated by adding fetal tissues and the redifferentiation can be avoided.

Fig. 129:
Explant-bone-marrow culture of white rats in nutritive solution. After a short while, fibroblasts as forms of redifferentiation will prevail.

Fig. 131:
Fibroblasts in the suspended culture with pure nutritive solution.

Fig. 130:
Addition of fetal cartilage to the nutritive solution multiplies derivatives of bone-marrow and extends the zone of migration.

Fig. 132:
Multiplication of fibroblasts in the suspended culture by adding placenta-lyophilisate (LANGER V. LANGENDORFF).

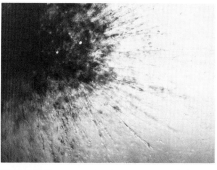
129

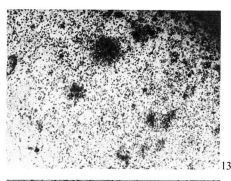
130

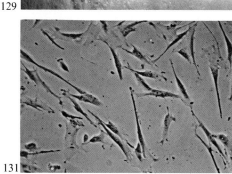
131

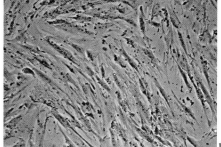
132

plantation and the experimentally or clinically seizable effect. The latency period lasts at least 3 days in mesenchymal organs and at most 2 to 3 weeks in specific organic tissues such as cerebral or renal tissues. Exceptions are various endocrine organs as placenta in that after implantations of these tissues by injection a remarkable influence on the peripheral blood circulation, on the general state of health in the form of general revitalisation can be observed already within a day or a few hours. In question are probably hormonal effects and influences of other cellular contents, which by release from the implanted cells can take effect at once.

STÜHLINGER (1979) has presented a number of impressive casuistics on the latency periods to the onset of the clinical (biological) action; they depend on the age and the basic disease, may amount to days or months. For most of the indications, the effect sets in subjectively and under objective parameters in the 3rd or 4th week after the implantation.

Tissue cultures of rat bone-marrow served for models so as to test the influence of heterologous, chiefly fetal, tissues on the growth of the tissue cultures in the absence of immunological defence. Eighteen tissues indicated various influences on extension, density and cytologic picture of the emigration zones. Most of the tissues exerted a distinct growth impulse but also inhibitions were seen. The kind of the added tissue influences the prevailing cellular form. Many circumstances seem to indicate that the heterologous tissular particles are dissolved in the nutritive medium and selected as additional nutritive substances. A detailed representation of the tests and results can be found in F. SCHMID and H. LEWALD (see also F. SCHMID, 1963).

Density and extension of the emigration zone in bone-marrow cultures after addition of dry tissues

Many of the 18 tested tissues revealed very distinctly a gradual influence on the emigration zone. Besides this extension of surface, the compactness of cells showed very differentiated changes. The results can be noted from tab. 8 and fig. 129–134.

A comparison between the averages of the control cultures in nutritive solution shows considerable growth impulses in certain tissues. The index of extension and compactness of the emigration zones e. g. of the hypothalamus exceeded the control figures by 66 %. These absolute maximum ciphers are followed by a group of about 40 % growth increase (liver 45 %, placenta 40 %, cartilage 37 %). The majority of the tissues, above all the lymphoreticular and cerebral tissues, registered a growth increase of 20 %–30 %. Striking was the absence of influence by fetal bone-marrow, which showed even a slightly negative tendency (-2%); the inactive osteoid fragments constitute a mechanical obstacle and dissolve very sparingly. There is no theory to explain the growth-retarding effect of testicles (-13%).

Identification and specificity of action

The about 1300 publications dealing with cell therapy comprise experimental and clinical papers, which are specified hereafter under relevant points of view:

Experimental data:

1. Physiological (biological) experimental studies –
2. Research of morphological elements –
3. Immunological studies.

1. Physiological (biological) experimental studies

Attention is drawn to the following, highly specified in part, experimental studies:

a) Biostatistical and methodical data (KMENT) –
b) Activity studies on rats by means of lyophilised organic preparations (KMENT, 1956) –
c) Tests on the activity of guinea-pig thyroid glands using radio-isotopes (J 131) after treatment with siccacell preparations (KMENT, 1958) –
d) Objective demonstration of revitalisation by cell injections in animals (KMENT, 1960) –
e) The substantiation of the revitalising effect on animals after cell injections (KMENT, 1963, 1967) –
f) Quantitative electron-microscopic studies on cardiac mitochondria of rats after cell injections from placenta or testicular tissues (KMENT, 1966) –
g) Studies on the revitalising effect of myocardial cells, myocardial nuclei and myocardial mitochondria in rats (KMENT, 1974) –
h) The dispersion of tritiated cardiac, liver and renal cells in old rats (KMENT, LEIBETSEDER and STEININGER, 1972) –
i) The analysis of the spontaneous activity of old and revitalised rats by means of electronic registration (KMENT and HOFECKER, 1972) –
k) Trace elements in heart, liver and brain of rats in various ages and after revitalisation by cell injections (KMENT, HOFECKER and NIEDERMÜLLER, 1973) –
l) Studies on the effect of revitalisation upon the absorption, dispersion and excretion of penicillin V in rats (KMENT and NIEDERMÜLLER, 1973) –
m) Article on the method of registering cinematographically the activity of rats as part of the research into revitalisation (JELENIK, 1971) –
n) The effect of organic extracts and sera on the metabolism of organic cultures (WRBA, 1961–1962) –
o) Experimental gerontological studies on the revitalization (KMENT, 1977).

These extensive experimental studies on the revitalizing effect, which are so far unique in gerontology, have demonstrated from various angles the possibility of influencing functionally aging tissues and organs. As in addition to the untreated controls, cellular suspensions (lyophilisates) of various organs were used, these results give also a relative explanation of the specificity of the effect.

2. Research of morphological elements

The following papers dealing with experiments on morphological elements relate to morphological effects of cell implantations:

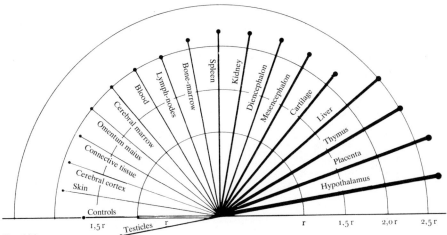

Fig. 133:
Extension of the zones of emigration in bone-marrow of rats on addition of fetal, heterological, lyophilized tissues as against the controls.

a) Growth impulses and prolongation of life of cell cultures (CARELL; LETTRÉ, 1954; SCHMID F., 1962, 1963, 1967; v. LANGENDORFF, 1974) (fig. 129–132, 133, 134) –

b) Increase of growth in corresponding organs (ANDRES, 1953, 1955, 1963); fig. 135 –

c) Morphological studies on the substantiation of a different effect of extracts of lymphatic organs (GOSLAR, 1959, 1969) –

d) Induction of the organic growth by implantation of hormologous tissues (NEUMANN, 1957, 1958, 1959, 1963, 1967) –

e) Influence of tissue injections on experimental hepatic lesions (NEUMANN, 1963, 1967) –

f) The organo-specific effect of implanted rabbit endometria on the uterus of castrated rabbits (BERNHARD and KRAMPITZ, 1958, 1959, 1960, 1963, 1967) –

g) Influence of placenta cells on the angiopathies of experimental angiosclerosis (DORNBUSCH, KLEINSORGE, 1956, 1963, 1967; WIETEK and TAUPITZ, 1957) –

h) Growing processes in mice treated with fresh cells (DITTMAR, 1956, 1963) –

i) Influences on leukaemia in animals (SCHMID F., 1963, 1967); fig. 289–294 –

k) The effect of cell injections on tumours in rats (HOEPKE, 1955, 1963, 1967) –

l) The effect of mast-cell substances on the growth of tumours (LANDSBERGER, 1963, 1967) –

m) Light- and electron-microscopic studies on cell therapy; studies on mitochondria (LANDSBERGER, 1974) –

n) Gerontological tests on mitochondria in the liver of rats (ADAMIKER, 1963; BURGER, 1965) –

o) Quantitative electron-microscopic studies on liver mitochondria of rats after injections of placental and testicular tissues (HARTMANN, 1964; LECHNER, 1965) –

p) Histological cross-sections of guinea-pig organs after injections of lyophilized placental cells (KLUDAS, 1954) –

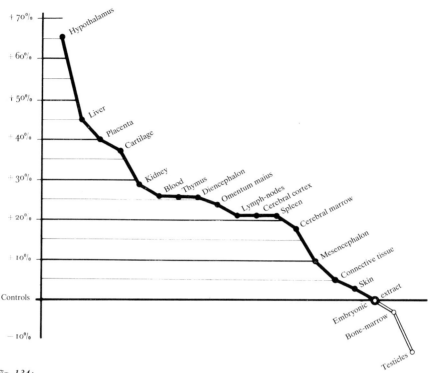

Fig. 134:
Growth indices from density and extension of the zones of emigration in explants of rat bone-marrow on addition of various heterological tissue as against the controls.

q) Studies on the vaginal epithelium of mice under lyophilised organic material (KMENT, 1958) –

r) Data and tests on animals respecting the therapeutic applicability of isolated mitochondria (LAUDAHN, 1956).

s) The effect of Fetal Mesenchymal Cells on a Hodgkins-like Lymphama culture (LANGENDORFF, W. v., 1978)

t) The effect of Fetal Mesenchymal Cells on the Morphology, Grouwth Characteristics and Function of an Experimental Wilm's Tumor culture (LANGENDORFF, W. v., 1979)

3. Immunological studies

Immunological viewpoints have been playing an increasingly important part during the last years, more so because cell therapy is concerned with the transplantation of heterogeneous tissue. The following experimental studies are worth mentioning:

a) The immunological reactions coming into question for cell therapy (H. SCHMIDT, 1963) –

b) Special immuno-biological problems of the implantation of heterological tissue (J. STEIN, 1963); this paper mentions also the immunologically interpreted complications known by that time –

c) The immunological mechanism of the cell (F. SCHMID, 1963) –

d) The dependence of the immunoreactions on the amount of blood in the implant (A. VALLS CONFORTO, 1963) –

Tab. 8: **Impulses stimulating the growth of heterologous tissues in the tissular culture**
(F. Schmid, 1963)

Test series	Extension	Density of cells	Growth	Promotion or delay of growth in %
Controls	1,6	2,2	3,8	0
Blood	2,0	2,8	4,8	+ 26 %
Bone-marrow	2,1	1,6	3,7	− 2,0%
Lymph-nodes	2,0	2,6	4,6	+21 %
Spleen	2,2	2,4	4,6	+21 %
Thymus	2,5	2,3	4,8	+26 %
Kidney	2,2	2,7	4,9	+29 %
Liver	2,5	3,0	5,5	+45 %
Cerebral cortex	1,9	2,7	4,6	+21 %
Cerebral marrow	2,0	2,5	4,5	+18 %
Diencephalon	2,2	2,6	4,8	+26 %
Hypothalamus	2,7	3,6	6,3	+66 %
Mesencephalon	2,2	2,0	4,2	+10 %
Skin	1,9	2,0	3,9	+ 2,6%
Testicles	1,2	2,0	3,2	− 13 %
Placenta	2,7	2,6	5,3	+40 %
Omentum maius	2,0	2,7	4,7	+24 %
Connective tissue	1,9	2,1	4,0	+ 5,3%
Cartilage	2,2	3,0	5,2	+37 %

e) The formation of antibodies after cell injections (Kanzow and Kindler, 1958) –

f) Change of the heterohemagglutination titre after injections of lyophilized organic cells (Möse, Wennig and Stein, 1957, 1958) –

g) Oncofetal antigens (Renner, 1973, 1974) –

h) Immunological effect of fetal cells (Renner, 1977) –

i) Interferon (Emödi, 1977) –

k) Methods of immunological identification (Seelig, 1977) –

l) Clinical aspects of a tumour-immunising therapy with lyophilized fetal cells (Renner, 1979)

m) Terapia celular con Resistocell e inmunidad en oncología (Fuente-Perucho, de la, A. et al., 1979).

n) Immunobiological synopsis (Schmid, F., 1980).

o) Regeneration, Immunstimulation und Interferon-Induktion (Landsberger, A; 1980)

p) Immunstimulation und Interferon-Induktion in der Tumortherapie (Hager, D., 1981)

q) Interferon-Induktion durch xenogenes Gewebe (Resistocell) (Wacker, A., 1982)

r) Immunmodulation and Restoration with Resistocell (Gianoli, A. C. a. Perez-Cuadrado, S., 1982)

A detailed representation of immunological questions will be given hereafter.

Fig. 133–135, legends and Tab. 8 comprise experimental examples of impulses stimulating the growth of heterologous tissues and the specific effect.

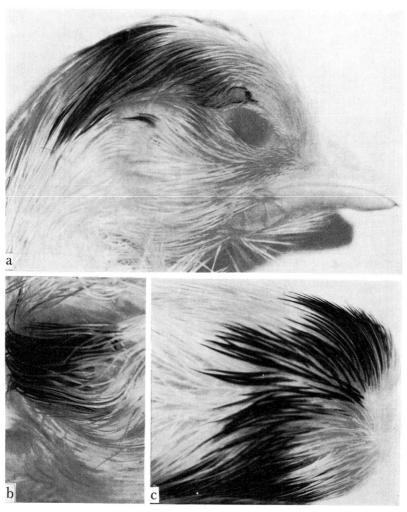

Fig. 135 (a–c):
Inoculated cell material is utilised in the areas of the body where it structurally belongs.
Intravenous injection of melanoblasts of a 2 days old donor (Barred Plymouth Rock and Brown Leghorn) into a 3 days old white Leghorn embryo shows an extensive deposition of pigment in the white hens. (From WEISS and ANDRES, 1952, from SCHMID and STEIN: Cell Research and Cell Therapy, Ott Publishers Thoune, Switzerland 1967).

Immunological synopsis

Man, like any other living being, is part of his environment and needs contact to and protection against this environment as a biological fundamental phenomenon. The interrelations – health/illness, survival or death – are results of inherited potencies (natural resistance), acquired capacities (immunity) and incidental events. Once one has studied the topographic organization, the functional processes and the life profile of immunity, many biological and clinical problems can be explained better and the connections will become clearer.

Immunological processes are initiated against substances «foreign» to an organism because it lacks the necessary (enzymatic) keys to incorporate them into their own structures.

«Natural resistance» is the sum of the innate, non-specific protective mechanisms of an organism, «immunity» implies the acquired specific measures for the maintenance of the individual integrity of the body. These specific processes developing immunoglobulin are an evolutionary event acquired during phylogenesis and becoming more complex as the differentiation goes on.

In the *life profile of immunity,* the following periods are distinguished:

– the immunological tolerance of the embryo and fetus;
– the immunological insufficiency of the baby;
– the immunological ripening during childhood to an optimum between the 10th and 12th years;
– the immunological maturity in adolescents and adults is followed, in the 5th and 6th decades of life, by the regressive phase, which leads to the senile immunological paralysis.

Immunological terms

Since VON PIRQUET introduced the concept of allergy in 1907, the definitions always difficult to interpret have been augmented by adopting plenty of concepts from the Anglo-Saxon literature. Concepts that can only insufficiently be defined and substantiated cannot be taught well either. In the field of immunology, the classical Central European concept of allergology and many recent versions from the Anglo-Saxon literature are now used simultaneously. Consequently, it may appear expedient to give a survey of the most frequent terms in alphabetical order and to try to make concise definitions.

Allergy (VON PIRQUET, 1906)
Changed reactivity after previous contact of antigens (= secondary response); the outcome is a specific hypersensitiveness, which appears as an immediate or as retarded type (tuberculin type).

Allogenous
homologous, originating from a genetically different individual of the same kind.

Anaphylatoxins
proteins released as fragments of complement factors (C_{3a} and C_{5a}) and thus releasing histamin substances.

Anaphylaxis (RICHET, 1902)
Allergic immediate reaction, dependent on reagin; the H-substances (histamin or histamin-like substances) released thereby may provoke urticaria, Quincke-edema or anaphylactic shock.

Anergy
Lack of hypersensibility reactions after previous sensitisation; a «positive» anergy is obtained by desensitisation, a «negative» one by illnesses, cytostatics, radiation (= largely identical with immunological paralysis).

Antigen
A heterogeneous substance or an autogenous substance with changed structures becomes an antigen by developing specific antibodies.

Antigenous determinant
Minimum reacting superficial unit of the antigen accounting for the specificity of the resulting antibody.

Antibodies
Specific proteins developed through stimuli from antigens (immunoglobulins; which see).

Autogenous
From the same individual (autologous); used for transfusions, implantations, transplants.

B-cells
GOOD (1962) divided the «immuno-competent cells» into B-cells (bone-marrow-derived cells, formerly referred to as «bursa»-derivatives) and T-cells (thymocytes). They can be differentiated by indirect methods, morphologically there are flowing transitions. In question are cell-derivatives of the reticulo-histiocytary system (histiocytes, monocytes, mesothelic cells, large lymphocytes), which have preserved the pluripotency of mesenchymal cells. Thus they can through stimuli from antigens rebuild the space of cytoplasm into a synthesis of highly specific macromolecules (immunoglobulins) and eliminate the latter by secretion (IgG) into the humoral system. They run through a phase of synthesis and a phase of secretion.

Chimerism
Chimaerae are living beings consisting of genetically different structures. Derived from chimaera, which is a fire-vomiting fabulous being of the Greek mythology, whose body was composed of parts of a goat, lion and snake.

Complement system
Compound system of 20 different protein fractions (referred to as $C_1–C_9$), which releases anaphylatoxin and leukotactic factors, promotes the opsonization and leads to cytolysis. The system working after the amplifier principle in the sense of a chain reaction needs essentially calcium (Ca) and magnesium (Mg).

Enhancement phenomenon
«Immune-enhancement» means the accelerated growth of malign tumours in test animals if preceded by a sensitisation with the antigen of the same tumour.

Fab-region
Part of immunoglobulin binding antibodies.

Fab-fragment
Monovalent fragment of immunoglobulin having a molecular weight of 50,000, isolated by enzymatic disintegration of immunoglobulin by means of papain or plasmin.

F(ab)₂-fragment
Bivalent fragment of antibodies, which comes into existence by enzymatic disintegration with pepsin; molecular weight: 100,000.

Fc-fragment
Fragment of the Fc-constituent of the immunoglobulin molecule, after enzymatic disintegration by means of plasmin or papain.

Fc-region
Complement-binding (constant) part of the immunoglobulin molecule.

Haptenes
Low-molecular antigen fragments, which cannot sensitise but can react with antibodies.

110

Heterotopic
at a topographically different site.

Immunbiology
The science of processes and mechanisms serving for the protection of the individual biological integrity against foreign substances.

Immuncompetent cells
Cells of the lymphatic and reticulo-histiocytary system, which can be stimulated by antigen contact to form specific antibodies.

Immunocytolysis
Dissolution of cells by antigen-antibody contact; the antibodies are cell-specific (IgM) or complement causes the cytolysis.

Immundeficiency
Deficient immunity by a deficit of immunoglobulins.

Immun-electrophoresis
Technique of identifying various serum proteins: the individual fractions are first separated electrophoretically, then precipitated with antiserum. The precipitation lines indicate the quantities and molecular sizes.

Immunglobulins
Highly molecular antigen-specific protein bodies, which are synthetized in mononuclear cells after contact with antigens. According to the size of molecules and site of formation they remain cell-bounded (IgM, IgA) or are eliminated into the humoral system (IgG, secretory IgA), then often called humoral antibodies. So far, IgA, IgM, IgG, IgE and IgD are distinguished. Low-molecular antibodies (IgG, gamma-globulin, gamma$_2$-fraction) travel electrophoretically the slowest. The molecular weight is 156,000–170,000, the sedimentation constant in the ultracentrifuge S_{20} = 6.5–7 × 10^{-13}, the size is 250–320 × 50 Å.
Higher molecular antibodies (IgM, beta$_2$-globulin-, gamma$_1$-fraction) are electrophoretically between the beta$_1$ and gamma-fractions. The molecular weight is between 500,000 and 1,000,000, the sedimentation constant S_{20} = 15 − 19 × 10^{-13}, the size somewhere between 500–900 × 50 Å.

Immuninsufficiency
Primary or secondary lack of immunoglobulins, with immuno-pareses resulting therefrom.

Immunity
To be immune from the sickening effect of foreign substances getting into the body, by means of synthetising autogenous proteins (immunoglobulins). A specific immunity is obtained by previous contact with the antigen (example: vaccinations).

Immunmodulation
(Arteficial) changing of the Immunsituation.

Immunocytes (F. SCHMID, 1963; DAMASHEK, 1964)
Mononuclear cells transformed functionally into cells synthetizing immunoglobulin. The morphological appearance depends on the maturing stage of the immunoglobulin. During the stage of synthesis they take up organic acids, become deeply basophile, pyronin-positive (RNA-concentration), the nucleus of the large-volume cells becomes peripherical as a compact ergastoplasm develops. This stage corresponds to the «plasma cell» in the classical meaning. In the stage of secretion, immunoglobulins (especially IgG) are secreted via cisterns (so-called vacuoles) into the humoral system.

Immunogenous:
causing the formation of specific antibodies.

Immunoparalysis
Failure (collapse) of the immunizing systems.

Immunoparesis
Deficiency of the immunizing system; the stimulation by antigens does not cause any adequate formation of antibodies.

Immun-reactions
Cellular or humoral reactions to antigens and antibodies. They include: sensitization, cytolysis, agglutination, precipitation. Common methods are: agglutination reaction, inhibitory test by agglutination, precipitation, neutralisation test (viral serum), complement-binding reaction, H$_3$-thymidin test, macrophages-migration-inhibitory test, etc.

Immunsuppression
Artificial suppression of the immunizing reaction of the organism by medicaments (cytostatics, antibiotics), radiation or immunologically (antilymphocyte serum).

Immuntolerance
Antigenic substances do not provoke the formation of antibodies; they are tolerated. The prenatal tolerance immunity is a prerequisite for the uninterrupted development of the fetus, which contains also foreign (paternal) protein structures.

Immun-Transfer
Immunoglobulins and their metabolites can be transferred « passive» with cells of sensitized organisms (peritoneal exudate cells, lymphocytes, meningeal, pleura cells, spleen cells, leukocytes, by exchange-transfusions). The recipient organism reacts within days to months as if it had been in contact with the antigen (example: passive transfer of tuberculin allergy with cells).

Interferons
Acid-resisting proteins, which are eliminated by cells in virus infections and blocks certain phases of the virus synthesis.

Isogenous
Syngenous = isologous, originating from a genetically identical individual (twin).

Killer cells
Macrophages with cytolytic functions; they may be identical with monocytes, which eat autogenous cells if these carry foreign substances (tumour substances) clinging to their cell membranes and thus give the body an impression of being foreign.

Mediators
Mediators (between chemical reactions).

Memory cells
Hypothetical vehicles of the «immune memory». The body forms antibodies (Booster effect, secondary response) faster and more intensively after second contact with antigens than after first contact.

Natural resistance
Individual, non-specific capacity to cope with heterogeneous noxae threatening the own existence or integrity.

Opsonization
Promotion of phagocytosis by the activated Fc-region of the antibody molecule.

Orthotop
= at an anatomically normal site.

Phagocytosis
«Eating» = ingestion of solid particles by cells.

Pinocytosis
«Drinking» = taking up liquids by cells.

Plasma cells (see immunocytes)
Deep basophile, mononuclear cells with marginal nucleus. Cells of the reticulo-histiocytary system (B-cells) in the synthetic stage of antibody formation.

Precipitation
Immunizing reaction provoking a sedimentary precipitate through contact of antigen-antibody. Demonstrable in test tube or by gel-diffusion test.

Reagines
Bivalent immunoglobulins (IgE) with strong ability of binding to cells (granulocytes, mast-cells). From the complex antigen IgE + cellular surface, vasoactive amins capable of provoking anaphylaxis are released with the loss of the basophile granules (= acid complexes).

Receptors
Areas (mostly cytomembranes) capable of specific stimulations and responses to stimulations.

Runt disease
The term is derived from the dwarf cattle (Runt) and means stunted growth caused by antigen-antibody antagonism in the maturing organism. The immunologically riper implant «terrorizes» the immunologically less ripe host tissue in the form of achronic auto-aggressional disease, which leads to «stunted growth» .

Thymosin
Thymus hormone

Transfer factor
Substances in cellular extracts capable of transferring passively and temporarily cellular properties such as the hypersensitivity to tuberculin.

112

Immunobiological phylogenesis and ontogenesis

The immunobiological differentiation and maturation takes place apparently in the course of the phylogenesis of the living beings. Whereas graftings in the vegetable kingdom and transplantations in the animal kingdom up to the avertebrates homologously are possible, they can be effected only in exceptional cases with mammals.

Customarily, antibodies are believed to form in the vertebrate organism after ingestion of antigenous foreign substances. There is, however, biological evidence (M. KRÜPE) that even higher plants such as cryptogames and phanerogames can form gammaglobulin though immunoreactions as observed in vertebrates are not known. Also proteins of viruses and bacteria can bind specifically with antigenous substances and cause agglutination or precipitation. These specifically reacting proteins are called *«lectines»* (fr. legere = select), as distinguished from the antibodies. The formation of gamma-globulin has been shown in lobsters and caterpillars of certain moths.

Of the poikilothermes studied so far (reptiles: tortoise; amphibia: frogs; fish: carp), agglutinins and lysins against bacteria, eryhtrocytes and sperm antigens have been found (KRÜPE). Quantitatively, the capacity of forming antibodies is lower than in birds, leave alone mammals, and depends on the temperature. Precipitines have so far not been provoked in cold-blooded animals.

Precipitating, agglutinating and lysing antibodies are sparingly formed in rats and guinea-pigs, but readily in rabbits and chicken. Horses are better producers of antitoxins than e. g. sheep or cattle. Gold hamsters and guinea-pigs are standard animals for sensitizing effects and anaphylactic reactions.

Homotransplantations can easily be obtained in coelenterates, planaria, earth worms, insects and echinodermes (CUSHING and CAMPBELL, 1957). Annelides take up homologous implants better than heterologous implants, the time of discharge depends on the mutual genetic distance.

Avertebrates cannot distinguish between autologous and homologous tissues, in certain cases not even recognize heterologous tissues.

Avertebrates do not show the characteristic consequence of the propagation of granulocytes → lymphocytosis → monocytosis when stimulated by foreign substances. The inflammatory process consists of phagocytosis and digestion of the foreign material. Indigestible material is sealed off.

Pigs and horned cattle have no gamma-globulins when born. Lactoglobulins contain high concentrations of antibodies, which are absorbed enterally within the first few days after birth.

The antibodies of the maternal serum in calves, lambs, mice and rats are transferred via the colostrum. The absorption is effected by pinocytosis.

Immunoglobulins in rabbits, guinea-pigs and rats are transferred via the fetal yolk-bag, not via the placenta. This membrane corresponds to the yolk-bag of chicken, which has long been known as the way of the immunoglobulin transmission in birds (GOOD and PAPERMASTER).

The existing fragments are too scarce for a phylogenetic synopsis. It is, however, certain that the immunological reactions differentiate in the course of phylogenetic evolution and develop fully in mammals.

The topography of the embryonic interrelations between mesodermic and ektodermic derivatives is found in man as a principle in many variations: layers of epithelial cells, which are filled with mesenchymal (lymphatic, reticulo-histiocytary) formations of tissue.

This principle is preserved the purest in the thymus.

The thymus

is an epithelial-lymphoid organ. Beginning from the 10th embryonic week, the epithelial thymus rudiment originating from the 3rd to 4th gill-arch fills with mononuclear (lymphatic) cells of mesenchymal provenance. The epithelial covering is preserved, but epithelial cells build in the lobes roundish formations of pavementlike epithelium, the Hassall's bodies. These epithelial cells have the characteristics of a secretory function.

Differences between the quantities of nuclei distinguish the cortex area from the marrow area. Compact clusters of lymphocytes with their quantitative superiority of nuclei are distinctive of the cortex. The third population of cells is represented by large mononuclears – reticulum cells, macrophages – which partly phagocytise the smaller lymphocytes and their fragments.

From the organogenesis and experimental findings (FORD and MICKLEM) it appears that mesenchymal parent cells migrate into the thymus and are apparently necessary for the function. The lymphocytes developed in the thymus can live from 3 to 4 days and only a small part of them (about 1%) are eliminated.

The thymus answers autonomously the influences from outside. Sterile breeding of animals does not influence the cell population. Stimulation of antigens makes lymphocytes decrease and activates the macrophages within 24–28 hours. Well-fed babies have usually a large thymus, which dwindles rapidly after infections, doses of cortison and X-ray radiation (the formerly customary radioscopy). Hyperplasia of the thymus in babies is a symptom of a good defence rather than expression of an illness.

Thymectomy in new-born animals causes a loss of cellular immunity, tolerance to foreign tissue antigens, in case even to Runt disease (stunted growth); the effects are small in adult animals, except lymphopenia.

Thymectomy and agenesia of the thymus may provoke regeneration after thymus implantations. Autogenous mononuclear cells colonize the implant and induce the function.

Much as the thymus was neglected in former studies, its importance seems to have been overestimated in recent years; he certainly plays a decisive part for the colonization of peripheral lymph-nodes and in cellular defence. Owing to the increasing numbers of interesting individual findings of recent past, the organismic connections have too much been neglected.

Bursa?

A substantial arsenal of mesoepithelial derivatives is found in the body-cavities of the warm-blooded animals. There is a large reservoir of lymphatic tissues (Payr's plaques, mesenterial lymph-nodes) of the abdominal cavity, besides an extensive net of mesothelial tissues. These mesothelial cells of the omentum, peritoneum, mesenterium have epithelial forms and mesenchymal functions, which originate from a typically reticular unit.

To explain the verbal significance of the B-cells, much has been philisophized on the possible equivalent of Bursa Fabricii of the birds in the warm-blooded animals. In the «bursae» of the body, in its peritoneal, pleural, meningeal and synovial spaces, the human organism has an extensive, functionally efficient system that can react locally (e. g. in perityphlitic abcesses, peritonitis) or generally (e. g. polyserositis).

The reticulo-histiocytary system (RHS)

The mesenchyme develops from the mesoderm. The originally prevailing epithelial units dissolve increasingly and are replaced by loose cellular masses. The latter constitute the rudiment of all organs and formations of the connective tissue and are called mesenchymes (fr. Gr. enchein = to fill in). The *embryonic mesenchyme* (HERTIG, 1881) is a syncitium, whose protoplasmatic cell framework contains a mucous tissue-fluid. It promotes the fetal forms and is the matrix of all supporting and connective tissues (fig. 136).

As an organismic system, the mesenchyme has penetrated into the medico-biological thinking while our knowledge of the morbific agents increased. After the fundamental observations by WYSSOKOWICH (1886) and METCHNIKOFF (1892) on phagocytosis, ASCHOFF (1924) was the first to point with the concept RES (reticulo-endothelial system) to the organismic connections. SIEGMUND (1927) added with the term *«active mes enchyme»* the functional-phylogenetic consideration to the purely morphologico-topographic idea. Largely adopted

has been the term *«reticulo-histiocytary system» (RHS)* as the endothelia are mainly predifferentiated elements and do not belong to the mesenchyme proper with pluripotent qualities (FRESEN).

Outside the uterus, the tissular formations originating from the mesenchyme are divided into the shaped and shapeless supporting tissues. While the shaped supporting tissues e. g. bones, cartilage, tendons, muscles, blood vessels have defined functions and perform special tasks, part of the mesenchymal tissue has retained pluripotency, the fundamental property of mesenchymal parent tissue. These mesenchyme derivatives with fetal potencies include the loose and reticular connective tissues and the terminal capillary net (fig. 136).

Main centres of reticular connective tissue are: bone-marrow, thymus, spleen, lymph-nodes, Kupfer's cells of the liver. The loose connective tissue is found chiefly in the peritoneum, omentum, mesenterium, pleura, meninges, interstitium, subcutaneous connective tissue. Of the shaped supporting tissues, only parts (e. g. metaphysis, periosteum

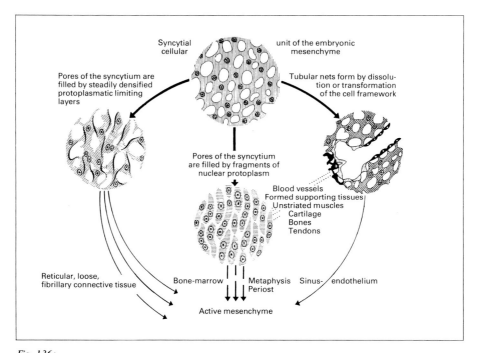

Fig. 136:
The «*active mesenchyme*» of the growing and adult organism.
The embryonic mesenchyme originating from the mesoderm has progressed or changed in 3 directions (see arrow). The active mesenchyme strictly speaking includes the reticular (thymus, spleen, lymph-nodes, bone-marrow, etc.), loose (omentum, peritoneum, mesenterium, pleura, meninges, articular and subcutaneous connective tissue) and fibrillary connective tissue. The formed supporting tissues (cartilage, bones, tendons, unstriated muscles, vessels) have special supporting and conducting functions and preserved only part of the pluripotency of their parent tissues (e.g. bone-marrow, periost, metaphysis).

and bone-marrow on the skeletal system) have physiologically preserved some of the fetal capacities.

The cells of the reticulo-histiocytary system have the following functions vital for the existence of a living being:

1. They are pluripotent. The developmental potencies dormant in them are the more numerous the less the cells are differentiated.
2. They are capable of effecting amoeboid movements.
3. They can take up, disintegrate, rebuild, build up substances and eliminate the products synthetised in the mesenchymal cells. This quality comprises the entire intermediary metabolism, moreover the intake of infectious morbific agents, the storage of organic foreign substances and the formation of proteins including the antibodies (fig. 137).

The intake of solid substances is called phagocytosis, the intake of liquid substances pinocytosis (= drinking).

As to the form and function, the so-called immuno-competent cells comprise 2 categories:

1. Large mononuclears with a comparatively small nucleus and larger space of cytoplasm, which alone by the proportion of space can better synthesize.

116

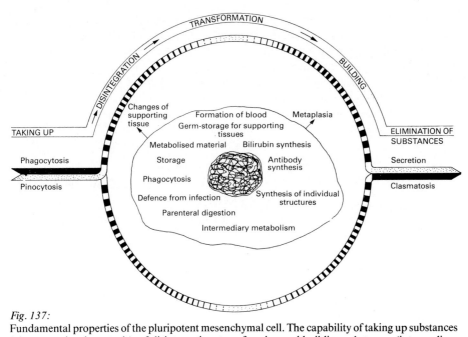

Fig. 137:
Fundamental properties of the pluripotent mesenchymal cell. The capability of taking up substances (phagocytosis, pinocytosis), of disintegrating, transforming and building substances (intermediary metabolism, storage, parenteral digestion, synthesis of proteins, lipoids and carbohydrates as well as their complex formations) accounts for the part that the mesenchyme plays in the germ-storing function of the supporting tissues, in the formation of blood, bilirubin synthesis, defence from infection, formation of antibodies, and for immunity.

The histiocytes, monocytes, reticular cells and mesothelium cells belong to them.

2. Small mononuclears with a comparatively large nucleus and little cytoplasm, capable of migratory and transporting functions rather than of synthesis owing to their small space of cytoplasm and their poor equipments for synthesis; the «small» lymphocytes of the lymphatic tissues belong to them.

The trite term of the B-cells and T-cells has deliberately been dispensed with in this classification. As the cellular form depends on the function rather than on the site of origin, a categorisation as to the origin is more hindering than of didactic use. The flowing functional transitions alone give a clear understanding of the biologically – dynamic connections.

Life profile of immunity

The innate defensive potencies *(natural resistance)* and the *acquired defensive capacities* (immunological processes) amount to a biological total achievement. Well though, theoretically, these concepts are separable, difficult to im-

possible in biology and clinic is the quantitative estimate of resistance and immunity. The sum of these processes serving for the integrity of an individual depends on many factors such as age, sex, general condition, climatic circumstances and accidental events. In spite of the latter, clinical experience as well as statistical and epidemiological recognition permits comparatively reliable conclusions about the life profile of the immunity. Like all biological processes, immunity is a developing, maturing, aging and disappearing phenomenon.

Embryo and fetus are, biologically, well tolerated homologous implants. Although proteins, chiefly in the liver, are formed in early stages of development, it has so far not been possible to win in any species traceable quantities of immunoglobulins during the normal fetal life (R. A. GOOD and B. W. PAPERMASTER). Through passive transmission from the mother, the new-born has first more gamma-globulins in the blood of the umbilical cord than the mother. But these quantities diminish rapidly in the absence of own synthetic performance.

Immunity is insufficient immediately after birth. In man and in most of the warm-blooded animals, immunological defence begins in the second week of life and is probably not sufficient before the 2nd to 4th years of life. The clinical observations are substantiated by

a) the absence of the plasma cells producing antibodies during the first 10 days of life,

b) symptoms of quantitative and qualitative insufficiency in the spectrum of the immunoglobulins,

c) comparatively weak mononuclear reactions in the new-born as a cellular response to non-specific inflammatory stimuli (SHELDON and CALDWELL).

The immunological maturation

follows the periods of immunotolerance of embryo and fetus and of insufficient immunity of the baby. The more the growing child gets into touch with his domestic and, later, extra-domestic environments, the more the antigens, against which antibodies are produced, will multiply. Immunoglobulins against most of the civilization diseases are acquired by natural infection or vaccination.

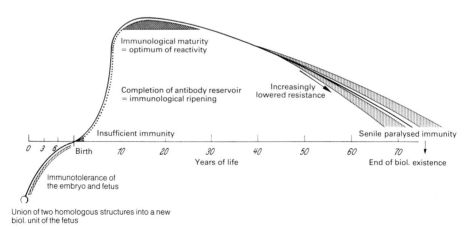

Fig. 138:
Scheme of the immunobiological life profile

The immunological maturity

is attained between the 7th and 12th years of age. Taking into consideration the immunoglobulin levels in the serum and the rates of morbidity and mortality, the maximum adaptability and power of defence are attained between the 10th and 12th years.

On the other hand, this period of life is the age during which preferably many diseases originating from antigen-anti-body reactions occur. They include: scarlet fever, rheumatic fever, glomerulonephritis, anaphylactoid purpura and hyperplasia of the lymphatic apparatus (hyperplasia of the tonsils, adenoids, lymphonodulitis mesenteralis).

Individually different transient depressions during puberty interrupt the period of maturity, which continues usually into the fifth decade of life.

The immunological regression

runs a slow course and sets in, individually different, in the 5th or 6th decade of life; it is characterised by an increased susceptibility to infection and by a decreasing protection of the integrity of autogenous tissular structures as the neoplasms are increasingly more endangered. The power of resistance to infections subsides at the end of biological existence as the senile immunoparalysis advances.

Natural resistance / Immunity

«Immunobiology» implies all processes serving for the protection of autonomous life and its integrity. Terminologically, it is divided into the «natural resistance» and the «immunity». By «natural resistance» we understand the individual, non-specific capacity to cope with heterogeneous noxae threatening the own existence. Components of «natural resistance» are the innate reactivity and responsiveness of the mesenchymal (reticulo-histiocytary) system, properdin, complement, opsonin, lysin, leukin, conglutinin and C-reactive protein.

«Immunity» is the acquired specific capability of preserving the own existence against certain foreign influences. The biological differentiation, however, is not as clear as the definition can distinguish the two phenomena because both elementary processes serving for the protection of the organism work into each other and even depend on each other.

Heterogeneous substances such as foreign proteins or infectious morbific agents that get into the organism by avoiding (as e. g. by vaccinations) or breaking through (e. g. lesion, failure owing to illness) the epithelial protective surface,

a) either are infiltrated (as far as suited) into the own metabolic cycles as working substrates

b) or (as far as unsuited to be disintegrated metabolically by homogenous enzymes) must be rendered biologically inert by protective globulins.

The latter process comprises the disintegration of the foreign substance to the antigenous determinants, which, as they cannot be broken down further, are palliatively enveloped by high-molecular globulins, which must specially be made to measure. The process is biologically circumstantial, takes from 4–6 weeks and comprises various phases.

The rapid evolution in the field for which in clinical usage the term «immunology» has been adopted, makes one sometimes believe that the defense of the body is a problem of the lymphocytes, thymus or «plasma cells», according to the experimental schools to which the authors may adhere. The more, however, the considerations draw nearer to the clinical problems and are confronted with practical decisions, the clearer the gaps of such one-sided interpretation of the highly differentiated and ingeniously arranged safety devices of the body will appear.

The following survey is to outline the arrangement and organisation of the organismic immunobiological system. The topographic «abstraction» is continued by the functional interrelations of importance for practical and clinical questions.

Specific or non-specific?

The classical science of immunity has been inclined to associate the processes of specific defence with *«immunity»* and to categorize the non-specific processes for the protection of the organism under the term *«natural resistance»*. Like in other fields of medicine, the question of specific or non-specific has lost importance also in immunology since it has been known how closely the processes are connected and work into each other.

The body-own defense preserves the individual integrity by means of «non-specific» and «specific» measures. The processes caused by a penetrating antigenous foreign substance are first non-specific. Among them are phagocytosis (LANGHANS, 1870; WYSSOKOVICH, 1886; METCHNIKOFF, 1892; F. SCHMID, 1967) and «parenteral digestion». If the latter cannot or not quite be effected because the body is inadequately provided with enzymes, the macroorganism must in another way bring about the biological inertia of the foreign substances (antigens, antigenous determinants): *it develops specific proteins for the palliative binding of the antigens, the antibodies (immunoglobulins).* Only from this moment, the components of the process, antigen and antibody, become specific. Specific actions are necessary when the organism cannot degrade and incorporate a foreign substance by means of non-specific mechanisms i.e. with its metabolic potentialities.

The following chapters are to show how accurately these processes work into each other.

Organisation of the immunological system

The immunological system in man is divided into three zones:

1. *the epithelial surface of contact and defense (against the exterior);*

2. *the thymolymphatic defense zones;*

3. *the organismic, pluripotent active mesenchyme (= reticulohistiocytary system).*

The biological and pathological reactions of the interdependently arranged systems are intimately implicated into each other.

The division into the three systems has a fundamental importance beyond the didactic value. The epithelial defense surface is the phylogenetically oldest, the thymo-lymphatic interface the youngest mechanism of defense. The systems differ not only in the morphe of their cells but also in many other respects. The most conclusive confirmation of this division into three parts is the fact that in each system special immunoglobulins are formed. Tab. 9 gives a synoptic survey of the theoretical and clinical significance of this division.

The attention of the immunologists has centered on the reticulo-endothelial system for decades. Thymus and the lymphatic system have been main topics of consideration during the last two decades. The importance of the surfaces of contact, which physiologically carry most of the burden in the fight with the environment, has hardly been discussed from the immunological point of view so far.

The epithelial surface of contact and defense

Every living being is part of its environment and needs absolutely the contact with and the defense against it to maintain its biological existence. Surfaces of contact have the function to take in substances that can be utilized by the organism and to keep away from the interior of the body all substances that have no biological functions or even harm the organism. During the phylogenetic development, these functions were first performed by the cell membrane, which takes up and secretes substances from the environment. In the higher developed organism, the surfaces of contact are formed by epithelial groups of cells; the most important surfaces of contact in man are the spaces of the mouth, pharyngeal cavity and nose as space of intersection for the ingestion of foreign substances from the respiratory air, from the digestive tract and for the fight against microbial noxae. In a wider sense, these surfaces of contact include the lining of the gastro-intestinal tract and of the urinary passages.

The air-passages and upper digestive tract lined with epithelium are connected closely with parts of the lympho-reticular connective tissue chiefly in the area of the Waldeyer's lymphatic glands of the fauces. Whereas the epithelial cells are physiologically suitable for the contact with foreign substances and even tolerate – and partly need as metabolic symbionts – microorganisms on their surfaces, the connective tissue below them reacts with regular defense measures if the areas of contact are exceeded.

The epithelia of the respiratory passages and of the digestive tract with their metabolic function are of great importance for the measures of defense against the environment. Usually, noxae are kept off already at this first barrier; they penetrate only in case of a failure and can thus provoke illnesses. The superficial epithelial cells must decide on the necessity of the intake and output of substances. Vital substrates as water, oxygen, carbohydrates, proteins, fats, vitamins and minerals are released by the epithelial cells to be transported on into the interior of the body. Ballast substances of the food shall be recognized at the limiting surfaces and not be taken in.

121

Tab. 9: **Organization of the immundefense-system. Survey of the guiding symptoms, the use and failure of the defense zones in the human body.**

Defense zones	Immunological principle	Immuno-globulin	Immunological reaction	Immunological depression
I Epithelial contact and defense surface			**Catarrhal**	
Skin Mucosae of the respiratory passages, of the gastrointestinal and urogenital tracts	The *epithelial* contact and defence surface is represented by the skin and the mucosae of the rhino-pharyngeo-oral cavities, conjunctiva and digestive, respiratory and urogenital tracts. These contact surfaces have an ambivalent function: substances likely to be of use to the body are taken up, substances that have no physiological functions or even may be harmful, must be kept away from the interior of the body, and metabolites of the own metabolism must be secreted through the same contact surfaces.	IgA	Dermatitis Rhinitis Sinusitis Pharyngitis Tracheitis Bronchitis (pneumonia) Enteritis Colitis Pyelitis Cystitis Urethritis	Necrobiosis of the skin Dermatitis bullosa exfoliativa toxica necroticans *(Stevens-Johnson syndrome Lyell syndrome)* Mucosae: necrotising inflammation noma
II Lymphoreticular defense area			**Proliferative**	
Thymus Lymphatic system Lymph-nodes Adenoids Tonsils Lymphplaques Bone-marrow Spleen, liver Lymphocytes (so-called T-lymphocytes)	The *lymphoreticular* defence areas constitute a colonisation family deriving from thymus, which, fully developed, comprises: lymph-nodes, tonsils, adenoids, lymphplaques, bone-marrow, fragments of tissue from liver and spleen. The lymphoreticular tissues react with proliferation i. e. multiplication of cells, hyperplasia of the thymus, hyperplasia of the tonsils, adenoid vegetations, swellings of lymph-nodes, hepato- and spleno-megaly are the clinical equivalents for the use of this defence area.	IgM	Thymus hyperplasia Lymphonodulitis Hyperplasia of the tonsils Adenoids Region. ileitis (termin.) Leukocytosis Splenomegaly Hepatomegaly	necrobiotic inflammation Pyemia Leukopenia Agranulocyto-sis
III Mesenchymal defense system of the organism			**Exudative**	
Serous membranes (Lepto-) meninges Pleura, pericardium Peritoneum Omentum Mesenterium Articular teguments Interstitium Loose connective tissue, endothelium Monocytes Histiocytes Cells of the mesothelium (= so-called B-lymphocytes)	The *organismic mesenchymal defense* system comprises the cells dispersed over the whole organism that have preserved the mesodermal pluripotency; the most reactive cellular units are in the fluffy connective tissue of the interstices and in the so-called serous membranes i. e. those mostly flat networks of fluffy connective tissue, which line the body-cavities: meninges, pleura, pericardium, omentum, peritoneum, mesenterium and synovia.	IgG	Meningitis Pleuritis Pericarditis Peritonitis Arthritis Arteriitis Angiitis Inflammation of the connective tissue	Empyema Polyserositis Sepsis

Fig. 139: Epithelial zone of contact and defence. ▶

1. Physical mechanisms
   film of secretion
   ciliary movement
   roofing-tile formation
   lipoid layer of cytomembranes

2. Biochemical mechanisms
   pH electrolytes
   (Na, K, Mg, Ca, J, Zn, S)
   mucopolysaccharides
   lysozyme
   glucosidases

3. Immune reactions
   IgA
   IgA secretory
   IgM
   IgG
   IgE

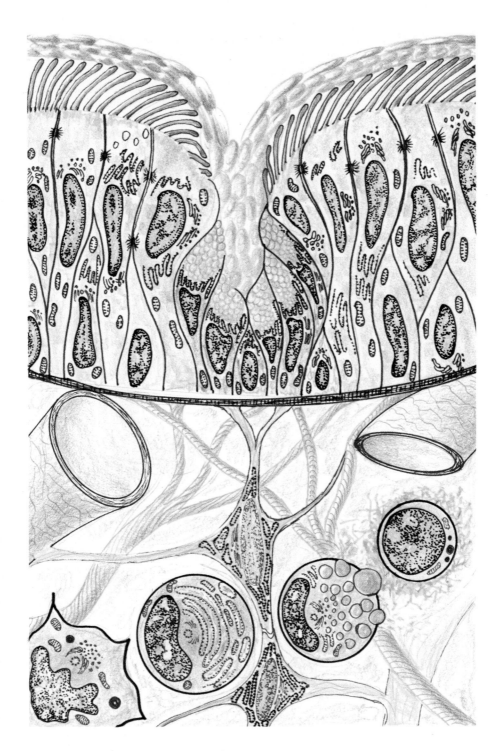

Fig. 139: Epithelial zone of contact and defence.

Metabolic end-products are secreted as e. g. carbon dioxide through the lungs or protein metabolites through the urine.

The upper epithelial cells of the oral and pharyngeal cavities constitute a limiting surface of the organism and are moreover initial links of the metabolic chains. Smears of the pharyngeal or oral mucosa show their various functions when the obtained preparations are subjected to a methodical cytochemical evaluation. Spatula smears of the superficial layer of epithelial cells reveal bizarre, imbricated cells of large volume, with a centrally located nucleus (fig. 140). Even in healthy individuals the surface of the cell membrane shows bacteria, and very frequently each epithelial cell seems to determine both the quantity and the kind of bacteria on the cytomembrane. All variations from individual bacteria to dense lawn of bacteria are found here (fig. 141).

The constituents of these epithelial cells can be prepared by cytochemical

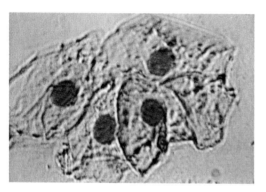

Fig. 140:
Cells of the pharyngeal epithelium arranged like roof-tiles (protective formation). Panchromatic colouration, 1:600, contrast of phases.

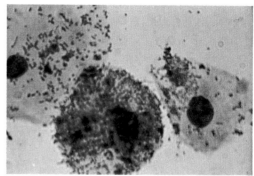

Fig. 141:
Various *settlements of bacteria* on the cells of pharyngeal epithelium; bacteria on the cytomembrane.

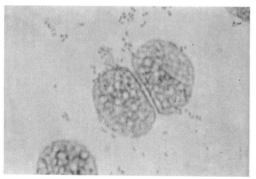

Fig. 142:
Interrelation between the (DNA-)nuclear metabolism and growth of bacteria. Inside the cells, the bacteria multiply with and at the expense of the nuclear substance (DNA); the more bacteria occur in the cell, the greater the chromatin defects in the nuclei. Panchromatic staining.

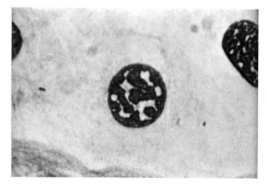

Fig. 143:
In *virus infections,* only indirect conclusions can be drawn on the interrelations between the nucleus and microorganisms. Fine to coarse structural defects of the nucleus may be indications. Panchromatic staining.

124

methods. Especially in activated epithelial cells (in infections) a dense system of channels can be detected very frequently within the cytoplasm, in which various groups of substances obviously transported there can be noticed. Thus glycogen or ribonucleic acid can be demonstrated whereas the fatty substances are seen chiefly on the nuclear membrane and the membrane of cytoplasm (fig. 146–149).

Lesions of the cytomembrane by phy-

sical or chemical noxae (fig. 145, 150) or injuries to the cytoplasm by chemical noxae or infection make the defensive function of the epithelial cells fail and interrupt the initial link of the metabolic chains. Whereas e. g. in normal epithelial cells the system of channels is filled with RNA, the destruction of the tube-system with a coarse precipitation of the RNA particles (fig. 144–147) is seen in inflammation (tonsillitis, phlegmon of the ground of the mouth, pneumonia).

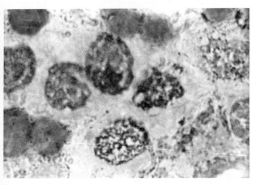

Fig. 144:
Different lesions of epithelial cells in bronchopneumonia. Panchromatic staining.

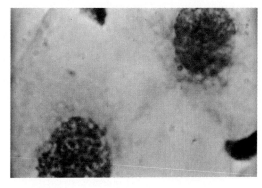

Fig. 145:
Broad-spectrum antibiotics intervene in the cellular metabolism; diffusion of nuclear substance into the perinuclear cytoplasm after treatment with ampicillin-chloramphenicol. Panchromatic staining.

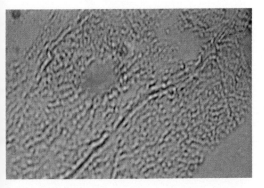

Fig. 146:
Intracytoplasmatic «metabolic channels» in cell of pharyngeal epithelium. Staining: methyl-green-pyronin. DNA = green; RNA = red.

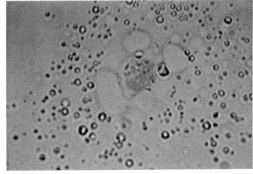

Fig. 147:
Destruction of the intracytoplasmatic metabolic transport-system by infections: phlegmon on the ground of the mouth; coarse particles of RNA. Staining: methyl-green-pyronin; DNA = green, RNA = red.

125

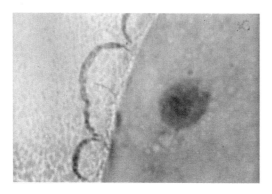

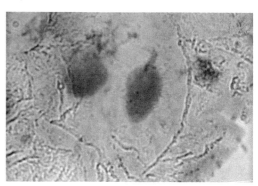

Fig. 148:
Detachment and conglutination of the cellular membrane (oral epithelium) by 44% *alcohol (whisky)*, tested in non-alcoholics immediately after drinking whisky. The cellular membrane rich in lipoids is injured. Best-carmine staining.

Fig. 149:
Synthesis of the cells of oral epithelium. Intracellular polysaccharide complexes (glycogen) occur already a few minutes after absorption of floracit. Best-carmine staining.

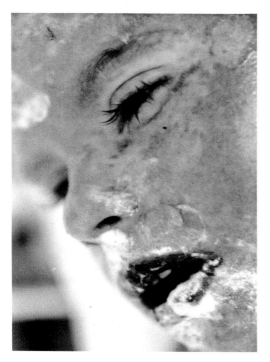

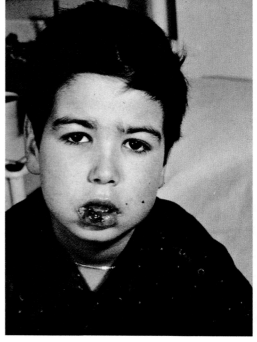

Fig. 150:
Generalised lesion of the epithelial protective surface as part of a *Lyell-syndrome* (by long-term sulphonamide); the layers of the oral mucous epithelium are afflicted more than others.

Fig. 151:
Terminal collapse of the epithelial defense surfaces in *leukemia*.

126

There is apparently a very close biological connection between the bacterial flora of the oral and pharyngeal epithelia and the epithelial cells as such. As long as the microorganisms are on the surface of the cells, they seem to have a symbiont effect and to support the cellular metabolism. If however microorganisms are in the space of cytoplasm, this will usually cause the destruction of the epithelial cells. As for bacteria, the connection can be seen direct whereas in the case of viruses only the defects in the nucleus, which contains DNA, can be detected (fig. 142, 143). In the cytological pictures, an antagonism will arise in that the nucleus gets increasingly low in chromatin whereas the lawn of bacteria becomes denser.

This antagonism between the microorganisms and the cells of the macroorganism reveals the essence of an infectious disease as a concurrent problem. Normally, the epithelial cells utilize the metabolic effects of their superficial bacteria, which they even may use as sources of nucleic acid. If the morbific agents transgress the cytomembrane, the economic relations between the bacteria and the macroorganism are reverted: the microorganisms multiply at the expense of the epithelial cells, especially the nucleic acids, and thus cause the destruction of the cells and injure the surfaces of contact and defense.

The general symptoms of the so-called prodromal stage of infectious diseases are due to these changes of epithelial surfaces of contact. On the other hand, many conditions of lacking immunity are accompanied by a pathological colonization of the epithelial surfaces; just to think of the candidiasis on the mucous membrane in the mouth of dystrophic babies, and of a collapse of the defense against infection in immunity paralysis (terminal stage of leukosis in children, gastrointestinal radiation syndrome, therapy with cystostatics). Also noxae due to medicaments (antibiotics, antiepileptics) can provoke serious aspects in the form of diffuse lesions of the mucosa, or of the skin and mucosa (Stevens-Johnson syndrome, pluriorificial ektodermatosis Glanzmann, Lyell's syndrome; fig. 145, 150, 151).

The thymo-lymphatic defense-zone

If as a result of lesions, injuries or evasion the organism lacks physiological surfaces of contact, foreign substances, chiefly morbific agents, can penetrate into the ducts of blood and lymph. For such cases, the organism is provided with the lymphatic system beneath the epithelial surface of contact. Especially in the pharyngeal cavity, the *Waldeyer's lymphatic glands* constitute a considerable zone of defense, but also the entire gastro-intestinal tract is secured with them (*Payr's lymphoid patches* of the intestine, mesenteric lymph-nodes). Adenoid vegetations, hyperplasia of the tonsils, swellings of cervical and mesenteric lymph-nodes are clinical equivalents of this permanent or relapsing struggle of the lymphatic ring of defence with infectious noxae.

The lymphatic apparatus of defense develops by *colonization from the thymus*. In the absence of the thymus or if it is malformed, this zone of defense will fail or offer insufficient defense. Vehicles of the cellular defense are small lymphocytes (so-called T-cells), which chiefly contain the cellular IgM. As the cytoplasm space of these lymphocytes is comparatively small and does not suffice to form any substantial quantities of immunoglobulins, immunological use of the lymphatic system causes always a multiplication of lymphatic cells (lymphatic hyperplasia). Unlike the reticulohistiocytary system, which reacts with the secretory processes (exudation), this system responds by proliferation. The differences between these two systems are shown synoptically in tab. 9.

The *lymphatic system* of defense is phylogenetically the youngest. in the course of life it experiences a stage of ripening between birth and an optimum between the 9th and 12th years of life, a stage of maturity and a stage of regression after the 40th year of life. An initial reactive organ after birth is the thymus, which can swell into a large organ owing to the struggles during the first weeks and months of life. Later, the peripheral and inner lymph-nodes take essentially the function of the thymus, which atrophies and beyond puberty loses much of its central function within the lymphatic system.

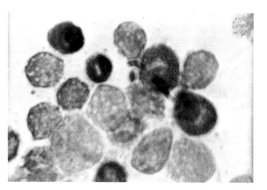

Fig. 152:
Normal *tonsil cytogram* (swab cytogram from middle of tonsils) in 3-year-old child. Abundant intact cell material, lymphocytes, lymphoblasts. Panchromatic staining.

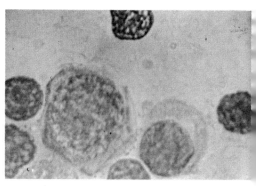

Fig. 153:
Tonsil cytogram in subacute *tonsillitis* of 6-year-old child; rich in cells. Panchromatic staining.

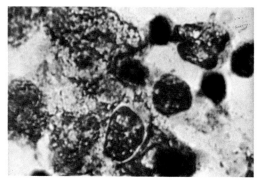

Fig. 154:
Tonsil cytogram of 15-year-old girl; abundance in comparatively small lymphocytes. *Cytolysis.*

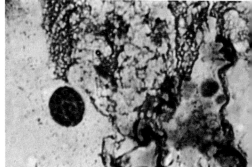

Fig. 155:
Tonsil cytogram of 30-year-old woman. Chronic tonsillitis. Abundance in cytolyses, despiralled chromatin substance.

128

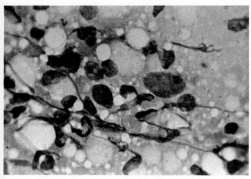

Fig. 156:
Lymph-node smear preparation in proliferative lymph-node *tuberculosis*. Matrix, epitheloid cells, fibres. Panchromatic staining.

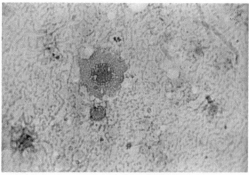

Fig. 157:
Lymph-node tuberculosis, smear from section as in fig. 156. Two minutes after effect of a tuberculin dilution (1:20) all structure elements have dissolved. *Cytolytic effect* between antigen and cellular immunoglobulins M. Panchromatic staining.

The importance of the tonsils in cellular respect is shown by various cytological smears taken at serveral ages of life (fig. 152–155).

As the immunoglobulins remain in the lymphatic cells, a contact of antigens and antibodies in the lymphocytes provokes a cytolysis i.e. disintegration of cells. Cytolysis is a prerequisite for the necrobiotic processes in the lymphatic organs and for the formation of focuses outside the immunological regularities.

Once a focus has formed – e.g. in a tuberculous lymph-node – immunological processes are maintained from there by swept-out antigens whereas the necrobiotic focus cannot be protected by these immunizing processes because he has no intact cells and therefore no aviable immunoglobulins M. These conditions are the basis for the origin of chronic diseases deriving from focuses of necrobiosis (fig. 156, 157).

The reticulo-histiocytary (mesenchymal) defense-system

The 3rd line of defense protecting the organism is a deeply echeloned system that chiefly coats the abdominal cavities and consists of loose connective tissue; it reacts when the 2nd i.e. the thymo-lymphatic line of defense is overcome.

Morphologically, this system includes: serous teguments, leptomeninges, pleura, pericardium, peritoneum, omentum, mesenterium, coats of joints; interstice and the loose connective tissue spread over the entire organism. Cellular representatives of this system are monocytes,

histiocytes and mesothelic cells. These cellular derivatives of bone-marrow, loose connective tissue and serous teguments are much identical with the so-called B-cells. The well-known term «B-cells» is ill-suited and cannot express the functional and morphological extent of the system.

Pluripotency is the functional mark of the cellular derivatives of the reticulo-histiocytary system. As part of the immunizing response of an organism, these cells produce immunocytes. In the days

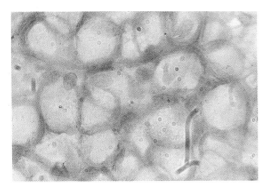

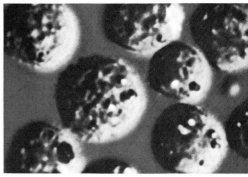

Fig. 158:
Omentum (guinea-pig, fetal) as an example of a *reticulo-histiocytary tissue*.Most of the figures of the immunological section represent derivatives of this tissue.

The methyl-green-pyronin staining provides a good reproduction of the reticular unit. The nuclei rich in DNA (greenish-blue) are located at the intersections of the network rich in RNA (red).

Fig. 159:
«*Autonomous cells*» of the peritoneal exudate with membrane activity during observation in vivo. The membrane activity expresses the taking (phagocytosis, pinocytosis) and the secretion of material (clasmatosis, secretion).

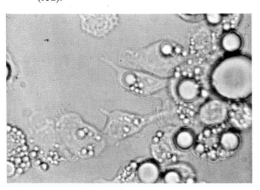

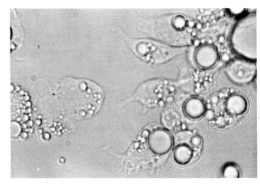

Fig. 160:
Elimination of mononuclear cells from the reticular unit. Observation in living tissue culture. Contrast of phases, 1:600.

Fig. 161:
After separation of the cytoplasm bridges, the large mononuclear cells grow round in the liquid medium and show symptoms of high metabolic activity on the membrane.

after the supply of antigens, organic acids accumulate in the cytoplasm of the mononuclear cells. The cytoplasm is deeply stained by basic dyestuffs. The development of a dense net of ergastoplasm within the cellular body is an electron-optical equivalent of this process. The immunoglobulins are synthetised on the ribosomes of these tubes of ergastoplasm and then eliminated into the interstices of the ergastoplasm. These widen into cisterns, which get into contact with the surface of the cells and there eliminate the synthetised immunoglobulins into the humoral system. The process of ripening and secreting immunoglobulins takes more than 3–5 weeks, probably according to the kind and quantity of antigens.

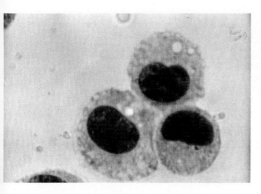

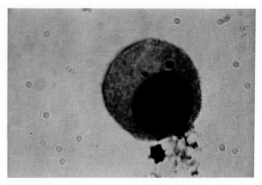

Fig. 162:
Panchromatic staining makes the mononuclear discharged from the reticular unit show the picture of the monocytes: large, loosely structured nucleus, grey-reddish-blue cytoplasm. Peritoneal exudate cells before immunisation, panchromatic colouration.

Fig. 163:
After sensitisation (here with BCG) the monocytes transform into immunocytes within 3–7 days. The deep-basophil cytoplasm is evoked by accumulation of organic acids. Panchromatic staining. Stage of the synthesis of the immunocytes.

Phases of this development of the *immunocytes* from large mononuclear cells are shown in the fig. 160–189. From these pictures it appears that a morphological uniform pattern of the immunocytes does not exist but that the shape depends on the momentary functional condition. Exaggerating, one may ask whether plasma-cells (immunocytes) produce immunoglobulins or immunoglobulins plasma-cells. The morphological changes and the various phases of the immunocytes depend on the cytochemical processes during the synthesis and secretion of the immunoglobulins.

The synthesis and secretion of the immunocytes produce above all the immunoglobulin G (IgG). As a secretion is in question, the reaction of the system is exudative i. e. the fluid is augmented. Clinical sequelae therefore are meningitis, pleuritis, pericarditis, peritonitis, arthritis, arteriitis, angiitis and interstitial inflammation. Overstrain provokes suppuration, empyema, polyserositis and sepsis (tab. 9).

Immunobiological cytobiology

To characterize cellular mechanisms in immunological processes, three fundamental points of view must be pointed out first:

1. Like any synthesis, the formation of specific antibodies (immunoglobulins) is a purely cellular process.
2. Immunizing cells i.e. those able to synthetise antibodies are unpolar cells, which have kept the pluripotency of mesenchymal cells in morphological and functional respect. Only this pluripotency makes possible to «work» «unknown» metabolic problems as constituted by antigens. Antigens are substances for the metabolization of which the organism lacks the enzymatic outfit.
3. The morphological condition of a cell depends on its function. According to the function, therefore, cells of equal origin form various morphological and functional = biochemical variants with flowing changes. The rigid

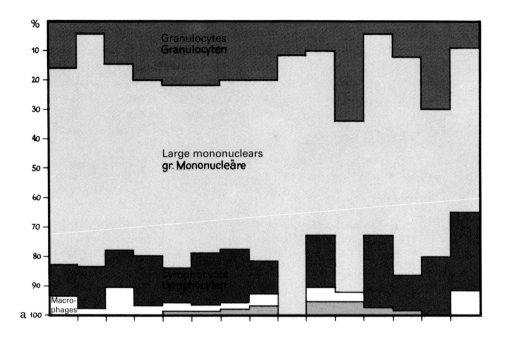

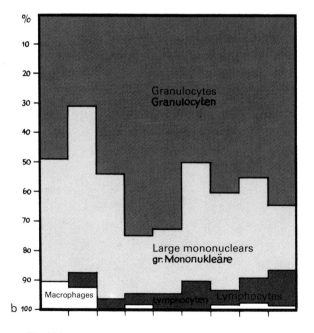

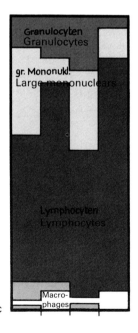

Fig. 164:
Differences of the cell-differential picture of the peritoneal exudate of guinea-pigs (a) after BCG sensitisation, (b) in non-sensitised controls and (c) in animals infected with virulent Mycobacterium tuberculosis; predominance of the mononuclears in the immunized animals.

132

division after indirect methods, as resulting from the conception of B-cells and T-cells, has didactic advantages but inhibits the development of cognition.

The immunologically competent cells form a deeply echeloned system, which covers the entire organism and has closely linked functions.

As an example, the course of the immunological change at the first contact with antigen can be demonstrated with the functional interplay of mesothelial and lymphatic tissues in the abdominal cavity, which constitutes the largest reservoir of immuno-competent cells. The production of cell material by puncture permits longitudinal observations in the living organism. The author (SCHMID F., 1955–1963; HAGGE W.) obtained the following results when provoking non-specific and specific stimulations in guinea-pigs and mice.

By evoking a non-specific stimulation with paraffin-glycerin, the cellular response in the peritoneal exudate will be different. Differentiations of 200–500 cells, 48 hours after injections of paraffin, revealed:

in healthy animals:
    50% granulocytes,
    35% monocytes,
    6% lymphocytes

in tuberculin-positive, BCG-sensitised animals:
    18% granulocytes,
    62% monocytes,
    17% lymphocytes,
    2% fibroplasts

in guinea-pigs with generalized tuberculosis (infected with human mycobacteria):
    13% granulocytes,
    23% monocytes,
    62% lymphocytes,
    2% fibroblasts.

This means that the cellular response to a non-specific stimulation depends on the biological starting situation of the organism.

Immunocytes

The antibodies are formed by cellular derivatives of the reticulo-histiocytary system, which show distinctive morphological changes parallel to the functional stage.

The term « plasma cell» goes back to WALDEYER (1895), the formal characterization to UNNA (1891). The development has been described in detailed, more modern studies by GOWANS and McGREGOR, FAGRAEUS, BRAUNSTEIN-ER, BESSIS (1972), the cytochemical findings were treated by F. SCHMID (1963, 1966); KRÜPE discussed the biological importance.

The difficulties with the morphological classification of transitional forms, on the one hand, and the understanding that «other» mononuclear cells e. g. the lymphocytes play a part in the formation and transmission of antibodies, on the other hand, have called in question the monopoly of the plasma cells to form antibodies. These difficulties are essentially due to the fact that defined functions are ascribed to defined forms. The supposition that the form is virtually patterned by the function clarifies the interrelations as the same kind of cells can show different morphological properties in different functional phases.

Controversy has been carried on for decades. MAXIMOW (1928, 1932) as well as DOWNEY and STASNEY (1936) considered the plasma cell as a functional form of a lymphoid cell. Others, as e. g. UNNA

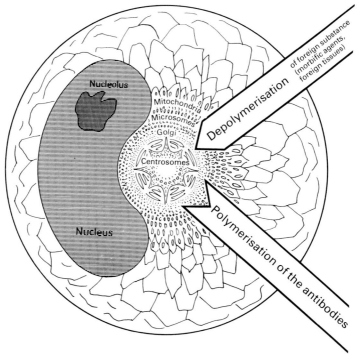

Fig. 165:
Principle of the immunological change of mononuclear cells: the depolymerisation of foreign substances (microbes, proteins) is followed by the polymerisation of new compounds (antibodies).

(1891), DOMENICI (1920), ROHR (1940) and BESSIS and SCEBAT (1946) see direct transitions from reticulum cells and «perithelial» cells to plasma cells.

As the *functional* ability to form antibodies is much more specific for the «plasma cells» than for the form, F. SCHMID suggested in 1963 the name «immunocytes»; the same term was favoured by DAMESCHEK (1964).

Morphologically, plasma cells are described as medium-sized to large (9–20 microns in diameter) mononuclear cells with the following characteristics:

a) marginal or eccentric, oval to flattened nucleus. The spoke-like form of the nucleus is an electron-optical phenomenon of the dispersion of chromatin;

b) dark to deeply basophile cytoplasm by panchromatic staining;

c) marked endoplasmatic reticulum.

This description relates only to «ripe» plasma cells. Functionally, the immunocytes (plasma cells) are characterised by the biological capability of

d) reacting to stimulations from antigens;

e) proliferating through these stimulations;

f) synthetising antibodies;

g) keeping a memory of previous contacts with antigens.

Extensive studies conducted from 1950–1966 on peritoneal exudate cells of the guinea-pig after sensitization with various antigens – BCG bacteria, human gamma-globulin, human Mycobycteri-

134

um tuberculosis, coli and proteus – gave the following summary. The course depends on the form and dose of antigens, the principle remains the same. The tests in the peritoneal space allows a dynamic observation by current differentiations of cells (cells obtained by puncture) instead of the mostly static findings in sections of thymus, spleen or lymph-nodes. The following phases respond regularly to stimulations by antigens:

Activation of microphages

Every stimulation by antigens is followed first by a multiplication of the polynuclear leukocytes. They perform the initial phagocytosis but later fall victims of phagocytosis by macrophages (within 24 to 48 hours) when their membranes have been loaded with antigenic substances (fig. 119–124).

The stage of mobilization

of the mononuclears is initiated few hours after the antigenic stimulation. The cells eliminated from the reticulo-histiocytary and mesothelial tissues round off into monocytoid forms (fig. 159) with loosely structured nucleus and neutral cytoplasm. Mitotic and amitotic divisions increase the cellular potential (fig. 166–169).

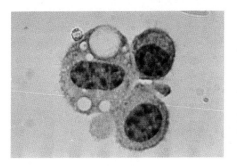

Fig. 166:
Mononuclear cells (monocytes, lymphoid cells) from the peritoneal exudate of guinea-pigs; 116th day after immunization with human gamma-globulin.

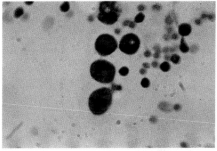

Fig. 167:
Mitosis of plasma cells in the peritoneal exudate after BCG-immunization. The cellular potential is increased by mitosis in the free exudate.

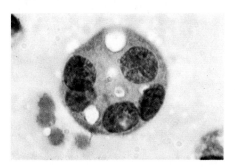

Fig. 168:
Amitotic processes cause formation of giant cells (peritoneal exudate of guinea-pigs after BCG-sensitisation).

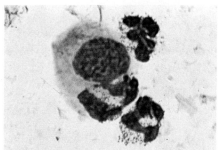

Fig. 169:
Direct elimination of polynuclear granulocytes from mesothelial cells of the peritoneal exudate increases on acute stimuli the potential of microphages.

135

Stage of transformation

The transformation of the mononuclear cells begins on the second or third day after the stimulation by antigens. The volume of the cytoplasm of the mononuclears grows. The cytoplasm becomes basophilous from the middle of the cell, the structure becomes more compact.

Electron-optically, these processes are characterized by the formation of dense structures in the middle of the cells (fig. 188) with abundant numbers of mitochondria, extended Golgifield and a growing endoplasmatic reticulum (fig. 186, 187).

The stage of maturity

is dominated by deeply basophilous cytoplasm (fig. 173), which covers the marginal, comparatively small, nucleus often to such an extent that it can barely be seen. Electron-optically, a dense endoplasmatic reticulum interlaces substantial areas of the cytoplasmatic space (fig. 186–189).

The stage of maturity is reached with the first contact with antigens, between the 7th and 10th days after the supply of antigens, according to the latter's quantity and quality

The stage of secretion

sets in already on the summit of the stage of maturity and lasts for 2–3 weeks (from the 8th to the 25th day). Light-optically, the homogenous-basophilous cytoplasm is interrupted by small «vacuoles» or vesicles filled with fluid; these proliferate and grow as the secretion goes on till at the end of the phase of secretion a large cell results, dominated by a system of vacuoles (fig. 29, 128, 176, 177, 178, 179, 181, 189).

Electron-optically, this process takes the following course: the spaces between the tubes of the endoplasmatic reticulum grow wider (fig. 187). The spaces between the lamellae, turned first in the direction of the lamellae, round off. The enlargement, probably pressure filtration, effects the evacuation of the synthesis products of the ribosomes into the cisterns filled with fluids (vesicles = vacuoles).

Fig. 170:
Monocytes of the non-sensitised animal.

Fig. 171:
On the 4th day after sensitisation: increased cytoplasmic space (in proportion to the size of nucleus), basophil consolidation in the Golgi-area of the cell.

Fig. 172:
Emission phase of a plasma cell from the mesothelial unit.

Fig. 173:
Mature plasma cell (immunocyte) with compact, deep-basophil cytoplasm, marginal nucleus (2nd-3rd week after sensitisation).

Fig. 174:
Consolidation of basophil products in membrane bulges.

Fig. 175:
Evacuated membrane bulges with direct channels into the interior of cytoplasm, the probable way of antibody extrusion. After extrusion of the basophil (= acid) material, the cell has re-adopted the character of monocytes.

Fig. 176:
Ageing secretory plasma cell (immunocyte) speckled with cisterns («vacuoles»).

Fig. 177:
Old immunocyte with large cisterns (vacuoles) and rigid cytoplasmatic structures, flattened nucleus, 3 months after sensitisation.

Fig. 170–181:
Maturation and ageing of immunocytes (plasma cells); characteristic examples of a longitudinal study of 3 months (peritoneal-exudate cells of guinea-pigs after sensitisation with xenogenous protein; 0.5 ml of human gamma-globulin or bovine serum).

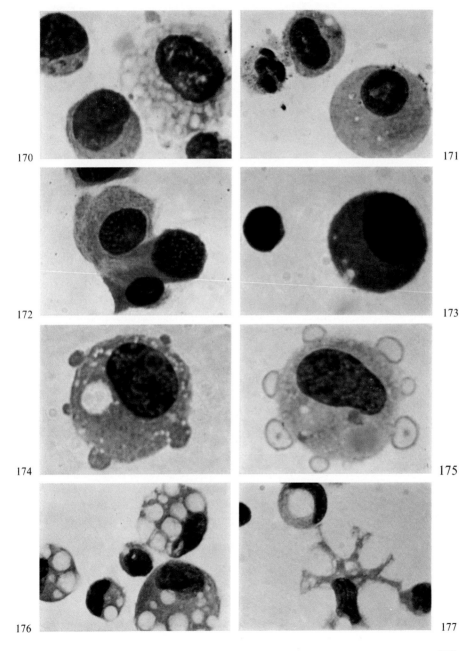

170

171

172

173

174

175

176

177

These intracellular ecological spaces follow a centripetal course and eliminate the synthesis products (including the antibodies) into the humoral system.

The elimination of the acid synthesis products seems to follow geometrical laws (fig. 174, 175); in the interest of the biochemical balance, it takes place at diagonally opposite sites.

The redifferentiation

occurs apparently in contrary direction. After the elimination of the antibodies and metabolites accompanying the synthesis, the cytoplasm decreases, takes a neutral colour, the nucleus gets mellow and less eccentric. Direct transitions to monocytes or reticular cells can be observed. Striking are the groupings of small lymphocytes on the membranes of excreting immunocytes; they seem to have transport functions (fig. 177).

Processes accompanying the synthesis of immune bodies

The transformation of mononuclear cells into immunocytes is accompanied by a concentration of *nucleotides* and *ribonucleic acid* (fig. 178) in the cytoplasm. The degree of polymerization of the RNA rises in the course of the first two weeks after stimulation of antigens. Lipoids and carbohydrates are there, cytochemically, in ripe plasma cells in small concentration but appear in the stage of secretion by higher quantities. The *acid mucopolysaccharides* (fig. 179) concentrate in the cytoplasm from the 3rd day after the sensitization and appear as interior lining in the cistern of the immunocytes, extracellularly, from the 7th to the 12th days; a net-like connection of the mucopolysaccharides to the cell membrane can nearly always be proved. The synthesis of antibodies is accompanied by a concentration of *non-specific esterases* (fig. 180, 181) whereas the alkaline phosphatase of leukocytes is completely absent in the mononuclear cells.

Little attention has so far been paid to the inorganic quantitative and trace elements in connection with the immunological change though particularly elements as e.g. *calcium, magnesium, zinc* and *aluminium* have always played an important part in practical immunology.

The *calcium* localized chiefly in the nucleus (fig. 182, 183) concentrates in the cytoplasm during the ripening of the plasma cells and can be demonstrated extracellularly in substantial quantities in the second week after sensitization. Amorphous, crystalline and crystallised formations are found here; they indicate that the cells lose ample quantities of calcium while the immunological process goes on. This applies specially to the cytolysis caused by antigens, which explains also the therapeutic effect of the calcium in conditions of allergy and anaphylactic shock.

Magnesium is concentrated in the plasma cell, chiefly in the cell membrane (fig. 184, 185) and along the cisterns. In the stage of secretion of the immunocytes, substantial quantities can be traced also outside the cells where it forms bizarre forms of crystals under experimental conditions. Moreover, aluminium and phosphates concentrate especially in the cell membranes whereas mainly concentrations of iron, copper, lead, zinc and sulphur compounds occur in the cytoplasm.

Examples of these concomitant processes are illustrated in fig. 166–185.

138

Kinetics of the immunoglobulin synthesis

Measured on titres of antibodies after the first contact with antigens, 4 phases can be defined (BRANDIS):

1. No antibodies can be traced in a *latent phase* of 2–3 days;
2. During an *exponential phase* (from the 3rd to the 7th day), the antibody titre increases rapidly up to a maximum;
3. From the 6th–7th day the titre remains on the same level for 2–4 weeks (= 2nd–5th week after the sensitization): *stationary phase;*
4. During months to years, the antibody titre will slowly decrease: *phase of reduction.*

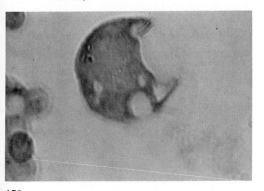

178

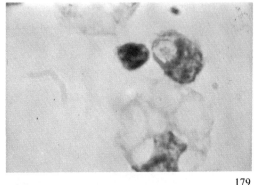

179

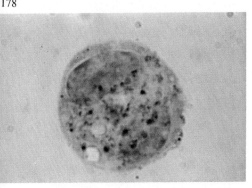

180

181

Fig. 178:
RNA concentration in the cytoplasm of an immunocyte at the beginning of the secretion (pyronin-positive cell). The synthesis of immunoglobulin depends on an increasing concentration of RNA. Methyl-green-pyronin staining; RNA = red, DNA = green.

Fig. 180:
Non-specific esterases take up mitochondria in the synthesis stage of the immunocytes. Esterase staining after LÖFFLER, esterase brick-red.

Fig. 179:
Acid mucopolysaccharides on the cellular membranes of immunocytes in the stage of secretion. Turquoise staining with alcian blue.

Fig. 181:
After the synthesis of immunoglobulin, the *esterase* is found chiefly in the cisterns, often in the form of crystals. Secretion stage of an immunocyte, esterase staining.

The cellular antibodies (IgM) attain a maximum late on the third day or on the fourth day, humoral antibodies appear on the fifth day. While the IgG level rises rapidly, the IgM level drops.

Latency-phase

The *phase of latency* corresponds to the transformation phase of the immunocytes. Transitional forms from mononuclears to «plasma cells» (often referred to as plasmablasts, fig. 171, 186) are found in the spleen, lymph-nodes and peritoneal space. As the direct method of cell differentiation from the perito-

neal exudate provides more exact kinetic aspects than autoradiography with 3 H – thymidin or the arrest of mitosis with colchicine, the phase of latency can be subdivided in a polynuclear episode of about 24 hours and a mononuclear phase, provable as from the second day after the exposition of antigens.

The indications of the rebuilding to the protein synthesis appear cytochemically and electron-optically. The cytoplasm becomes gradually basophile, pyronin-positive (= takes up RNA), the Golgi-apparatus grows, the mitochondria multiply, the endoplasmatic reticulum takes shape.

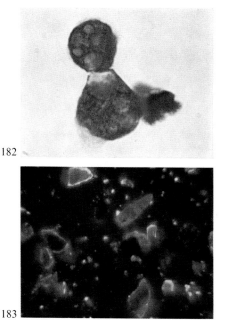

182

183

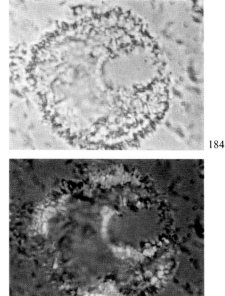

184

185

Fig. 182:
Concentration and extrusion of *calcium* from monocytes: cells of peritoneal exudate 2 weeks after sensitisation. Calcium-red coloration.

Fig. 183:
Extracellular calcium deposits in the peritoneal exudate, 3rd week after sensitisation.

Fig. 184:
Concentrations of *magnesium* on the cellular membrane of an immunocyte in the secretory stage and along the membrane of a cistern (vacuole); peritoneal exudate, magneson staining.

Fig. 185:
Cell as in fig. 184: under crossed nicols of the polarization microscope, the accumulations of magnesium membranes appear in a *crystaloid arrangement*.

140

The exponential phase

results from the quick rise of the titre of antibodies in the serum. The rapid division (fig. 167) of the mononuclears changed into immunocytes makes the antibody-producing cell potential go up rapidly till the 4th–6th day after the exposition of antigens. The numbers of cells and the titre of antibodies double in this phase within 6–12 hours (BRANDIS).

The exponential rise of the titre reflects the IgM production. Two cellular processes act together: the multiplication and ripening of the cells. The interference of the cell multiplication with a doubling rate within 9–12 hours and the doubling of the synthesis rate of the single cells every 9 hours make the production of antibodies double within 4.5–6 hours.

Cytochemically, basophilia and the expansion of the volume of cytoplasm as well as the pyronin positivity (= high concentration of RNA) characterize this phase; electron-optically, a dense ergastoplasm rich in ribosomes prevails (fig. 163, 173, 186–188).

Stationary phase

From the 6th to 7th day after the antigen stimulation, the titre of the antibodies remains steady for 2–4 weeks. This level is maintained within the classes of antibodies as the IgG values rise and the IgM concentrations decrease. The secretion during this phase could not be supported better than by the rise of humoral antibodies at the expense of the cellular antibodies. The IgG titres keep in this way rising till the end of the 3rd week,

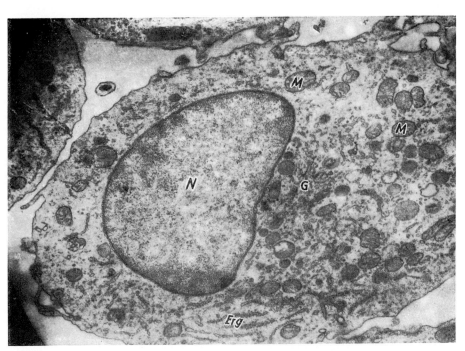

Fig. 186:
Early stage of plasma-cell (problasmoblast). Still oval but already eccentric nucleus (N), consolidation of the Golgifield (G), beginning formation of ergastoplasm (Erg). Abundance in mitochondria (M). Electron-opt. 1:15,000.

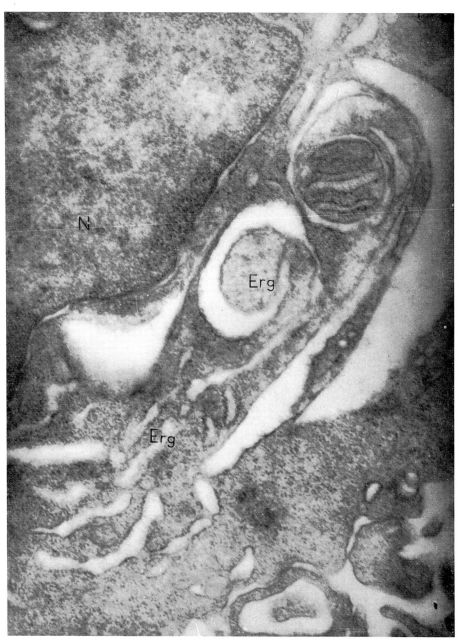

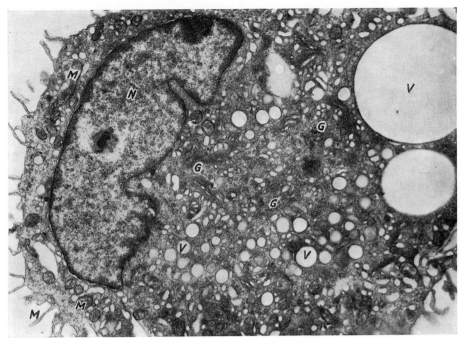

Fig. 188:
Mature plasma cell of the loose connective tissue. Marginal flattened nucleus (N), extended Golgi-area (G-G), consolidated, irregular cytoplasm; small to medium vacuoles (V) surrounding the Golgi-field, small mitochondria (M). Electron-opt. 1:12,000.

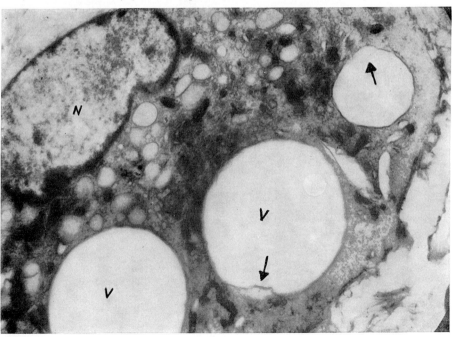

189

followed by a real stationary condition of about 2 weeks, during which the production of IgG and the disintegration of the immunoglobulin are equal.

The morphological equivalent of the stationary phase is secretory plasma cells with increasingly more vesicles and cisterns (fig. 174–177, 178, 181, 184, 189).

Phase of reduction

As the cellular potential producing the antibodies diminishes, the level of antibodies drops for months or years according to the stimulations by antigens. For this time, and longer, cells (memory cells) resuming after another contact with the same antigen the production of antibodies faster than at the first contact (secondary response) will remain.

Within wide outlines, this principle equals the immunokinetics. The spaces of time change according to the quantities of antigens. The more antigens, the faster and more intense the synthesis of antibodies will take place.

Eosinophils

An essential part in the defense mechanism of the body is ascribed to the eosinophilous leukocytes with a polymorphous nucleus. This kind of blood cells known since 1879, whose multiplication in diseases so different as asthma, parasitosis and in the monocytary-eosinophilous phase of overcoming after infections concealed the biological common denominator, have virtually been clarified as to their form and function. They are no longer classified under the collective name «leukocytes», at least since it has been known that more eosinophils than neutrophils can be found in the bronchial secretion of patients suffering from allergic asthma.

Morphology

Eosinophilous leukocytes have a diameter of 12–17 m i m and are found mostly in the area of the large-sized leukocytes. The main volume of the membrane-enclosed cell is formed by 2 (–3) roundish-ovoid nuclei. The distinctive fundamental capability of selecting acid dyestuffs from a panchromatic mixture (PAPPENHEIM, MAY-GRÜNWALD, GIESMA) detected by P. EHRLICH accounts for the separation from the neutrophilous and basophilous leukocytes. The space of cytoplasm contains several, usually twenty, roundish, oval or elliptical granules; their refractive power is due to the axis crystals, sometimes referred to as «cores». The basic protein of the granule accounts for the acidophilia; it contains an unusually high percentage of arginin (KOENIG, GLEICH, etc.). The granules are covered by a simple cytomembrane. The densities of the axis-crystalloids and matrix in a cell are considerably different (ZUCKER-FRANKIN, 1978).

The electron-optical fixation methods define the optical picture of the granules. Whereas the fixation of osmium makes appear the crystalloids denser (darker) than the matrix (fig. 190), phosphorus-molybdane or hypertonic fixation methods produce a negative picture showing the matrix black and the crystalloid as a bright, rectangular space, with ground-off ends. The elements of the basic structure of the crystalloid have a periodicity of 40 Å (fig. 191).

The crystalloids may derive their importance from inorganic substituents. The high percentage (15%) of zinc, which probably originates from the Charcot-Leyden crystals growing from the eosinophils, makes believe that the crystalloid axes of the granules owe their

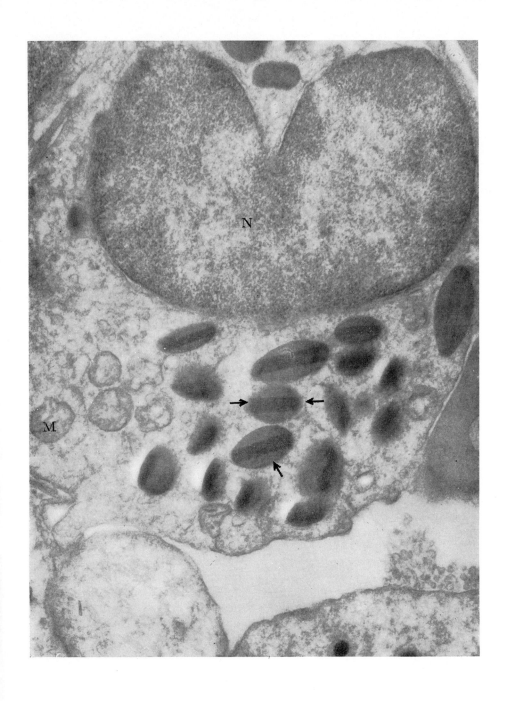

N

M

Fig. 190:
Eosinophilous granulocyte. In the (more compact) granules the axis crystalloids (arrows). N = nucleus; M = mitochondria 1:20,000.

crystalline form to a zinc complex compound, more so because zinc (Zn^{++}) inclines to form tetraedic complexes. For the inorganic order of crystals speaks the fact that the crystalloids are sparingly soluble in biological media and resistant to mechanical, osmotic and enzymatic influences. Even during the foudroyant destruction in digestive vacuoles of macrophages, the crystalloids resist the longest.

The *Charcot-Leyden crystals* (CHARCOT: 1853 for leukocytemia; LEYDEN 1872 for bronchial asthma) are found in the neighbourhood of accumulations of eosinophils. They can be produced in vitro by destruction of eosinophils (by detergents, Na-dihexyl-sulphosuccinate) (AYRES). The granules contain zinc, iron, copper, ubiquinon. Of the metals, zinc is likely to form the nucleus of the crystallization; in the crystal occur proteins and amino-acids, specially arginin, tyrosin and tryptophane.

The cytoplasm of the eosinophils contains more mitochondria, abundant quantities of small to medium, often grouped, vesicles, abundant numbers of ribosomes and a well marked Golgi-apparatus (fig. 15–18). «Microgranules» are dumb-bell-like or ring-shaped structures of the endoplasmatic reticulum, 100–150 Å in length.

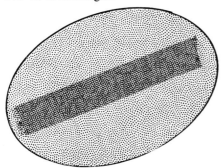

Fig. 191:
Scheme of the eosinophilous granules with the axillary crystalloids and the matrix surrounded by the membrane (see text).

Biochemistry

Histochemically, most of the lysosomal enzymes were traced in the eosinophils. The quantity of peroxidase is larger than in the granules of the neutrophils and moreover seems to function in a somewhat different way (ZUCKER-FRANKIN). The myeloperoxidase has a highly bactericide potency, the peroxidase of the eosinophils evidently not. Regarding the eosinophil granules there is the remarkable fact that Zn^{++} (and $Fe^{++,+++}$) take part in the formation of peroxide from plasmalogenes in the tissue (OHNISHI, F.).

The arylsulphatase B, too, is more concentrated in eosinophils than in neutrophils. This enzyme is said to have a function inactivating the «slow reacting substance» of the anaphylaxy (SRS-A). Another two substances are of importance though the site of their origin has so far not been located: bradykinin neutralises histamin; a factor denoted as EDI (inhibitor of histamin release) prevents the release of histamin from tissue mast-cells and basophilous leukocytes. In tissue mast-cells, histamin is bound to heparin in the form of a ternary complex (KERP G. and STEINHAUESER G.).

Origin

The general supposition that all granulocytes originate from the common mother cells (myeloblasts) of the bone-marrow, conflicts with certain objective observations. Patients suffering from agranulocytosis can have increased eosinophil numbers in the absence of ripe neutrophils (ZUCKER-FRANKIN D.). In congenital neutropenia, the myeloblasts do not ripen fully, the development of the leukocytes with polymorphous nuclei is arrested on the step to the myelocyte; then ripe eosinophils cannot only be normal but even multiply. From mother cells of the human blood originate in agar cultures either neutrophils or eosinophils, no mixed populations.

The formation of eosinophils in the thymus of rats has been proved safely (YOKE M. S. and SAINTE-MARIE G., 1965). As for the human thymus, J. SCHAFFER described the occurrence of eosinophils already in 1891.

Eosinophils circulate in the Ductus thoracicus lymphaticus where neutrophils are rare (ZUCKER-FRANKIN D.). The narrow relations between the thymus and the production of eosinophils have been proved repeatedly by the lack of eosinophils in thymic insufficiency of various species of animals. On the other hand, individuals suffering from agammaglobulinaemia of the Swiss type can show considerable increases in eosinophils in dysplasia of the thymus.

Function

Clinical and experimental findings have substantiated the supposition that the eosinophils play an important part in the immune-defense. Studies on parasite eggs of schistosoma (MACKENZIE et al.; MCLAREN et al.; KÖNIG W.) have shown that eosinophils effect a membrane adherence with pseudopodia after «palpating» the parasite membrane. By accumulating enzymes in the neighbourhood of the site of contact, the active ingredients – specially peroxidase – injuring the parasite membrane are produced; they start the destruction of the parasites as the usual way via the phagocytosis is not feasible owing to the dimensions.

The following factors account for this no doubt most important function:

The eosinophil chemotactic factor (EFC) is a peptide favouring (besides other powers) the contact of the eosinophils with immune complexes; it is released from lymphocytes and neutrophils (KÖNIG). Another factor of lymphocytary origin, the eosinophil stimulating factor (ESP) controls the migration and does not depend on immune complexes.

Eosinophils are chemotactically attracted by immune complexes (specially after complementary activation) and bacteria.

Anaphylactic reactions are always associated with eosinophils, ruptured mast-cells are surrounded by eosinophils. Histamin seems to have a special «affinity» to eosinophils. Owing to the nearly regular correlation between IgE and the multiplication of eosinophils, a direct relation between the two components is postulated.

Basophils

Basophilous granulocytes and tissue mast-cells have as a common characteristic basophilous, or rather, metachromatic granules. Metachromatic means that toluidine-blue or giemsa does not stain the granules blue but in gradations of violet. *Basophilia* represents highly acid structures taking up greedily the basic constituents from a colour mixture.

The blood of healthy persons contains 25–50 basophils/mm^3. There are no regular quantitative relations between the blood basophils and the tissue mast-cells. In the bone-marrow, the basophils make about 0.33%, in the tissue, the tissue mast-cells make 0.001–0.02 (BESSIS, 1972; BRAUNSTEINER and ZUCKER-FRANKIN, 1962; WOLF-JURGENSEN, 1968; FREDERICKS and MOLONEY, 1959).

The basophils multiply in hypothyreosis, after splenectomy, in cirrhosis of

147

the liver; they decrease after an anaphylactic shock, in thyreotoxicosis, in rheumatic arthritis.

Morphology

In granulocytopoiesis, the first metachromatic granules appear in the stage of the promyelocytes; they become more distinct in the myelocytes. The granules originate in the Golgi-apparatus and unite gradually to form larger structures.

The (metachromatic) basophilous granulocyte is the smallest granulocyte offshot (∅ 10–14 microns). The granules, 0.1–1.0 (up to 1.7) microns in size, are roundish, oval or angular; frequently, they are placed in cisterns (vacuoles). The granules, covered by a simple membrane, include a marginal matrix, and a parallel layered or hexagonally structured compact interior mass (see fig. 193); DVORAK, 1978; ZUCKER-

FRANKIN, 1967. The particles are not separated sharply from the matrix and vary between 113 and 260 Å in diameter. The granules can comprise particles of varying size and membrane structures. Smaller peroxidase-negative granules are found in the vicinity of the nucleus.

The cytoplasm is pale, grey to reddish in the ground tone, contains abundant quantities of vesicles and of glycogen deposits. A small Golgi-apparatus, few mitochondria, few ribosomes and scarce rough endoplasmatic reticulum, microtubuli and microfilaments have been detected. The nucleus is «S» or «J»-shaped, less segmented than in the segment-nuclear cells or eosinophils and has compact chromatin structures.

Cytochemistry

Basophilous granulocytes and tissue mast-cells contain many bioactive, bio-

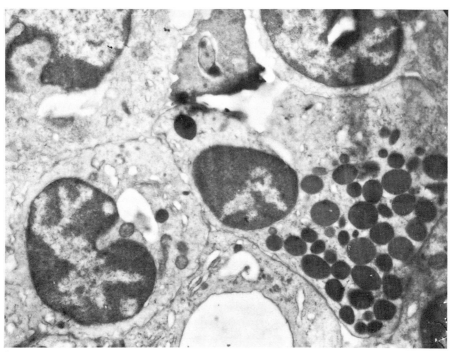

Fig. 192:
Basophilous granulocyte from the peritoneal exudate of the guinea-pig; 1:10,000.

chemical substrates and enzymes (Ac-
KERMANN, 1963).

Acid mucopolysaccharides

The phenotypical basic property
–metachromasia, basophilia– is due to
acid mucopolysaccharides of the granules. Blue dyestuffs like toluidine blue,
methylene blue, methylene violet provoke colours in red (positive metachromasia), red dyestuffs (neutral red, safranin, pyronin) yellow to yellowish-greenish
shades (negative metachromasia). OR-
ENSTEIN et al. found 85% of chondroitin
sulphate and dermatan sulphate, 15%
were heparan sulphate (not heparin, as
supposed earlier).

Histamin

Whereas in various animals only part
of the body-histamin occurs in basophils / mast-cell reservoir, the entire depot of histamin seems to be located in the
basophilous cells in man. The human basophils include 1–2 pg of histamin, mast-
cells of the peritoneal exudate of rats up
to 20 pg (DVORAK). Histamin is bound to
the granular fraction.

The synthesis takes place through a
cytoplasm enzyme, the histidin-decar-
boxylase. In tissular cultures of guinea-
pig basophils tagged with 3 H histidin,
the increase of histamin was registered
after 1 hour already, the maximum of
production is attained after 24 hours.

Platelet-activation factor

The accumulation of blood-platelets
around degranulated basophils suggested a connection. The aggregation-pro-
moting factor (PAF) is found especially
in «sensitized» basophils and anti-IgE
antibodies. PAF is a low-molecular protein (molecular weight = 1,100), which
forms rapidly compounds with albumin
and cell membranes. It does not cause
contractions of unstriated muscles but
improves the permeability of vessels and
cannot be influenced by antihistamins or
antiserotonins.

Further substances

In contrast to the sparingly soluble
crystalloid axes of the eosinophils, the
basophilous granules dissolve readily in
water and glycerin; this makes the cytochemical analysis more difficult. Nevertheless, quite a series of further substances has been detected.

The positive PAS-reaction proves the

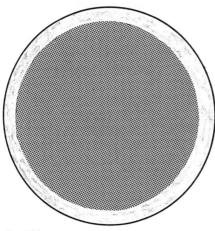
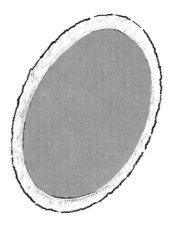

Fig. 193:
Scheme of the basophilous granules (see text).

presence of *glycogen (or glycoprotein) aggregates* located outside the granules, with particles up to 300 Å in diameter. The presence of *lipids* has been demonstrated with Sudan-black-B.

The enzyme pattern of the basophils is not quite clear. The most important enzyme seems to be the *histidin decarboxylase,* which transforms histidin to histamin. Neutral *esterase-proteases* have been found. Oxydative enzymes such as *diaphorases* and various *dehydrogenases* are ascribed to the mitochondria fraction of the basophils. The *activity of the peroxidase* seems to differ in various species. There are some deviations from the normal lysosomal enzymes as e.g. the *absence of the lactate-dehydrogenase.* Phosphatases, aminopeptidases, phosphorylases seems to be absent. The *non-specific esterases* – unlike the mast-cells – have not been proved in blood basophils. A *plasminogen-activating factor* has been detected in the membrane of basophils, not however in the purified granular fractions (summaries by DVORAK, 1978; BESSIS, 1972; ACKERMANN, 1963).

Human mast-cells and basophils of leukemic patients contain the *eosinophilous chemotactic factor (EFC-A)* and the *slow-reacting substance (SRS-A).*

After the influence of microradiations or distilled water, needle-shaped crystals will grow in the granules.

Function

Basophils move like amoebae, their phagocytic power is inferior to that of other species of leukocytes; they can phagocytose complexes of antigens and antibodies as well as sensitized erythrocytes. Their main function, possibly, is to act as a histamin reservoir of the body. In spite of certain differences in granule-chemistry, the blood basophils and the tissular mast-cells constitute a functional unit, with the basophils representing the transport system and the tissular mast-cells the depot system.

One of their most important properties is the degranulation. Whereas, physiologically, the degranulation can eliminate the granular contents when required, the evacuation of the granules takes place in the form of explosion under immuno-pathological conditions. After the elimination of the compact contents, vesicles rimmed with membranes will remain and disappear gradually. Electron-optical observations have shown that the contents of the granules are directed into the extracellular space through a «cytoplasma canal» (DVORAK), or that a partial evacuation takes place after fusion of the granular and cytoplasmic membranes. This process is initiated by immunity reactions mediated through cellular membranes and IgE (fig. 192, 194, 204).

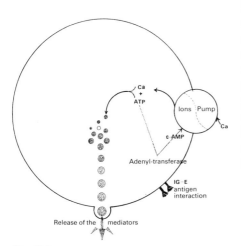

Fig. 194:
Degranulation of a basophils.

150

Immunological constituents

Antigens

The concept «antigen» cannot be interpreted by an absolute definition but is associated with the complementary antibody. A foreign or an endogenic substance with a changed structure becomes an antigen by provoking the formation of antibodies as its structure is heterogeneous to the organism. Antigens have macromolecular structures and are found in the many categories of the biochemical substances of the animal and botanic kingdoms. In contrast to earlier views that only albuminoids had an antigenous effect, it is now taken for granted that polysaccharides, proteins, lipoids and complex compounds of these classes of substances can be antigens. Another point, however, is the macroorganism, which marks these substances as «foreign» and reacts with the formation of antibodies.

The *antigenicity* of a substance depends on its molecular weight. Substances with a molecular weight of less than 500 are usually not antigenic. Haptenes and weak antigens have molecular weights of between 5000 and 30,000, antigenic proteins however between 34,000 and 5,000,000 (KWAPINSKI). Antigenic molecules of 200–700 Å can bear up to 23 antigenic determinants.

Much as the *macromolecular vehicle* influences the antigenicity, it does little to contribute to the structure of the antibodies; the macromolecular association accounts probably for the invulnerability of the foreign substance by the enzymes of the contaminated organism. Decisive for the specificity of the resulting antibody is the smallest reacting superficial unit of the macromolecule, the so-called *«determinant group»*. The antigens occurring in nature are multivalent i.e. have several different determinant groups.

Whereas the antigenicity *(capacity of*

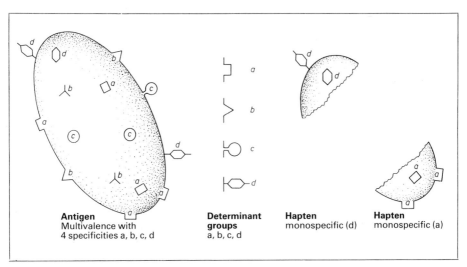

Antigen
Multivalence with
4 specificities a, b, c, d

Determinant groups
a, b, c, d

Hapten
monospecific (d)

Hapten
monospecific (a)

Fig. 195:
Antigen – determinants – hapten

sensitizing) requires the macromolecule as a biochemical unit, dissociation products (or natural substances of similar structure) suffice for the reaction with the formed antibodies. These lower molecular, not antigenic but reactive, fragments of antigens (fig. 195) are called *haptenes* (from Gr. haptein = to stitch). In biochemistry, the haptenes have an analogue in the prosthetic groups of the ferments that have no fermentative activity themselves but cause the specificity of the ferment.

If the *depolymerisation* of the antigenic proteins or polysaccharides is continued i. e. if they are broken down into peptides, amino-acids, oligosaccharides or monosaccharides, they can only fill and thus block the «ecological niche» in the antibody. Thus they are capable of inhibiting the reaction between antigen and antibody.

Endogenic cells discern antigens as foreign if the enzymes of a cell have no

key to «open» and to disintegrate the foreign substance. The cell as the smallest unit of organization in the higher organisms must detect the «foreign character». However, it has to be realised that the immunological process involves cells and tissues but takes place in the molecular domain.

Origin and affinity to the organism have led to the following subdivision of antigens:

Tab. 10: **Division of the antigens according to their origin:**

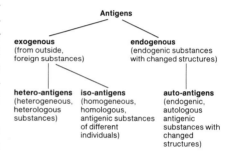

Antigenic determinants

Polysaccharides as antigens

The knowledge of the antigenic character of groups of polysaccharide molecules is much based upon the research into pneumococci. The specificity of the now more than 70 serologically differentiable types of pneumococci is defined by the sugars of the capsule polysaccharides. Capsule polysaccharides isolated from large cultures of pneumococci turned out to be highly antigenic i. e. they provoke the formation of antibodies (AVERY and GOEBEL, HEIDELBERGER, KABAT). This refuted, already decades ago, the dogma that only proteins could be full antigens. The determinant group in the highly molecular unit is restricted to 1–3 (–6) terminal, «disponible», glucosidically bound sugar molecules.

The abundance of the polysaccharides is restricted among the antigenic to certain few but more frequently occurring substances of terminal groups, socalled «antigen communities» (KRÜPE). These communities «bridge» even the boundaries of species. Such communities exist e. g. between

pneumococcus type II, Friedländer bacteria B, richettsial fever, proteus OX 19, pneumococci polysaccharide type XIV, degraded blood-group substance A. The determinant group contains glucose, glucuronic acid and rhamnose.

The specificity of antigens relies on the chemical structures of the terminal groups so to speak on the molecular profile. It explains also the affinity of such terminal groups with the human blood-group substances. There is, consequently, even for the polysaccharide antigens a bridge between the capsular substance of bacteria and cellular antigens.

The *ABO and Lewis blood-group* substances of man are *glucopolypeptides*. The specificity-determining polysaccharide has a molecular weight of 300,000–350,000 and consists of the following 4 sugar elements:

L-fucose
N-acetyl-D-glucosamin
D-acetyl-D-galactosamin
D-galactose;

the latter is coupled to non-antigenic polypeptides of 11 amino-acids, which make about 20% of the volume. In the blood-group A the N-acetyl-D-galactosamin, in the group B the D-galactose, in the group 0 the L-fucose are terminal. The Lewis-(a)-substance (MORGAU) is characterized by a determinant group – trisaccharide from N-acetyl-D-glucosamin, D-galactose at the 3rd C-atom in a beta-glucosidic compound, L-fucose at the 4th C-atom in an alpha-glucosidic compound (fig. 196).

The specificity-determining area of antigens is controlled by genes and formed from a mother substance containing all 4 sugars, which is called «*H-substance*» for its heterogeneous origin. This mother substance is found mostly in the blood-group 0.

For specificity, the following items seem to be of importance:

a) the alpha- or beta-glucosidic binding of the terminal sugar-molecule;

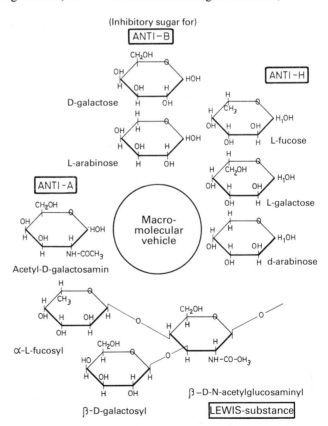

Fig. 196:
Ring-shaped structures of pyranose from monosaccharides blocking specifically anti-A, anti-B, anti-H; below: trisaccharide or Lewis-(a)-property.

b) the sugar must be ring-shaped (as pyranose) like in nature;
c) the cis/trans-configuration of the OH groups;
d) the d- or l-stereoisomere structure.

For salmonellae and coliform bacteria, a new class of desoxy-sugars, the 3,6-di-desoxy-sugars were found to be specificity-determining (WESTPHAL et al.). The mucous substance from Leuconostoc mesenteroides, the dextran (glucose-polymerisation product), much used in the therapy, has probably an antigenic effect through the glucoside bridges, which do not correspond to the glucogenous structure.

Lipoids as antigens

Lipoids occur in the living nature mostly as complex compounds with proteins and polysaccharides. In the cells of warm-blooded animals they are accumulated in the cellular membrane and in the Golgifield, in viruses (e. g. mixoviruses) and bacteria (e. g. tubercle bacilli) chiefly in the coats of morbific agents. Purely isolated lipoids are not full antigens, have usually the character of haptenes but can «borrow» the character of antigens before the injection by a mixture with proteins. Whereas the trailing function of the proteins increases the antigenicity of the lipoids, we know many tuberculo-immunological tests raising the antigenicity of the bacteria or bacterial proteins by mixing with lipoids. Between the two groups of substances, therefore, a completing antigenicity seems to exist.

A known lipoid haptene is the phosphatide acid «cardiolipin» (isolated from ox hearts) used specially in the diagnosis of lues.

Proteins as antigens

Thanks to the variabilities in the sequence of their building elements (24 amino-acids) and the binding, pleating and clewing of the polypeptides, proteins are structurally much more variable than polysaccharides or lipoids. However, also in this case, not the macromolecular proteins but the terminal group is the vehicle of the antigenic quality and specificity. These antigenic determinants are oligopeptides from several (probably up to 12) amino-acids. The order of the binding of amino-acids seems to be decisive, and the terminal molecules of the ends of the proteins determine the specificity more than the central amino-acids of the antigenic oligopeptides. As an example, H. E.-SCHULTZE has assembled the conditions among the serum albumins of various mammals (tab. 11).

As the protein structure is bound to the species and controlled by genes specific to individuals, the number of the potential protein antigens is incalculably

Tab. 11: **Amino-acid-sequences on the C-ends of serum-albumins**

Kind	NH$_2$ end	COOH end
Man	Asp-Ala	Gly-Val-Ala-Leu
Ox	Asp-Thr	Asp-Glu-Lys-Ser-Val-Thr-Leu-Ala
Horse	Asp-Thr	Val-Ser-Leu-Ala
Ass	(Asp-Thr)	Ser-(Val-Lys-)Leu-Ala
Mule	(Asp-Thr)	(-Leu-Ala)
Rabbit	Asp-	Leu-Ala
Wether	Asp-	(Glu-Asp-Thr)-Ser-Val-Lys-Leu-Ala
Monkey	Asp-	(Asp-Glu)-Ser-Lys-Val-Leu-Ala

high. Whether a protein really acts as an antigen depends on the individual readiness of the recipient, on the affinity, the «maturity» and on the biological situation.

Ferments and hormones bear their enzymatic potencies in peptide areas, which show the same sequence of amino-acids in the various species of animals. This constant sequence of the amino-acids is a prerequisite for the therapeutic efficiency of ferments and hormones from the animal kingdom in man. The biologically active areas are located in lateral chains of the protein structures specific to each species. Aberrations from the sequence of amino-acids are seen in the best analysed insulin from animals (horned cattle, pig, sheep, horse, whale) only in the 8th, 9th and 10th links of the glycyl chain whereas the terminal groupings are identical for the species mentioned. In long use, the hormones (e. g. ACTH, insulin) may certainly become antigenic, which receives expression in hyperergic symptoms and in the loss of the therapeutic effect (by disintegration or binding).

Nucleic acids – macromolecular polymerisation products of the nucleotides – are not complete antigens in spite of their high molecular weight up to 10 million although they bear the marks of species and individuals. The organism of mammals contains the highly molecular DNA (mol. weight 6–10 million) in the chromatin substance of the nuclei, the RNA is located in the nucleolar system and cytoplasm; it occurs soluble (mol. weight 20,000–40,000) and bound to the structure (500,000–2 million). Considering the high constituents of nucleic acid in the microbes (viruses consist of RNA, bacteriophages of DNA, higher microorganisms of both), this statement of lacking antigenicity surprises. The findings of antigenic effects of nuclear material in so-called autoaggression diseases (LE-phenomenon) are no convincing proof either. An explanation is difficult because highly antigenic substances form at once when nucleic acids are bound to proteins, and such bindings are usual in biological structures.

Antibodies

Antibodies are immunoglobulins formed by antigenic stimulation; they can form complex compounds with the antigenic determinant by stereo-chemical complementarity. Sized about $34 \times 12 \times 7$ Å, only a small part of 0.1 to max. 1% of the surface falls to the niche capable of effecting a specific binding (fig. 201). The specificity of antibodies depends on the sequence of the amino-acids of the variable segment (see fig. 197) of the H-chains whereas the variable segment of the lambda-chains seems to serve rather for formal functions of the secondary and tertiary structures. Free amino-groups are apparently essential for the reactivity of the antibody molecules.

So far, 5 classes of immunoglobulin have been characterized by antigen analyses: IgG, IgA, IgM, IgD, IgE. The important data have been stated in tab. 12. Antibodies are dispersed about uniformly over the intravasal and interstitial fluid space of the body as far as they are not in cells; about 1/4 of their quantity is regenerated every day (KWAPINSKI, 1972; KABAT, 1960). A healthy person can synthetize 2–5 g of immunoglobulins daily, and 7 times more on immunization and infection stimuli.

If the molecular differences between

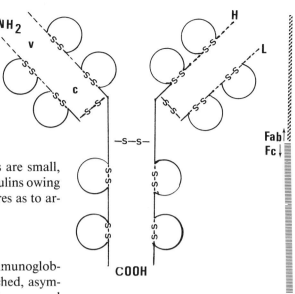

Fig. 197:
Diagram of an antibody molecule

various classes of antibodies are small, these are called immunoglobulins owing to their common main features as to architecture and function.

Form and structure

In a liquid medium the immunoglobulins have the form of stretched, asymmetric rotation ellipsoids. It is supposed that, unfolded, the IgG molecule takes a Y-shape (fig. 198), the IgM molecule a radial formation (fig. 200). The specifically reacting area makes less than 1% of the total molecular surface and is localized in a pouch-like cavity (niche) formed by the pleats of the peptide chains. The niche relief is complementary to the surface structure of the determinant group on the antigenic molecule (fig. 201–203).

The complementary molecular regions on the antigenic and antibody molecule fit into one another like a key into the lock. They are fixed by hydrogen bridges, coulomb powers and intermolecular-active van-der-Waal attractive powers (Krüpe). As the groupings of molecules on the antibody can evidently not become the motive of antigens as long as they have not changed, it can be supposed that the antibody includes cavities depending on the structure or relief. This rule, however, has considerable exceptions (Rother, 1979).

Two kinds of polypeptide chains form the common ground structure of the antibody molecules. Owing to the

different lengths of chains, heavy chains (= eta-chains) with molecular weights of 50,000–70,000 are distinguished from light chains (= lambda-chains) with a molecular weight of about 23,000. Every antibody molecule consists of 2 eta- and 2 lambda-chains (fig. 197) connected by disulfide bridges. The immunochemical differences owing to a different sequence of amino-acids in the eta-chains account for the classification of the 5 main classes. Immunoglobulins M are characterized by mi-chains, IgG by gamma-chains, IgA by alpha-chains, IgD by delta-chains and IgE by epsilon-chains. Of the lighter lambda-chains, 2 types, type kappa (kappa-chains) and type lambda (lambda-chains) are known.

Minor molecular changes induced the subdivision of the main classes; IgG has 4 subclasses namely IgG_1, IgG_2, IgG_3 and IgG_4 whereas IgA falls into IgA_1 and IgA_2. Genetically fixed antigen structures (e. g. Gm-, Am-factors) on the eta-chains, Inv-factors on the lambda-chains provide an additional differentiation of this subdivision (Brandis).

Tab. 12: **Characteristics of the immunoglobulins and complements factors**

Protein class	Plasma concentration (mg/100 ml)	Molecular weight	Sedimentation constant	Biological half-life period (days)
Immunoglobulin G (IgG)	800–1600	150.000	6,5–7,2	23
Immunoglobulin A (IgA)	90–420	180.000 (+ polymeres) secretory: 390.000	7; 9, 11, 13, 15, 17 11,4	6
Immunoglobulin M (IgM)	60–250 ♂ 70–280	950.000	18–20	5
Immunoglobulin D (IgD)	0,3–40	155.000	6,2–6,8	3
Immunoglobulin E (IgE)	0,01–0,14	196.000	7,9	?
C_1	2–3		18	
C_{1q}			11,1	
C_{1q}			7	
C_{1s}			4	
C_2	1		6	
C_3	80–140		9,5	
C_4	20–40		10	
C_5	3–5		8,7	
C_6	1		5–6	
C_7			6–7	
C_8			8	
C_9			4	

The two main sections of the antibody molecule are referred to as Fab-region and Fc-region, respectively. The molecule can be split at different sites by papain, plasmin and pepsin. Within the Fab-region, the terminal part has a variable structure and is therefore called variable region (v) as distinguished from the constant region (c).

The function of the Fab-regions is to bind the antigenic determinant in the complementary variable niche. As a consequence, an antigen-antibody complex will be formed namely

a precipitation in the fluid medium,
an agglutination in antigens with corpuscular carriers (erythrocytes, viruses, bacteria),
a neutralisation when the antigen is wrapped up (neutralized) by the antibody.

With the antigens bound to the Fab-region, the structure of the Fc-region will change so that the Fc-region becomes effective to cellular (membranous) or humoral systems (complement) (fig. 204).

The chains are divided into several homologizing regions or domains. The site of the antigen binding in the Fab-region consists of 3 segments of each of 5–10 remainders of amino-acids and is very variable as to structure. This site ac-

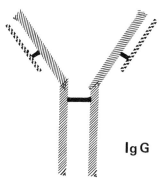

Ig G

Fig. 198:
Diagram showing structures of an IgG molecule

counts for the specificity of the antibody. The complement is bound in the domain C_{H2}, the interaction with the Fc-receptor on cellular surfaces depends on C_{H3} (RIESEN and BARANDUN). IgM and IgE contain C_{H4} as a further domain.

Biology and biochemistry of the antibodies

Antibodies are palliative structures «wrapping up» foreign substances and estranged endogenic substances so as to render them biologically inert. They appear when appropriate enzymes lack in the body so that the antigenic substance cannot be disintegrated and conveyed into the body's metabolic tracts.

The daily rate of transformation of the gammaglobulins is estimated by KRÜPE at about 35 mg/kg of body-weight; but this figure is probably a very approximate value. The rate of transformation is certainly lower for the baby and higher for the school-child than this rough estimate applying to the adult.

The expectation of life for the gammaglobulins is expressed by the following half-life periods:

23   days in man,
21   days in cows,
8   days in dogs,
5   days in rabbits,
4.5 days in guinea-pigs;
2   days in mice.

The essential biochemical and physical data have been summarized in tab. 12.

Immunoglobulin G (IgG)

With a share of 80% in the total depot of immunoglobulins, IgG is the most important; IgG occurs preferably in body fluids and placenta and is taken up by the new-born via the intestinal mucosa from the colostrum. It can form compounds with complement, bind to macrophages and seems to have special affinities to bacterial toxins.

Immunoglobulin A (IgA)

IgA, with a share of 13%, is the second important of the immunoglobulins. It occurs in the serum as a 7S-monomer, but with a polypeptide rich in cystein, the so-called xi-chain, it forms polymers. IgA is synthetized by immunocytes and

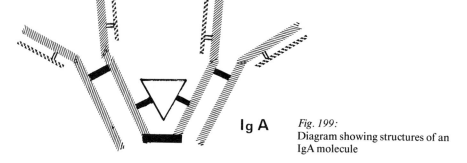

Ig A

Fig. 199:
Diagram showing structures of an IgA molecule

excreted in a dimeric form. It is found concentrated in the secretions of the body's epithelial interfaces, especially in the saliva, lacrimal fluid, nasal secretion and in the mucous layers of the respiratory and gastrointestinal tracts. It is supposed that a synergism exists between IgA, lysocyme and complement for the destruction of colibacilli. Aggregated IgA is capable of binding to polymorphic nuclear leukocytes and, unlike the classical complement-activation (fig. 204), of activating the so-called C^3-sideway (ROITT).

Immunoglobulin M (IgM)

Owing to its high molecular weight of 900,000 and 19 S sedimentation constant, IgM is also called macroglobulin-antibody. The polymerisation of the basic unit depends, also in this case, on the presence of a xi-chain. In small antigens, the binding valence is 10, in larger antigens 5. Thanks to their high binding valence, these antibodies tend very much to agglutination and cytolysis. Topographically, the location in the cells of the lymphatic tissues must be mentioned. The IgM-antibodies include: the isohaemagglutins (anti-A, anti-B), antibodies against the typhoid-0-antigen (endotoxin) and the antibodies in Wassermann's lues reaction.

Immunoglobulin D (IgD)

The percentage of IgD is about 1% of the immunoglobulins. The biological

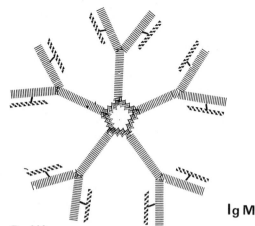

Ig M

Fig. 200:
Diagram structures of an IgM molecule

function is not yet clear. IgD was found on the surface of lymphocytes in the venous blood of the umbilical cord. It is believed that receptors, which are later conveyed to other immunoglobulins, may be present.

Immunoglobulin E (IgE)

IgE, making 0.002% of the globulin reservoir and concentrated 17–450 ng/ml, seems little important as to its quantity but belongs to the most notable immunoglobulins with regard to the clinical effects. IgE makes receptors on the cellular membrane bind to the complement system and thus initiates the output of histamin from basophils and mast-cells (fig. 194, 204). Large quantities are found in parasitosis, especially worm diseases, in allergic rhinitis (pollinosis) and bronchial asthma.

Theories of the formation of antibodies

As the exact course of antibody-synthesis is not known because it takes place beyond optically controllable molecular sizes, much has been theorized about this subject. Beginning from Ehrlich's «side-chain» theory, many versions of instruction-, selection- and seed-leaf the-

ories came and disappeared. The mental substance of those theories will be outlined hereafter.

The instructive theories

maintain that the antigen (or its determinant) acts as a stencil, around

159

which a normal globulin molecule forms in such a way that a niche complementary to the stencil results. This globulin molecule, specifically transformed on an area making less than 1% of the globulin surface, is stabilized by disulphide and hydrogen bridges and keeps the specific capability of binding when detached from the stencil.

The selective theories

suppose that certain antigens respond to special cells within a population, which are capable of answering specific stimulations. It is taken for granted that the information for the synthesis of certain antibodies exists already in the genetical material of these reacting cells. The code contained in the gene is said to be just called by the antigen so that the cells are selected by this code to form certain antibodies (Klon's selection theory).

The germe-layer theory

presumes that the genomes of the antibody-forming cells have the code for all antibody specificities so that these need just to be called by an antigen stimulation; this theory relies on pluripotent cells.

The quantum theory

of the immunogenesis (KWAPINSKI, 1972) regards the immunogenous stimulation as a transmission of an energy quantum from an inductor molecule to a growing globulin molecule, which is more flexible than ripe globulins.

The selective theories favoured in recent years offend against a fundamental immunological law: antibodies are produced against substances that an organism cannot process metabolically for lack of appropriate enzymes (= genes). EHRLICH's papers already have shown that antibodies are formed against substances (such as dinitrobenzol or sulphanilic acid) that do not occur in the living nature; consequently, a genetic basic information resulting from phylogenesis can hardly exist. The mobilized potential of immunocompetent cells depends on the quantity and kind of antigens rather than on other factors. Needless to say that transformed cells form a functional unit upon an antigenic stimulation. The cellular clonus does not exist primarily, it comes about through the functional community.

The following must be stated:

1. Antibodies are formed by pluripotential cells, which have a special synthetic function.
2. The cell transformation goes through a ripening phase and a longer secretion phase.
3. The production of antibodies is associated with an increase in RNA.
4. The synthesis is induced through m-RNA.
5. The light (lambda-) chains are formed on small ribosomes, travel to large poly-ribosomes where the heavy eta-chains are formed slowly.
6. Antibody synthesis is a cellular «de novo» synthesis.

Antigen-antibody relations

Only fragmentary knowledge exists about the many relations between antigens and antibodies. It is supposed that the higher molecular antibodies (e. g. 7-S-antibody-gammaglobulins) carry at

best 2 reactive molecular groups, which can correlate with the antigen determinants. The reactive areas are probably distant, perhaps at the ends of the globulin ellipsoids. Antibodies with one reac-

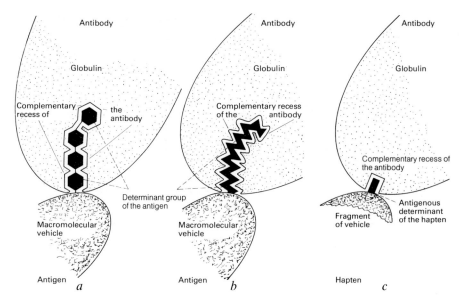

Fig. 201:
Spatial relations between antigenous determinants and antibody-globulins; (a) symbolizes an oligo-saccharide, (b) a peptide chain, (c) a hapten with determinant.

tive surface are called «monovalent», those with two reactive surfaces «bivalent».

The reactive area is estimated to measure 700–1000 Å, which corresponds to about 1% of the surface of a 7-S-antibody-gammaglobulin. The supposed shape is a pouch-like, peripheral dent in the peptide clusters of the globulin molecules, which is stereochemically complementary to the superficial profile of the determinant group on the antigen molecule. The spacious complementarity is fixed in the antigen-antibody reaction by hydrogen bridges, *coloumb powers* between NH_2- and COOH-groups as well as intermolecular *van-der-Waal's electric* powers. The binding condition, however, can be dissolved by many chemical and physical effects.

As long as the antibodies are strictly specific, they probably cover the entire determinant group of the antigen (1–12 molecules), later sometimes only the terminal molecule. This «blurs» the specificity, hyperergy and immunity (so-called cross-immunity) are extended i. e. involve several antigens. In clinical immunopathology, this phenomenon becomes important in the increased sensitisation of the adult allergic patient.

Gammaglobulins carry one (monovalent) to two (bivalent) reactive areas. It has not yet been proved whether the higher molecular beta$_2$- globulins carry more reactive areas and more specificities, but their multiplication in chronic diseases accompanied by polyvalent hyperergia suggests so.

Antigen-antibody complexes

When antigens and antibodies meet in a solution with equal or similar complementary reactive areas, a specific complex will arise. This antigen-antibody complex is the basis of the definitions and of the customary serological and immunological methods. The antigen-antibody compound takes place at an incredible speed. Tests by SINGER using a simple haptene and a purified

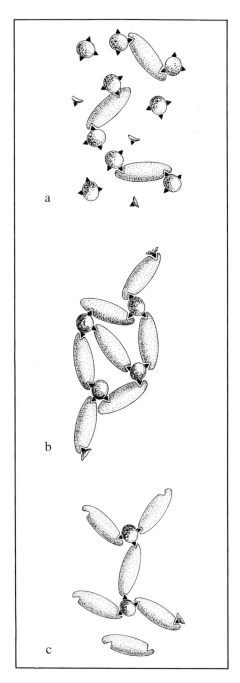

rabbit antibody showed a reaction at a speed of K = 1 × 10⁸ M⁻¹ sec. This bimolecular reaction is one of the most rapid known in biochemistry (CAMPBELL). Even the chain reaction, which provokes lesions of cells, occurs like an explosion if cellular antibodies are involved (fig. 156, 157).

The antigen-antibody complex depends on profile qualities of the reacting components (number and kind of the determinant groups and specificities) and environmental factors (temperature, solubility, electrolytic conditions). The secondary processes following the molecular compounds –on the molecules or cells, tissues and proteins– such as lysis, agglutination, precipitation, depend also on environmental conditions. Of decisive importance, however, is the quantitative proportion between antigen and antibodies (reacting components) from which the following possibilities result (CAMPBELL, SINGER, CUSHING and CAMPBELL):

1. Antigen is abundant, not all antigen-reactive areas are bound. The situation is similar for haptene or abundance of antigen-haptene (fig. 202a).
2. The quantities of antigen and antibodies are equivalent and form a saturated complex (fig. 202b).
3. The antibodies are abundant; all antigens and haptenes are bound, excessive antibodies still free (fig. 202c).

In precipitational reactions of dissolved antigens and antibodies in vitro, these quantitative reactivities appear in 3 zones (CAMPBELL). The antibodies have 2 reactive areas so that usually 1 antibody molecule binds 2 antigen molecules. This proportion $Ag_2 : Ak$ is a biologically inactive complex. Also in molecular groups, the number of the antibody molecules is smaller than the antigenic molecules ($Ag_x > AK_y$). The com-

Fig. 202:
Quantitative proportions of antigen/antibody.
a: Surplus of antigens.
b: Ideal, well poised proportion.
c: Surplus of antibodies.

plex is dissociable at pH 3.5. Even a proportion of $Ag_3 : AK_2$ is biologically active and binds complement (ISHIZAKA). Changes of the optical rotation (increased levorotation) suggest structural changes (stretching? plastic deformation?) of the antibody molecule, by which probably the toxic biological effects are caused.

The conditions are more complicated in vivo. Considerable quantities of soluble antigen (e. g. bovine S^{35}-labelled serum-albumin in rabbits) were found in the liver at least one year after the injection (GARVEY and CAMPBELL). The antigen persists as a small polypeptide fragment about the size of an «antigenic determinant». These fragments of the original antigen molecule are bound to soluble ribonucleic acid (Ag + s-RNA) and probably play a decisive part for the further production of antibodies, more so because they carry some protein. Whereas the polypeptide fragments alone (= antigenic determinants) do not provoke a formation of antibodies, antigen fragments + RNA compound are highly immunogenic.

The effects of the antigen-antibody complex on cells and tissues (= biological activity) are the strongest if the antigens abound. Details of the mechanism are not known, it is supposed that serum reactions likely to activate enzymes and to form pharmacologically active substance take place (DIXON). This explanation remains unsatisfactory as injuries can be caused also to washed plasma cells containing antibodies (F. SCHMID, 1953). The site, size and duration of the antigen-antibody relations are of importance for the clinical effects; especially plasma cells, serous membranes, unstriated muscles and endothelia are sensitive.

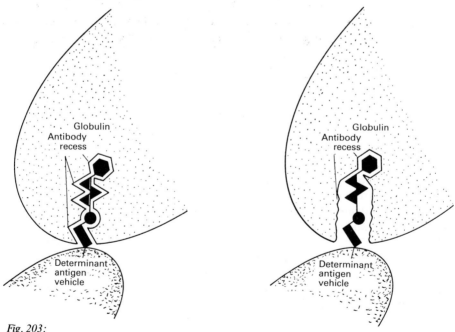

Fig. 203:
Plastic transformation of a complex determinant by the antibody (a); «enlargement»of the specificity. As the relief of the recess flattens, the antibody remains specific only for the terminal sugar molecule but can now respond also to all other antigens possessing such a terminal sugar ring.

crease of the immunoresistance is, symptomatologically, unimportant but constitutes a partial symptom of the whole illness.

Transitory immunodeficiencies

Nutritive influences

The synthesis of immunoglobulins requires a hardly surveyable number of cellular metabolites, which partly go into the balance and become structural elements, in their majority have a temporary, but essential, importance as catalysts. Among them are nucleic acids (RNA), magnesium, calcium, iron, zinc and phosphorus compounds. Lack of these substances necessary for the formation of antibodies prevents a sufficient synthesis. A deficit, therefore, may result if the supply is insufficient, the absorption does not suffice, the intracellu-

lar metabolism is disturbed and excessive quantities of metabolites are lost. Tab. 16 gives a survey of the clinical forms.

Infectious influences

The immunoresistance, which depends on the age and individual properties, can be overstrained by casual infection or artificial infectional strain (inoculations). The result of such a coincidence of illnesses is transitory immunodebilities as incidental occurrences. Three basic constellations must be distinguished:
1. Intact systems of defense are overcharged by the coincidence of infections and become insufficient. The coincidence of a chronic disease (tuberculosis) with an acute infectious disease (e.g. measles, influenza, chickenpox) is the clinically most

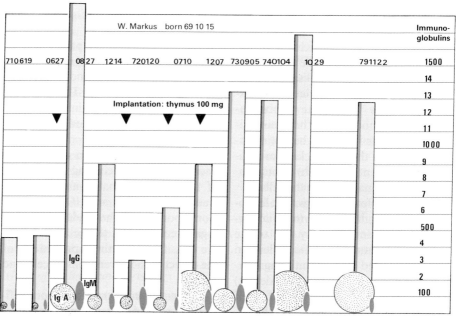

Fig. 205:
Syndrome of innate antibody-deficiency; development of the immunoglobulins after implantation of xenogenous, fetal, immunocompetent tissues. The antibody-deficiency is repaired by 3 series of implantations for many years. A subsequent control (800318) showed high values: IgG 2000, IgA 250, IgM 194.

170

conspicuous example. The resistance to infection by the chronic disease (e.g. miliary tuberculosis) may collapse.

2. A temporarily not fully efficient defence system against infection is exhausted even by «trivial» infections. Lack of protein, malnutrition, avitaminosis, accumulated infections, diseases of the haematopoietic system and extended neoplasms may cause such depressions of the immunological potency.

3. Vaccinations meet with an organism already overloaded by infections (see 1) or not fully efficient owing to other causes (see 2). This may lead to «inoculating complications» in the form of

   a) insufficient formation of immunoglobulins against the inoculated antigen,
   b) provocation of acute infections,
   c) exacerbation of a chronic or latent basic disease (e. g. tuberculosis)
   d) an abnormal sequence of inocula-

tions increased to an «vaccination disease».

Immunodepressions by chemical substances

External influences on the cells of immunocompetent tissues can diminish or even abolish the capability of synthetising immunoglobulins. As the formation of antibodies on the basis of RNA takes place in the immunocytes, an immunodepression is effected by processes that

a) change the biochemical qualities of the cell, specially to RNA metabolism,
b) inhibit the mesenchymal proliferation of the cell,
c) bring about a non-physiologically enhanced cytolysis.

Corresponding noxae are provoked by many chemical substances, drugs and physical influences (radiation).

Immunoinhibitory effects of chemical substances have been detected first in alkalizing substances (benzene, toluene, 1916; dichlorethylsulphide, 1916). The

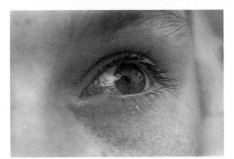

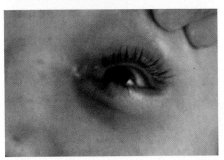

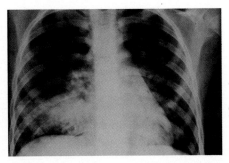

Fig. 206:
Ataxia teleangiektatica (Louis-Bar syndrome) as a typical example of a mesenchymal-epithelial insufficiency: IgA deficiency, dysfunction of thymus, infections of the respiratory passages, cerebellar ataxia; here a) typical dilation of the conjunctival vessels; b) chronic herpes of the lower eyelid; c) bronchiectasis.

formation of antibodies was suppressed by these substances if they were administered together with the antigen or 4 days earlier. On this principle depend now several groups of substances with immunoinhibitory effects (tab. 17).

Most of the antibiotics (the wider the spectrum of therapeutic effect the more distinct) influence strongly not only the bacterial but also the nucleic acid metabolism of cells; this property is a prerequisite for the effect on microorganisms that also consist of nucleic acids but applies just as well to the cells with a high synthesising activity such as the immunocytes. For the duration and dosage of antiphlogistic drugs, antirheumatics, cortisone derivatives, phenothiazines, antihistamin products, certain sedatives and antiepileptics, this immunoinhibitory effect on the formation of antibodies ought to be taken into account same as for the dosage and duration of broad-spectrum antibiotics.

Tab. 17: **Immunodepressory chemical substances**

1. **Alkylising substances** (e.g. *trenimon, endoxan, honvan, myleran*) 2. **Antimetabolites** a) folic-acid antagonists (aminopterin; *methotrexate*) b) purin antagonists (6-mercaptopurin; *purinethol*, and others) c) pyrimidin antagonists (5-fluoruracil)	3. **Mitotic poisons and blockers of mitosis** (colchicine, vincaleukoblastin, podophyllotoxin) 4. **Antibiotics** (actinomycin C and D; mytomycin C) 5. **Antiphlogistic medicaments** (antirheumatics, cortison derivatives, antihistamines)

Artificial immunosuppression

For excessive immunizing reactions, the therapy uses increasingly the so-called immunosuppression; the same principle is applied in cases of unwelcome immunizing reactions. In such cases, specially the above chemical substances and physical insulti (rays) are used.

Immunological effects of irradiation

The effects of ionizing irradiation on immunobiological processes depend not only on the dose but also on the volume of influence (irradiation of part of the body or whole-body irradiation). Whole-body irradiation influences the production of antibodies according to the dose and stage. Doses up to 400 r are sublethal, those between 400 and 900 r are lethal, and those over 1000 r supralethal.

Lethal and supralethal doses of irradiation provoke immunoparalysis, whose clinical effects constitute the panmyelophthisic syndrome (collapse of the lympho-reticular zone of defense) or the gastrointestinal radiation syndrome (collapse of the epithelial protective surfaces) (tab. 18).

Tab. 18: **Radiation syndromes**

1. **Syndrome of panmyelophthisis** (bone-marrow syndrome); by eliminating universally the areas of haematpoesis, a «haematological death by radiation» is caused.	2. **The gastrointestinal syndrome** caused by destruction of the epithelial protective surface of the gastrointestinal tract. 3. **The neurological radiation syndrome**

plex is dissociable at pH 3.5. Even a proportion of $Ag_3 : AK_2$ is biologically active and binds complement (ISHIZAKA). Changes of the optical rotation (increased levorotation) suggest structural changes (stretching? plastic deformation?) of the antibody molecule, by which probably the toxic biological effects are caused.

The conditions are more complicated in vivo. Considerable quantities of soluble antigen (e. g. bovine S^{35}-labelled serum-albumin in rabbits) were found in the liver at least one year after the injection (GARVEY and CAMPBELL). The antigen persists as a small polypeptide fragment about the size of an «antigenic determinant». These fragments of the original antigen molecule are bound to soluble ribonucleic acid (Ag + s-RNA) and probably play a decisive part for the further production of antibodies, more so because they carry some protein. Where-as the polypeptide fragments alone (= antigenic determinants) do not provoke a formation of antibodies, antigen fragments + RNA compound are highly immunogenic.

The effects of the antigen-antibody complex on cells and tissues (= biological activity) are the strongest if the antigens abound. Details of the mechanism are not known, it is supposed that serum reactions likely to activate enzymes and to form pharmacologically active substance take place (DIXON). This explanation remains unsatisfactory as injuries can be caused also to washed plasma cells containing antibodies (F. SCHMID, 1953). The site, size and duration of the antigen-antibody relations are of importance for the clinical effects; especially plasma cells, serous membranes, unstriated muscles and endothelia are sensitive.

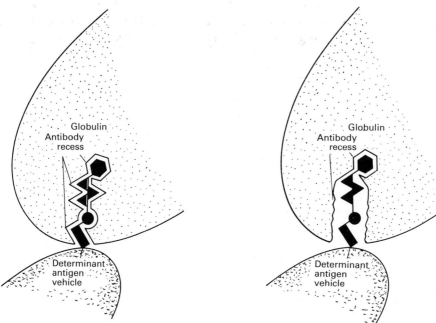

Fig. 203:
Plastic transformation of a complex determinant by the antibody (a); «enlargement» of the specificity. As the relief of the recess flattens, the antibody remains specific only for the terminal sugar molecule but can now respond also to all other antigens possessing such a terminal sugar ring.

163

The complement system

Besides the cellular synthetic system and the humoral transportation and distributing mechanisms, the complement system forms the third characteristic chain of reactions of the immune system; cellular and humoral factors concur in a cascade-like chain reaction. As part of the antigen-antibody interrelations, the complementary system has a complex relay function. As the components are known, the former definition as «cytotoxic activity» of the serum has turned out to be a partial aspect, but there are more effects and secondary processes. Besides the cytotoxicity with subsequent immunocytolysis, the complement has the capacity of dissolving bacterial walls. Intermediary products and split fractions perform during the chain reaction essential immunobiological functions such as phagocytosis, immune adherence, chemotaxis, formation of anaphylatoxin.

Complement is a colloidal, heat-labile complex of euglobulin, carbohydrates and phospholipids. It belongs to the components of the «natural resistance», of the non-specific constitutional power of defense, and cannot be increased by immunisation processes. Complement cannot only unite with any antigen-antibody system but can just as well become antigenic itself. Complement occurs in fresh serum and plasma, and can be inactivated by many chemical agents at 51° in 35 minutes, at 55° in 12 minutes, at 61° in 3 minutes.

The reaction phases referred to as complement factors C_1–C_9 (fig. 204) of substrates and enzymes contain not less than 20 serum proteins. The most important is C_3, which is activated in the classical way (fig. 204) via C_1, C_2, C_4 but can just as well act through a short circuit. C_3 decomposes into the active component C_{3a} and the component of continued activation C_{3b}. The latter has multidimensional effects: it promotes the integration of C_5–C_9 into the complex of cytolytic effects, but also activates the formation of serum proactivators and can split into the fragments C_{3e} and C_{3d}, which are said to have the function of inactivators in the complement regulation. The enzyme activities C_5–C_9 can, in this completion, break defects of substance into the cellular and bacterial membranes and thus enable the cellular contents to extravasate into the extracellular fluid spaces.

The main function of the complement is «to break holes into the membranes» i. e. membranes foreign to the body (bacteria) or endogenic, antibodies carrying cell membranes. With the cell membrane lost, the bacterium (or the cell) is deprived of the protective wall of its own integrity and falls a victim to the enzymatic activity of lysosomatic enzymes. This positive effect is completed by the negative action i. e. the release of enzymatic and vasoactive cellular contents (mediators) (fig. 194). The complementary factors are macromolecules of the gammaglobulin fraction, which are formed in the liver and in macrophages.

The components may be characterized as follows:

C_1 is an esterase-active macromolecule with a molecular weight of 900,000 – 1 million and a sedimentation constant of 18–19 S. The influence of sodium ethylene diamin acetic acid (Na₃ HEDTA) or oxalate or citrate makes it break down into the fragments C_{1q}, C_{1r} and C_{1s} (LEPOW et al., 1963). This splitting is effected by uniting with calcium (Ca^{++}); the 3 fragments can be recombined only by the intervention of calcium. C_1 unites with an antibody molecule of the cellular surface.

Activated C_1 has the function of an activated esterase, which starts up the components C_4 and C_2. The acting factor is the fragment C_{1s}, the substratum is C_4. With the essential participation of magnesium (Mg^{++}), C_2 is formed. C_2 disintegrates rapidly and initiates the complement-fixation reaction to C_9. $C_2–C_4$ set a complex enzyme of C_3 convertase, which cata-

lyses the adsorption of C_3 to the cell membrane.

The C_3 component consists of at least 4 fragments: C_{3b}, C_{3c}, C_{3e}, C_{3f}. C_3, C_5, C_6 and C_7 form a thermostable intermediary product, the membranolytic effect comes on only with the completion by the factors C_8 and C_9. The terms $EAC_{1a,4,2a,3}$, which are used frequently, mean complement erythrocyte complex (E = erythrocytes of sheep; A = antibody; C = activated complementary factors), whose reaction product is $EAC_{1a,4,2a,3,5,6,7}$.

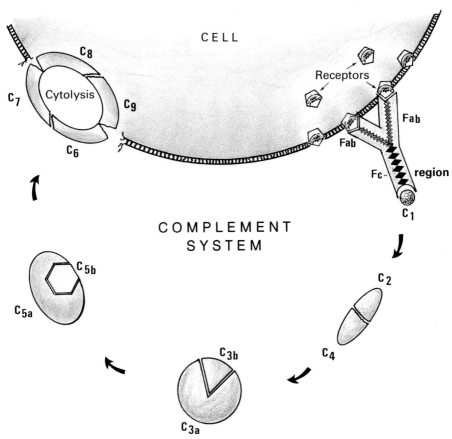

Fig. 204:
Complement system (for particulars see text)

Immun-deficiencies

Immunobiological mechanisms serve for the preservation of the biological character and integrity, and therefore are obligatory properties of independent life. Rudiments of a cellular immunity occur in the human fetus after the 10th week of pregnancy, humoral antibodies about the 20th week of pregnancy, immunological maturity is reached about birth till 9 days thereafter. Physiologically, the fetus (which consists of maternal and paternal tissular structures and is regarded as a foreign implant according to immunological cliché interpretations and ought to be discharged) is tolerated and even gets a privileged treatment from the host, the mother. The end of the immunotolerance in the embryonal and fetal time is the immunobiological ripening of the fetus, which is likely to initiate birth i. e., physically, the discharge of an implant.

Although immunocompetence (the capability of producing or transporting immune bodies) is an autochthonous property of the cells, immunology has worked for long epochs chiefly at secondary and tertiary mechanisms (humoral reactions of antibodies and complement, precipitation, agglutination, cytolysis).

The production of the immunoglobulins is a function of the endoplasmatic reticulum of immunocompetent cells; like in other products of synthesis, the production of proteins is readjusted in the ribosomes specifically to an antigenic stimulation so that antibodies ready to function are available within 7–12 days. Whereas ribosomes, mitochondria, Golgi-apparatus and cytoplasm take part in the production, the functional preparation is completed through the membrane of cytoplasm.

The properties of the human blood-groups (A, B) are coupled to the membrane of the erythrocytes; here, foreign blood-groups are discerned, antigen-antibody reactions take place, as agglutination or as haemo- (better: erythrocyto-) lysis.

Other antigens are discerned and answered by the mononuclear cells (usually referred to simply as lymphocytes). Best known and characterized is the so-called HLA (human lymphocyte antigen) system. The most important of these more than 60 antigens known so far (D. NIETHAMMER, 1979) is the major histocompatibility complex (MHC system), which is coded on 4 genes of the chromosome 6. Even if there were not more than 60 antigens, the prospects of finding a donor of identical tissue would be extremely low. The compatibility is more likely in brothers and sisters with usually 4 different combination factors, best in twins.

These then are the limits of the tissue and organ transplantations, though however without an important additional factor, which is often forgotten. Even well corresponding tissular properties become antagonistic when organs are transplanted as the living conditions of the transplant till the integration into the organism of the recipient are unfavourable. The initial problems of transportation (blood circulation, evacuation of the metabolites through the lymph ducts) cause secondary changes of the tissular properties, which imply considerable additional antigenicity. The negative experience made in grafting surgery is surely due to these circumstances rather than to the original antigenicity. The suppression of the immune response from the recipient, immunosuppression, is a necessary though not the best conclusion from this situation.

166

Forms of the cell implantations

The clinical application of cell implantations in innate immunodefects has kept abreast of the development of the oretical knowledge. According to a survey by D. NIETHAMMER, 1979, implantations in 69 children with serious combined immunodefects had been conducted by that time. Table 13 contains a summary of the tissues used, complications and rate of survivals.

It appears that so far mostly HLA genotypically identical bone-marrow, HLA phenotypically identical bone-marrow, HLA-D-identical and non-identical bone-marrow, fetal tissue of the liver, of the thymus or of both were used. As far as can be judged from results obtained and from the discharging reaction, the compatibility of fetal tissues, which need not be identical, is not more unfavourable than in genotypically identical bone-marrow, and more favourable than in phenotypically identical bone-marrow and non-identical bone-marrow.

As the possibility of obtaining genotypically identical tissues from brothers and sisters, other members of the family or twins is rather restricted, the problem can be solved by means of fetal tissues from the liver and thymus. Recent experience has shown that the fetal tissues are tolerated the better the earlier the stages of fetal growth from which they originate.

Immunobiological life-profile

The physiological development of the immunocompetence in man is characterized by lacking or insufficient immunity before birth, by a maturing period of immunological defense during childhood

Tab. 13: **Cellular implantations in severe combined immunity defects** (after NIETHAMMER, 1979)

Group/transplant	Transpl.	Graf-versus-host-reaction[a]				Survival after 6 months
		Survival < 6 months		Survival > 6 months		
	Transpl.	0−+	++−+++	0−+	++−+++	
I HLA-genotypically identical bone-marrow (brothers and sisters, other relatives in inbreeding) 16 18		1	3	8	2	10/16 = 63%
II HLA-phenotypically identical bone-marrow 4 4		2	4	3	2	5/13 = 38%
III HLA-D-identical bone-marrow with incompatibility of the HLA-A and/or HLA-B-locus 9 23						
IV HLA-D-non-identical bone-marrow with/without incompatibility of HLA-A and/or HLA-B-locus 19 27		3	7	1	0	1/19 = 5%[b]
V Fetal organs 21 30		3	2	7	2	9/21 = 43%[c]
Fetal liver 8 14						
Fetal thymus 11 14						
both 2 2						
Total	69 102	−	−	−	−	25/69 = 36%

167

Type	Supposed location of the cellular defect in		
	stem cells	B-cells	T-cells
Severe combined insufficient immunity			
a) autosomal-recessive	+	+	+
b) x-bound	+	+	+
c) sporadic	+	+	+
Insufficient immunity with generalised hematopoietic hypoplasia	+	+	+
Insufficient immunity with short-membered nanism	+	+	+
Insufficient immunity with thrombocytopenia and eczema (Wiskott-Aldrich-syndrome)		+	+
Insufficient immunity with Ataxia teleangiectatica		+	+
Insufficient immunity in thymoma		+	+
Insufficient immunity with normo- or hyperimmunoglobulinaemia		(+)	(+)(−)
Infantile X-bound agammaglobulinaemia		+	
Selective lack of immunoglobulin (IgA)		+(−)	
X-bound insufficient immunity with hyper-IgM		+/−	
Transitory hypogammaglobulinaemia in babies		+	
Thymus hypoplasia (Di George-syndrome)			+
Episodical lymphopenia with lymphocytotoxin			+

up to a biological culmination in the 9th–12th years, by a slowly declining plateau in adults and a growing decrease in higher periods of life. This profile includes:

1. the immunotolerance in the embryo and fetus;
2. the insufficient immunity in the baby, which is compensated towards the end of the second year;
3. the immunological ripening and period of maturity;
4. the increasing senility beyond the 40th and 50th years of life;
5. the senile immunoparalysis at the end of biological existence.

Division of the immunodeficiencies

Only innate defects of the immunosystem are often denoted as immunodeficiencies. The acquired immunodebilities, however, are certainly not only more frequent but, practically, more important. To meet the plurality, the immunodeficiencies must be divided into the following groups:

Immunodeficiencies

1. physiological immunodeficiencies
2. innate immunodeficiencies
   a) primary
   b) secondary
3. transitory immunodeficiencies caused by
   a) nutritive influences
   b) infectious diseases
   c) chemical substances
   d) physical noxae (radiation).

A special group must be mentioned:

4. artificial immunodegradation (immunosuppression)

Innate immunodeficiencies

Innate immunodebilities can result from a universal insufficiency of the mesenchymal defense mechanism or selectively influence various components of the same.

Tab. 15: **Organismic mesenchymal weakness and decrease of immunity**

1. Immaturity of the mesenchyme (immature new-born, premature children)	3. Decrease of the volume of immunocompetent tissues (osteosclerosis, marble-bones, storage-reticulosis, systemic malignoma of the bone-marrow)
2. General mesenchymal hypoplasia (general weakness of the connective tissue, Osteogenesis imperfecta, Down-syndrome)	4. Runt's disease

Tab. 16: **Defective material for the formation of antibodies**

1. Insufficient supplies
Qualitative false nutrition or quantitative insufficient nutrition; dystrophy, atrophy, kwashiorkor, nutritional faults by overfeeding infants with carbohydrates, lack of vitamins

2. Defective absorption
a) by lack or absence of ferments (mucoviscidosis)
b) by inflammatory (enteritis, enterocolitis) or allergic (Coeliakia, intestinal allergy) alteration of the intestinal epithelium
c) by mechanic lesions of the intestinal wall

in abnormalities (stenosis, atresia, megacolon)

3. Disturbed intracellular metabolisation
in enzymopathies and storage disorders, hypothyreosis, Diabetes mellitus

4. Increased loss
a) enteral syndrome of protein loss
b) loss of renal proteins (nephrosis)
c) loss of vascular proteins (extensive bleedings, subdural haematoma, transudates, Shwartzmann-Sanarelli syndrome, Waterhouse Friderichsen syndrome, haemolytico-uremic syndrome)

Selective innate insufficiency of the resistance to infection is due to an insufficient production or mobilisation of immunoglobulins. The stimulation of antigens provokes inadequate concentrations of antibodies in the immunocompetent cells or in the humoral system: either (a) through lacking or deficient cellular synthesis, or (b) through insufficient elimination from the cells.

Clinically, blood findings with leukopenia, anemia, thrombocytopenia suggest a general insufficiency also of the immunoapparatus, the deficiencies can be demonstrated by substantiating a deficit of humoral antibodies (IgG deficit) whereas the serum concentrations of IgM and IgA reflect only indirect the cellular deficiency.

The defense against infection (especially against extracellular microbes) is reduced, the surfaces exposed to the environment (respiratory passages, gastrointestinal tract, skin, urinary passages) tend to recurrent and, partly, serious and fatal infections. The degree of the lowered resistance to infection is decisive for the prognosis and thus for life expectancy.

The aspects shown in tab. 14 have been established according to a division of the primary innate immunoinsufficiency prepared by a WHO-committee. Corresponding to the modern immunological conception, the cellular defects are classified after the supposed site of the defect in the parent cells, B-cells and T-cells.

These primary innate immunoinsufficiencies should be regarded in contrast to the secondary immunoinsufficiencies. These forms summarized in tab. 15 are systemic dysfunctions of the vascular-connective tissue apparatus, and the decrease of the immunoresistance is, symptomatologically, unimportant but constitutes a partial symptom of the whole illness.

lar metabolism is disturbed and excessive quantities of metabolites are lost. Tab. 16 gives a survey of the clinical forms.

Transitory immunodeficiencies

Nutritive influences

The synthesis of immunoglobulins requires a hardly surveyable number of cellular metabolites, which partly go into the balance and become structural elements, in their majority have a temporary, but essential, importance as catalysts. Among them are nucleic acids (RNA), magnesium, calcium, iron, zinc and phosphorus compounds. Lack of these substances necessary for the formation of antibodies prevents a sufficient synthesis. A deficit, therefore, may result if the supply is insufficient, the absorption does not suffice, the intracellu-

Infectious influences

The immunoresistance, which depends on the age and individual properties, can be overstrained by casual infection or artificial infectional strain (inoculations). The result of such a coincidence of illnesses is transitory immunodebilities as incidental occurrences. Three basic constellations must be distinguished:
1. Intact systems of defense are overcharged by the coincidence of infections and become insufficient. The coincidence of a chronic disease (tuberculosis) with an acute infectious disease (e.g. measles, influenza, chickenpox) is the clinically most

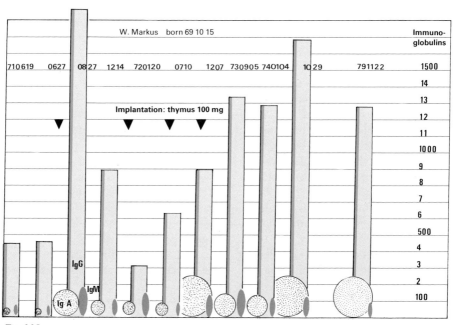

Fig. 205:
Syndrome of innate antibody-deficiency; development of the immunoglobulins after implantation of xenogenous, fetal, immunocompetent tissues. The antibody-deficiency is repaired by 3 series of implantations for many years. A subsequent control (800318) showed high values: IgG 2000, IgA 250, IgM 194.

170

For the sublethal radiation area in the whole-body irradiation and irradiation of part of the body (including most of the diagnostic and natural irradiation insulti) the moment when the rays meet with a formation of antibodies is of importance. Whereas the initial phase of forming the antibody is very radio-sensitive, irradiation during the first days after supply of antigens can even enhance the production of antibodies. The strongest stimulation sets in 60 hours after the administration of antigens.

In animals that got whole-body irradiation by doses of 200 r, the dropping of granulocytes in the peritoneal exudate attained the low mark after 36 days, at 400 r after 30 days, at 800 r already within the first week. The normal cell population in surviving animals reappears after 3 months (90–120 days).

Clinical data on immunizing reactions

Clinically, 4 forms of immunizing reactions are distinguished after the modern classification:

1st type	I	reaction:	immediate anaphylactic reaction of the reagin type
2nd type	II	reaction:	hypersensitiveness of the cytotoxic type
3rd type	III	reaction:	immediate reaction of the Arthus type
4th type	IV	reaction:	cellular immunizing reactions of the «retarded type».

The immediate anaphylactoid reaction

Through the intervention of IgE, a few minutes after the contact with antigens circumscribed vasculo-capillary reactions in the form of erythema, urticaria (wheals) or rush will be seen. The reaction reaches a maximum after 20–30 minutes and will subside after 1–2 hours without leaving any injured tissue. With the help of the IgE molecules, the antigens bridge the barriers of cell membranes and release contents of mast-cells over the complement bridge (fig. 204). The released «mediator» or «liberator» substances histamin, serotonin, bradykinin and SRS-A (slow-reacting-substance-anaphylaxis) dilate vessels, increase the permeability of the capillaries and contract the unstriated muscles.

Clinical sequelae of these morphological elementary processes are (tab. 19):

Hypersensitivity of the cytotoxic type

Antigen-carrying cell membranes combine with the corresponding antibodies through their Fc-part or by the mediation of complement, either from complexes or provoke cytolysis by rupture of membranes. A prototype of this form of reaction is erythrocytolysis in Rhesus-incompatibility and other hemolytic diseases. Drugs ments such as chloropromacine and phenacetine may cause in this way haemolytic anaemia, pyramidon and quinine lead to leukopenia, sedormid to thrombocytopenia (H. SCHNEIDER). Rapidly supplied antilymphocyte globulin may provoke equal reactions, and still more phenomena of autoimmunization can certainly be associated with this type of reaction.

Immediate reaction of the Arthus type

The structures of antibodies acquired after contact and circulating in the serum are changed by repeated contact with antigens; thus substances leading to «serum disease» are relased at the Fc-end of

173

Tab. 19: **Clinical symptoms and therapy of anaphylactoid reactions.**

Localisation	Symptoms	Therapy
Skin Mucosa	Local erythema Flush-rush Urticaria Oedema Cyanosis Salivation Sweating «Goose-flesh»	1. Dose corresponding to age *Suprarenin* or noradrenalin Aludrin Alupent Norphen subcutaneous or as inhalation for
Heart Circulation	Tachycardia Fall of blood-pressure Precapillary constriction of the arterial vessels Tissular hypoxia Tissular acidosis Circulatory arrest Respiratory-arrest	symptoms of respiratory passages 2. Dose corresponding to age of an *antihistamin preparation* *3. Glucocorticoids* oral, intramuscular or intravenous
Respiratory passages	Stridor Throat irritation with mucous discharge Spasm of the bronchi Dyspnoea	1–2 mg/kg of body-weight works after lapse of 20–30 minutes! 4. *Calcium*
Digestive tract	Vomiting Rectal tenesmus Intestinal colic Diarrhea	5. Substitutions of volume and catecholamines Strophantin for volume shock
Subjective disorders	Nausea Sickly feeling Headache- and back-pain Paleness Anxiety or heat-feeling	6. For seizures: phenobarbital chloralhydrate 7. For clotting disorders: heparin 150–200 U/kg of body-weight, in case substitution of clotting factors

the antibody molecules. This clinical picture has become known chiefly through the use of antidiphtheritic serum in recent decades. After injection of heterologous antidiphtheritic serum (from horses or other animals), antibodies are produced. Between the 6th–12th days after the injection, the serum disease will appear under the following aspect: erythema to urticaria to generalized oedema; fever, nausea, vomiting; generalized lymphonodulitis; arthritis, nephritis, myocarditis.

The morphological basis is an immu-

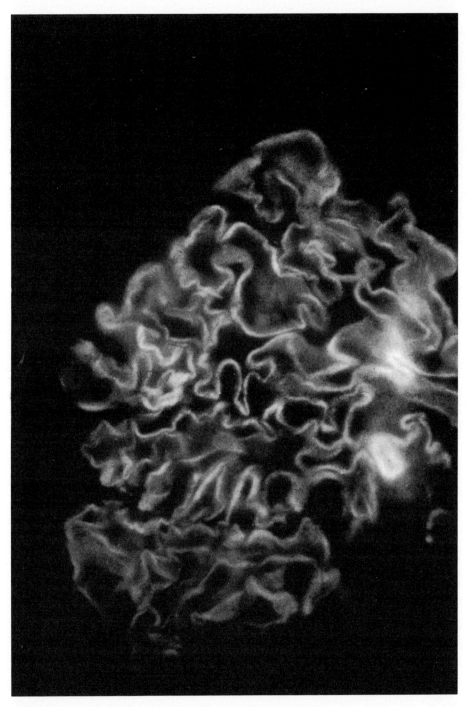

Fig. 207:
Sedimentation of immunocomplexes in the capillary loops of a renal glomerulus for Goodpasture syndrome. Immunofluorescence (SCHNEIDER H., BRUNNER P. and MEINL M.).

no-complex vasculitis, which, in contrast to the anaphylactoid reaction (type I), can cause and maintain lasting injuries to tissues. The intravasal antigen-antibody complexes clot and damage cellular constituents. Specially, aggregations of thrombocytes release substances damaging the vascular walls. Soluble immunocomplexes get into the elastica interna of the vascular walls or the basal membrane of the renal glomeruli (fig. 207). Here concentrated immunocomplexes bind complement, and the released anaphylatoxin C_{3a} may in addition affect the permeability and favour the formation of edema and vasodilation. This vicious circle is worsened by immigrating granulocytes with polymorphous nuclei, the lysosomal contents of which affect the vascular walls as their pH is low.

The inflammatory reaction subsides only after the elimination of the immunocomplexes. As the numbers of antigens grows steadily, the lack of antibodies will cause chronic diseases. Examples are «chronic glomerulonephritis» after infections with beta-hemolytic streptococci of group A and the extended alterations of tissue in Lupus erythematodes disseminatus.

Reaction of the retarded type

After preliminary sensitisation, certain antigens and haptenes elicit a retarded inflammatory reaction of the so-called «tuberculin type». In this phenomenon, described by R. KOCH and

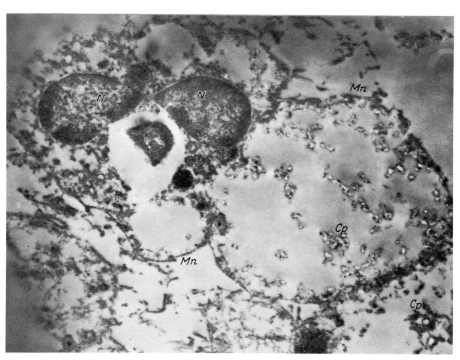

Fig. 208:
Explosive disintegration of a cell of peritoneal exudate (guinea-pig); shock elicited $88\frac{1}{2}$ hours after sensitisation. Fragmentation of the cytoplasm starting from the perinuclear space. N = nucleus, Cp = particle of cytoplasm, Mn = membrane.

176

Tab. 20: **Autoantibodies in human diseases** (after WARNATZ, 1979)

Disease	Antibodies against	% positive
Immunothryreoiditis (HASHIMOTO)	Thyreoglobulin	up to 90
	Microsomal thyroid antigen	100
	Border-cells	32
Primary thyreotoxicosis (long-acting thyroid stimulator [LATS])	TSH receptor of the thyroid cell	20–40
Pernicious anaemia with chronic atrophic gastritis	Intrinsic factor	70
	Border-cells	83
Idiopathic Addison's disease	Cytoplasmatic Ag of the NNR cells	50–70
Male infertility	Spermatozoa	rare
Myasthenia gravis	Skeleton-muscles	30–65
	Thymus myoid cells	–
	Acetylcholine receptor	–
Pemphigus vulgaris	Desmosomes of the prickle-cells	up to 100
Phacogenous uveitis	Lentil protein	–
Goodpasture syndrome	Basal membrane of the glomerulum capillaries	100
Immunohaemolytic anaemia	Erythrocyte antigens (mostly Rh-antigens)	100
Cold-agglutinin disease	Erythrocyte antigen (l-antigen)	100
Paroxysmal cold-haemoglobinuria	Erythrocyte antigen (P-antigen)	100
Active chronic hepatitis	Nucleoprotein	20
	Mitochondrial antigens	25
	Involuntary muscles	70
Primary biliary cirrhosis	Mitochondrial Ag	90
Colitis ulcerosa	Mucopolysaccharide of the colon cells	50–100
Lupus erythematodes disseminatus acutus (SLE)	Nucleoproteins	100
	DNA	100
	IgG (rheuma factor)	35
	Erythrocyte antigens	15–20
Mixed connective-tissue disease	Extractable nuclear antigen (enA)	100
Primary chronic polyarthritis =	IgG (rheuma factor)	75
rheumatoid polyarthritis	Nucleoprotein	10
Sjögren's syndrome	IgG	75
	Nucleoprotein	55
	Thyroid gland	45
	Epithelia of the salivary glands	–

C. v. PIRQUET, an immunological cytolysis is at the beginning of the chain of reaction.

Cellular immunoglobulins M respond, after another supply of antigens, with a cellular antigen-antibody reaction, which entails the instantaneous explosion-like destruction of the cell (see fig. 156, 157, 208). In the tuberculin reaction, best explained of all, a haptene i. e. the tuberculin (tuberculoprotein fraction) evokes this reaction. According to quantitative relations, vasculitis, which via the fibrinoid conversion may even lead to necrosis, will develop. Vasculitis is characterized after 24–72 hours by a reddening and infiltration of mononuclear cells (lymphocytes, monocytes, epitheloid cells) round the damaged vessels. This process causes necrobiosis and the caseation in tuberculosis and other chronic diseases as mycosis, leprosy, brucellosis, psittacosis and infection of echinococci. The contact dermatitis and the contact eczema rely on a similar mechanism.

Common denominator

Plausible though this division into 4 types of reaction may appear, it leaves many questions unanswered, many discrepancies remain dark. The common denominator of most of the reactions is the release of cellular contents by antigen-antibody relations. Intracellular substrates and enzymes, which have to perform metabolic special tasks in ecological areas surrounded by membranes (such as enzymes in lysosomes, transport substrates in vesicles) are suddenly released and cause destruction of the reactive, broad surfaces of contact of the terminal vessels. The pH necessary for the biochemical functions within the spaces delimited by membranes are probably of decisive importance because, suddenly set free into the fluid-stream, they can exert destruction by acid-alkaline corrosion.

Different and specific though the causes of immune processes may be, the reactivities of the organism are quantitatively different, qualitatively virtually equal. They run form the reactive chain of biochemical lesions of the small vessels – vasodilation – increased permeability – extravasation of fluids and cells from the vessels into the surrounding tissue. From this uniform primary process, the aspect of inflammation, various clinical pictures develop by secondary processes, according to localization and quantitative conditions.

Prophylaxis and therapy

Owing to the non-specific, after all, response of the body to specifically induced processes, prophylaxis and therapy use for all forms of allergic reactions the same therapeutic principles: (1) Withdrawal of antigens (2) Blocking of antibodies (3) Inhibition of the inflammatory reaction.

The essential data of practical use are stated in tab. 19 and 21.

Tab. 21: **Prophylaxis of anaphylactoid reactions especially by repeated administrations of heterologous foreign tissues or sera**

1. 5 – 15 min. before injection:
   single dose, corresponding to age, of
   a) a glucocorticoid preparation
      (0,5 – 1 mg/kg of bodyweight prednisolon)
   b) *an antihistamin product*
      best of all a combined preparation
      (e.g. a measuring spoon or 1 tabl. of celestamines)
2. Immediately after injection (implantation):
   a single dose (corresponding to age) of a catecholamin by drops (*Novadral, Norphen, Effortil,* Artenerol, or similar prep.)

CLINIC AND PRACTICE

Cellular defects as guiding principle of the therapy

Diagnosis and therapy in medicine have been and are reflexions of the momentary state of knowledge. The diagnosis, in fact, keeps better up with the theoretical knowledge than the therapy, which must usually, with difficulty and often over generations, fight for the practical consequences of really progressive knowledge.

The historic metamorphosis of occidental medicine ranges from the supernatural abilities (loans) of Cheiron and Asklepios to the molecular-biological details of our days – or from the God-priest medicine of the inconceivable in antiquity to the biology of atoms and molecules in the area of the no longer visible and no longer imaginable dimensions. Medical diagnosis approaches this field reluctantly, and the principles of therapy are still based upon the dimensions of the visible, controllable, objectively demonstrable, if possible measurable. The clinical findings on the body, on the organs, on parts of organs (tissues) or products of organs (secretions), which must be rendered visible, constitute the outlines of therapy.

These comparatively rough proportions necessarily make the therapy symptomatic rather than causal. The last sequelae of the long chain of causes are followed up so as to eliminate them if possible, and the beginnings and connecting links are often difficult to trace by scientific parameters and thus ill-suited to a therapy relying on control and objectivity.

We measure the immunoglobulins and divide the states of a disease by these final products of a long process of cellular synthesis, and observe the retarded sequelae, not the causes. The metabolic diseases are divided by groups of material, metabolic disturbances of proteins, lipoids, carbohydrates, instead of finding out whether the metabolism is disturbed in the mitochondria or ill-regulated in the ribosomes, inhibited in the cytomembranes or misprogrammed already in the nucleus.

If one submits to the cogent logic that every control or miscontrol in the body must originate from a biochemical reaction from cells or cell organelles, this origin of disease should be made the ther-

179

apeutic leitmotif where the origin is known. Possibilities and realities of a

causal therapy make the subject of the considerations given hereafter.

The diseases of the blood-forming system

are usually divided under quantitative viewpoints – anemia/hyperglobulinemia; leukopenia/leukocytosis – which direct the therapeutic tendencies automatically to the quantitative deviation; substitutions and destruction take place. As for anemia, a cogent relation to cellular and subcellular structures results here already.

The globin of the *hemoglobin molecule* shows characteristic innate abnormalities:

1. Deviations within the rate of synthesis in one of the polypeptide chains of the hemoglobin molecule provoke *thalassemia.*
2. Tissue defective through amino-acid, with an amino-acid substituted by another in the alpha-, beta-, gamma- or delta-chains (e. g. in *sickle-cell anemia/*fig. 297) or with an amino-acid lacking without substitution (e. g. in the *hemoglobin M-Freiburg*).
3. Disturbed sequence of amino-acids in the beta- and delta-chains provoking *lepore hemoglobins* and *thalassemia-like diseases.* 13 abnormalities in alpha-chains, 23 abnormalities in beta-chains have been differentiated, 2 dozen are not yet differentiable.

Anemia is the common result of the much differentiated abnormalities; in part of the cases, the changed sequence of amino-acids reduces the stability of the hem-group of iron. Hemoglobin S and hemoglobin C in a reduced condition are less soluble than hemoglobin A_1; when the oxygen saturation declines, crystals of hemoglobin will form, the shape of the erythrocytes changes to the sickle-cell phenomenon. The dispersion of the hemoglobin in the erythrocytes is disturbed in carriers of the hemoglobins C, E and in thalassemia; hemoglobin occurs chiefly in the center and periphery of the erythrocytes. The morphological outcome is the target cells, the clinical result is a reduced survival of the erythrocytes, hemolytic anemia.

Innate or acquired insufficiencies or depressions of the hematopoietic tissues – *thrombocytopenia, leukopenia, anemia, panmyelopathia*– have for decades come under the therapeutic axiom of substitution. Here, too, it is advisable though only in part of the cases possible, to implant or transplant bone-marrow for causal stimulation instead of symptomatic substitution at the end of the chain.

Immun-insufficiency – immun-depression

Insufficient immunity is identified serologically and immunochemically i. e. diagnosed by secondary findings (immunoglobulins in the serum) or tertiary mechanisms (method of precipitation, stimulation test). Of the division of primary immunoinsufficiencies estab-

lished by the WHO-committee, all are of cellular origin (tab. 13, 14).

Whereas the therapy has hitherto been based upon the idea of substituting lacking products of synthesis, the causal attack on the sites of cellular origin is more logic and more promising. Since

180

insufficiencies of tissue and organs are in question, a biological stimulation of the insufficient cellular units ought to be tried. Effective ways to the not tissue-identical implantations of fetal liver or thymus tissues via the HLA-identical transplantations of bone-marrow are approached just reluctantly (tab. 14, fig. 205, 206).

The neuralgic point of these insufficiencies declared as cellular lies in the ribosomes of the endoplasmatic reticu-lum. The cause may be alone a false information of DNA – like in the hereditary and sex-linked forms – or originate on the way: r-RNA → m-RNA → transfer RNA, or in the final processing of the protein structure.

As to the therapy, success can be anticipated for these ailments only if one does not rely on a substitution of the final products IgA, IgM and IgG but tries to repair the «manufacturing base».

Equal origin – different sequences

Let us consider the problems from another perspective. The manuals of medicine aiming at a systematizing order include clinical aspects as e. g.

enchondral dysostosis,
mucopolysaccharidosis,
sphingolipidosis,
disturbances of the glycoprotein metabolism,

i. e. groups of ailments comprising a total of 22 well defined nosologic pathological units in quite different chapters: disorders of the skeleton, metabolic diseases, affections of the central nervous system. The symptomatological variety can be brought to a common denominator: lysosomal defects (see tab. 22).

The *lysosomes* are cellular organelles serving with their oxyreductases and differentiated hydrolases for the rapid rebuilding and disintegration of superfluous structures; they play an important part in the quickly changing formations of embryonic and fetal life. As substrate is dammed up, storage cells with an extended cytoplasma space such as in Morbus Gaucher (fig. 209) grow, because the enzyme gluco-cerebroside-beta-glucosidase is lacking.

In mucopolysaccharidosis, the sulphatases, iduronidases and glucoroni-dases of the lysosomes (see tab. 22) are deficient.

The example of the relations between lysosomes and circumscribed aspects explains the causal nexus between cell organelles, their contents and the somatic and spiritual influences (tab. 22, lysosomal diseases). It appears that quite different clinical aspects have a common topographic denominator, the lysosomes, and that the therapy must centre on this conditions. Similar statements apply also to other cell organelles, especially to the large number of membraneous diseases. The clinical aspects, however, ought to be treated in the clinical chapters because only the correlation-principle has to be shown. The Fabry syndrome alone has been picked out for an example.

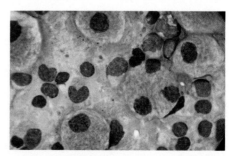

Fig. 209: Gaucher cells: spleen

181

Tab. 22: **Lysosomal diseases (genetic defects of lysosomal enzymes) Mucopolysaccharidoses**

• = *Leading clinical symptoms*

Disease (syndrome)	Enzyme defect	Metabolic disorder (affected substrate)
Mucopolysaccharidosis I (Pfaundler-Hurler-S., Dysotosis multiplex, Gargoylism)	α-L-iduronidase	Dermatan-sulphate Heparan sulphate

• *Skeleton symptoms – Storage symptoms – Mental retardation. Disproportionate nanism, thoracolumbal gibbus, macrocephalic dyscephalia, typical physiognomy («gargoyle face») hepatosplenomegalia, opacity of the cornea, steadily increasing backwardness of mental development*

Mucopolysaccharidosis II (Hunter's syndrome)	Iduronate-sulphatase	Dermatan-sulphate Heparan-sulphate

• *Symptoms similar to I, but milder. Skeleton changes and mental development impaired. Hepatosplenomegaly, no opacity of the cornea, defective hearing. Only male sex afflicted.*

Mucopolysaccharidosis III (Sanfillipo-syndrome, Oligophrenia-polydystrophica) Subtype A Subtype B	Heparan N-sulphatase (Heparan-sulphamidase) α-N-acetylglucosaminidase	Heparan-sulphate

• *Progressive mental reduction with disturbed behaviour, aggressivity Hypertrichosis; enlargement of the liver, no splenomegaly.*

Mucopolysaccharidosis IV (Morquio-Brailsford-S)	N-acetylhexosamin-6 sulphatase	Keratan-sulphate Chondroitin-6-sulphate

• *Disproportionate nanism due to platyspondyly. Projecting sternum. Angular knees. Normal mental development. Slight opacity of cornea, sometimes hepatomegaly.*

Mucopolysaccharidosis V (Ullrich-Scheie's disease)	α-L-iduronidase	Dermatan-sulphate Heparan-sulphate

• *Moderate skeleton changes like type I and slighter hepatosplenomegaly. Dense opacity of the cornea; normal mental development. Multiple articular contractions*

Mucopolysaccharidosis VI (Maroteaux-Lamy's s.) Syndrome of lacking β-glucuronidase	N-acetyl-galactosamin-4-sulphatase (arylsulphatase B) β-glucuronidase	Dermatan-sulphate Heparan-sulphate
Chondroitin-IV-sulphate mucopolysaccharidosis		Chondroitin-VI-sulphate

• *Intense nanism with chondrodysplasia-like proportions and, in certain circumstances, morquio-like changes of the spinal column. Hard features, hepatosplenomegaly, opacity of the cornea; normal intelligence.*

Sphingolipidosis

GM$_1$-gangliosidosis (generalised gangliosidosis; pseudo-Hurler's disease; Landing syndrome)	Galactosidase	GM$_1$-gangliosides Glycopeptides Keratan-sulphate

• *Hypotonia of muscles, motor regression, neurological deficiencies, skeleton changes, in case distended abdomen.*

Disease (syndrome)	Enzyme defect	Metabolic disorder (affected substrate)
GM$_2$-gangliosidosis (Tay-Sachs' disease, juvenile form)	β-N-acetylhexosaminidase A	AGM$_2$-gangliosides

- *Psychomotor retardation. limited motility of joints. Hepatosplenomegaly; red macular spots (50 % of the cases)*
  Macroglossy, gingivahyperplasia; coarse physiognomy. Vacuolised lymphocytes.

Sanhoff's syndrome (Tay-Sachs'-O-variant)	β-N-acetylhexosaminidase	GM$_2$-ganglioside Globosides

- *Storage of gangliosides in the brain with progredient deficiencies.*

AB-variant	GM$_2$-ganglioside-β-N-acetylgalactosidase	GM$_2$-gangliosides
Morbus KRABBE	Galacto-cerebroside β-galactosidase	Galactosylceramide; galactosylsphingosin monogalactosyl-diglyceride

«Slowly progredient encephalitis»

- *Cerebral-degenerative symptoms with seizures.*
  «Slowly progredient encephalitis». Beginning in the early infancy.

Morbus GAUCHER	Gluco-cerebroside-β-glucosidase	Glucosylceramide

- *Two forms: Infantile form with moderate hepatosplenomegaly, increasing bulbar deficiencies (dysphagia, strabism, opisthotonus); normal fundi*
  Adult form: splenomegaly more distinct than hepatomegaly.
  «Hypersplenism»: leukopenia, haemorrhages.
  Changes of bones (Perthes' necrosis), articular disorders.

Morbus FABRY	α-galactosidase (ceramide-trihexosidase)	Trihexosylceramide; digalactosylceramide

- *Angiokeratoma corporis diffusum; cornea-dystrophy; cardiovascular, renal degeneration.*

Metachromatic leukodystrophy	Cerebroside-sulphatase (arylsulphatase A)	Sulphatides

- *Steadily increasing mental retardation. Death mostly till the 10th year.*
  Disturbance of the statomotor development in early infancy with muscular hypertonia, hyperreflexia.
  Muscular atrophy with growing involvement of peripheral nerves, specially in the lower extremities.

Lack of polysulphatase	Arylsulphatases A, B, C Sterol-sulphatases Mucopolysaccharide sulph.	Sulphatides Mucopoly-saccharides Sterol-sulphates
Morbus NIEMANN-PICK	Sphingomyelinase	Sphingomyelin

- *4 clinical variants:*
  A. *Serious retardation of development, considerable hepatosplenomegaly, macula degeneration to blindness. Death in the first two years.*
  B. *Storage without involvement of ZNS.*
  C. *Most frequent form, manifestation in late infancy, survival 3 – 6 years. Progredient statomotor and mental deficiencies.*
  D. *Manifestation in mid-childhood, survival till 2nd decade of life*

Morbus FARBER	Ceramidase	Ceramides

- *Reddened cutaneous nodes to plaques, swelling and rigidity of the extremities. Dysphonia.*
  Rise in temperature. Articular, cerebral and cardiopulmonal symptoms possible.

Disease (syndrome)	Enzyme defect	Metabolic disorder (affected substrate)

Disorders of the glycoprotein metabolism

Fucosidosis	α-L-fucosidase	Glycoprotein fragments Glycolipids

- *Hypotonia, resulting in spastic tetraplegia and growing decerebration rigidity. Frequent infections of the respiratory passages, hyperhidrosis, cardiomegaly. Hurler-like phenotype, death mostly before the 6th year.*

Mannosidosis	α-mannosidase	Glycoprotein fragments

- *Muscular hypotonia, hepatosplenomegaly, opacity of the lens, abnormal bone-structure, vacuolised lymphocytes, accumulated infections of the respiratory passages, Hurler-like phenotype.*

Aspartylglycosaminuria	Aspartylglucosylaminase	Aspartyl-2-deoxy-2-acetamido-glucosylamin

- *Mental retardation, opacity of the lens, hepatomegaly Changes of bones like in mucopolysaccharidosis.*

Lack of β-xylosidase	β-xylosidase	Xylose

- *Mental retardation, spasm, vomiting, recurrent infections of the respiratory passages.*

Further lysosomal enzymatic defects

Pompe's disease	α-glucosidase	Glycogen

- *2 forms: infantile and adult forms Generalised glycogenosis; vomiting, anorexia, dystrophy, cardiomegaly with dyspnoea and cyanosis. Storage mostly in muscles, liver and nervous system. Infantile form: death within the 1st year*

Morbus WOLMAN	Acid lipase	Cholesterol-ester Triglycerides
Lack of acid phosphatase	Acid phosphatase	

- *Hepatosplenomegaly, blown-out abdomen, anaemia, vacuolisation of lymphocytes; no ZNS-symptoms! Vomiting, diarrhea. Adrenal calcination. Death from inanition within the first 4 years.*

Fabry's disease

(Angiokeratoma corporis diffusum universale, FABRY, 1898; referred to also as RUITER-POMPEN-WYERS syndrome (1939) after the discoverers of the relations to participations of inner organs.)

The X-chromosomal inheritable enzymopathy of lysosomal localisation is accompanied by storage of trihexosyl-ceramide through lack of alpha-galactosidase. Intarsia-like deposits of livid to blackish colour occur in the skin and mucosae. Paraesthesia, rheumatoid pain, subsidence of mental power, cardiovaso-renal symptoms (edema, dilatation of the heart, renal insufficiency) and ocular symptoms (ampoule-like conjunctival

184

veins, Tortuositas vasorum retinae, spot-like opacity of the cornea) indicate the extended deposits. This ailment occurs chiefly in the male sex.

The prognosis, serious especially if kidneys and eyes are involved, seems to be influenced with a longer lasting effect by implantation of fetal liver cells (TOURAINE I. L. et al., 1979) than by other measures such as transplantation of kidneys, steroid hormones or azothioprines. The authors discuss a «colonization» of lysosomal enzymes.

Membrane dysfunctions

Membranes are cell organelles separating ecological spaces, on the one hand, and assuring the necessary exchange of material and fluids, on the other hand. This is effected by a structure of 3 lipophile and hydrophile layers, an accordion-like elasticity, a special outfit of enzymes and the apparatus for the transport of ions, with calcium/magnesium and sodium/potassium taking a key-position.

Membrane defects and dysfunctions include pathological units of all age groups:

1. Innate metabolic disturbances;
2. Acquired membrane dysfunctions;
3. Responsibility for the control of immunological identity.

Any body-cell can have membrane dysfunctions if it is supposed that the erythrocytes without nucleus have the properties of blood-groups in their membranes. In pathology, the membranes in the kidneys, in the lungs and in the gastrointestinal tract are of greater importance because metabolic processes essential for the continuance in life take place.

The innate defects of the *renal-tubulus epithelia* cause aspects characterized by an increased loss of substrate through the urine, on the one hand, and by a corresponding lack of substrates in the body, on the other hand: amino-acids are secreted in the urine selectively or generally, the excretion of protein and sugar increases. The organism lacks these substances specially in the period of growth, which causes delays of growth and partly serious rickets-like changes of the skeleton.

Acquired nephrosis is accounted for by a similar loss of membrane function. In most of the chronic renal disorders, the changes of the basal membrane and of the tubulus apparatus are the essential pathological deviations.

An improper outfit of enzymes in the intestinal epithelia same as cases of lacking disaccharase or of intolerance to fructose cause delay of growth and emaciation just as immunological alterations of the intestinal epithelia in allergies to cow's milk, egg, fish and other nutritive allergens.

A decisive part in the aging process of the tissues is ascribed also to the rigidity, thickening and loss of functions of the cell membranes connected therewith.

185

Clinical principles
Cell therapy as biomedical fundamental concept

From the preceding chapters on the principles and experimental studies on cell therapy it appears that this therapeutic trend is far better founded both theoretically and experimentally than many other forms of therapy, and that the assertion that it «lacks scientific significance» can be explained only with the absence of corresponding experience and knowledge of literature.

The question whether clinic and practice have been equally verified and substantiated cannot be affirmed and substantiated unrestrictedly in spite of 4–5 million patients treated already with cell therapy. This is due chiefly to the insufficient documentation of the results obtained mainly in the practice so that knowledge transmitted by word of mouth and by individual experience rather than a systematology suited to serve for science has been developed. Questions like the dose of the implanted quantities, number of the tissues to choose, intervals of implantations can not be answered free from contradiction – which no doubt is true for many biological methods.

The following chapters try to systematize the clinical questions; owing to the situation described above they must be a side by side of «hard», clinically significant data and facts and casuistic individual results (individual experience).

First, a general introduction on technique, indications, basic tests and side-effects is given, then the clinic is subdivided after the 4 indications crystallizing from the variety of applications:

   I innate dysfunctions of organs and organic systems;

   II pathological dysfunctions of organs and organic systems;

   III impaired functions of organs, organic systems and of the whole organism as a result of ageing processes;

   IV concomitant therapy of tumours.

«*Cell therapy*» is a biological form of therapy. It is defined as an injection-implantation of fetal or juvenile cells and tissular particles in physiological solutions.

As a matter of principle, it must be pointed out that cell therapy like any other medical trend should be part of a comprehensive wholistic concept. Than more this therapy with biological components is embedded into a number of necessary concomitant measures, than more convincing the effect will be.

The opinion often expressed formerly that «if cell therapy then nothing else beside it» has never been founded and cannot be justified in the apodictic postulate. Of course, supporting procedures ought to be used – not such of contrary action. It is of minor value to apply some hundreds of mg (100–400) of fetal tissue for reconstruction of defective tissues, and to administer at the same time antagonistic tissue-destroying drugs by grams or kilogramms. It must be emphasized that cytostatics, anticonvulsives, a few antibiotics and electromagnetic short wave radiations counteract the constructive principle of cell therapy as they destroy structures. Except these groups and narcotics, however, there are hardly any other medicaments that, if necessary, could not be used as concomitant remedies.

Cell therapy should in all cases be the constructive part of a medico-biological therapeutic general concept.

Under this aspect, the doctor using cell therapy must proceed on a broader base than usually. The purpose of therapy is not to remove a conspicuous symptom but the elimination of the cause of the symptom. In other words, not only the affected organ, the entire complex of regulations of the organ should be taken into account also.

Choosing the tissues indicated in an individual case is an art in the strictest sense of the word, which requires a deep insight into the biological general condition of an affected body.

The effect of cell therapy depends not only on the selection of the proper tissue but also on the body's demand for the substrates and enzymes offered. Where there are no defective structures or want of enzymes, biological components can neither be built in nor take effect.

The demand for biological structures and enzymes is a presupposition for the effect.

Preliminary tests

By extensive preliminary tests the doctor should

a) gain a detailed picture of the individual clinical aspect, and
b) find out any possible risks of side-effects.

It is of less importance to establish an exactly defined scheme of laboratory data than to carry out the necessary clinical and biochemical tests relating to age, sex, and disease. These tests differ from each other according to whether a child with infantile cerebral paresis or a potency problem in a middle-aged patient or loss of vitality in old age are in question.

It is essential

a) to exclude acute infections, especially such of the respiratory tract, and
b) to treat chronic infections (otitis, mastoiditis, tonsillitis, sinusitis, cholecystitis, pyelonephritis).

Useful, if possible, is the knowledge of complement factors and of the IgE level as immunological side-effects may occur on this base.

The detailed biological general aspect (state of the illness, vitality status) is necessary because from this assessment primarily cell-type selection and concomitant therapies adjusted to the individual situation of life can be derived. On the other hand, it does not promise an optimal therapy to rely only on a clinical guiding symptom or on striking laboratory findings.

Besides the reasonable therapy, the preliminary test has the purpose to prevent avoidable risks. The injection-implantations are followed within the first, generally 2–3 but also even 7 days by a stress on the body, which is due to the high metabolic function of disintegrating and transporting the implanted tissues. Whereas an organism capable of bearing stress experiences this phase of stress objectively as an agreeable fatigue or lassitude, the stress on an already strained organism may provoke unwelcome side-effects. Three starting conditions must be taken into account:

a) Infectious stress by acute bacterial and viral infections, or stressing chronic infections. In either condition, the implantation may strain the reactivity of the body beyond the expected limit of stress. High blood sedimentation, high complement titres, high IgE or the proof of specific tissular antibodies give valuable contraindications.

b) The organism is stressed (exhausted) by the basic disease to such an extent that its reacting mechanisms – espe-

187

cially the reactivities of the adrenal glands and of the hypothalamus/diencephalic system – are reduced enough to allow a stronger influence of the «physiological» general effects of the stressing phase. Then the lassitude is frequently felt as an unwelcome side-effect.

c) In patients of advanced age, the conditions of vessels and blood circulation at the site of injection have often been worsened by degenerations of vessels to such an extent that the absorption and removal of the implanted material are impaired and intensive local reactions may occur. The same conditions apply to diabetics advanced in years and patients suffering from chronic hypertension.

In all situations mentioned, it must be found out whether or not a cell therapy is feasible. This question should be analysed critically as the stressing factors are high and

cell therapy remains often the only possible therapeutic alternative.

The decision lies between the extremes «no treatment because risk is high and perhaps not justified» and «the higher risk must be taken in order to try and stop the fatal course of the disease»; moreover, precautionary measures are indispensable.

Precautionary measures

Cell therapy requires perfectly sterile working as a generally necessary measure. The implant is tissue that, after resuspension, forms a substratum favourable for ingested microorganisms and those already existing in the body. The technical equipment and disinfection of the skin must be perfect, but bacterial or mycotic disseminating focuses cannot be excluded safely.

Technical equipment

The technical equipment (injection syringes, needles) must be sterilized immediately before use unless disposable articles in commercial packings are used. Wing canules offer the advantage of better handling when the syringe is changed i.e. they can be operated without touching the nozzle of the canule; on the other hand, there is the disadvantage that the metal cylinder of the needle is usually thicker.

The disinfection of the skin

at the site of injection ought to be double. Primarily, a sufficient area of the skin should be disinfected with a preparation containing iodine or an iodine substitute. After at least one minute of action the iodine must be cleaned away from the site with alcohol or ether. Besides the double disinfection, this method avoids traces of iodine getting into the body through the prick of injection and causing allergies. Disinfection with alcohol or ether alone – benzene should not be used – is not sufficient as the bactericidal effect of these agents cannot set in before the lapse of several minutes whereas the interval between the disinfection and injection uses to be shorter. Before the injection, the site must be dried with a sterile muslin tampon so as to avoid the penetration of even traces of alcohol or ether through the puncture channel.

After the injection, the puncture channel must be covered for 3 days with an adhesive tape to bar the invasion of germs. As the injections are preferably applied to the gluteal region, this subsequent measure is necessary specially for patients with insufficient hygiene. Among these persons are disabled children and persons advanced in years, for whom a contact of the site of injection with urine or faeces cannot be excluded. Consequently, the protective tape must be renewed after every bath on the first three days following the injections.

Immunological precautionary measures

The complexity of the immunological processes has for consequence that

a) interrelations with other immunological processes through the non-specific bridging links (complement factors) cannot be excluded
and
b) immunizations against partial components of the used tissues – specially cell membranes, connective tissue – may occur if the implantations are repeated.

Experience with 4–5 million cell implantations carried out so far has shown that the immunological side-effects are extremely rare in contrast to the rate of expectance postulated by certain immunologists. Many patients treated over a long time tolerate completely without reaction even up to 40 injections administered at intervals of 5–6 months.

On the other hand, intensive local or even urticarial reactions may occur already after the 3rd or 4th implantation in patients suffering from acute infections or chronic suppurative focuses (otitis, mastoiditis, tonsillitis, sinusitis). Special caution is indicated in acute infections of the respiratory tract because stenosing laryngitis is possible.

As all these responses provoke the unwelcome hyperergic reactions via virtually non-specific mediators, extensive precautionary measures are necessary.

Since the reactions of the vascular apparatus – irrespective of how they are elicited – are caused mostly by the release of mediators from the basophils and mast-cells, the following measures are advisable though allergic reactions may occur:

1. Single dose, according to patient's age, of a *cortison preparation* (prednisolon, triamcinolon, bedneson) and *antihistamine product* 5–10 minutes before the injection/implantation.
2. Single dose of an *adrenalin derivative* (epinephrin, suprarenin, novadral, norphen, effortil and similar derivates) immediately after the implantation.

A favourable combination of a cortison- and antihistamin preparation is *celestamine* in the form of syrup and tablets.

The cortison derivative covers generally the antiallergic effect, the antihistamin preparation the effect of histamin, the catecholamin derivatives answer the reactions by the IgE-Complement.

«Antiallergic» treatments several days before are not necessary. A single dose of the above groups of drugs is usually enough; in case of need, they may be given several days.

Together with chronic bacteremia – especially Otitis chronica, mastoiditis – retarded urticarial reactions may occur weeks later in extremely rare cases.

189

Then, one must not rest content with the antiallergic covering, for only the elimination of the focus calms down the relapsing urticaria. From his own experience relying on 3 cases in which urticaria helped to detect otitic complications with chronic osteomyelitic lesions, the author points to the rare sequence of combinations; the implantation plays the part of a non-specific stimulator in a labile-latent immunological structure.

If intense local reactions (fig. 219) or an urticarial general reaction (fig. 220) occur, the alternative of choice is a parenteral (subcutaneous) dose (according to the age) of suprarenin or of a related adrenalin derivate.

Cortison in the form of suppositories, tablets or injection can also be given simultaneously though it must be taken into consideration that its optimal effect occurs 20–30 minutes later and that cortison preparations alone are not a proper remedy to control an acute allergic reaction.

A cup of a *mixture of vitamin-C-calcium* sparkling effervescent tablets: Cal-C-Vita, Ce-Ca-bion) is for children a placatory end of the injection. It is difficult to answer or to refute the question whether this beverage has an essential antiallergic-antiphlogistic effect.

Implantation technique

Although the implantation by injection is an injection, in practice there are more problems than one should expect.

The resuspension

of the tissular lyophilisate extremely poor in water can be effected in the ampoule. As the surface of the lyophilisate forms a film difficult to penetrate when getting in touch with the resuspension liquid, the lyophilisate dissolves slowly. This becomes a time factor if several ampoules must be drawn up for a treatment.

It is therefore recommended to fill the contents of 1–3 ampoules of the lyophilisate from behind into the syringe barrel; for this purpose, the end of the syringe must be provided with a needle to prevent any loss of material. After putting the piston into place, the solution is drawn in and the resuspension effected by shaking the barrel (fig. 210–214).

As many tissues (e.g. cartilage, connective tissue, placenta) swell, it is expedient to let pass 5–10 minutes, not more,

between the resuspension and injection; if it takes longer, an injection canule with a wider calibre should be chosen.

Equipment for injection

The syringe should have a capacity of 10–20 ml. Syringes of 10 ml are easier to handle and hold well 3 × 100 mg of lyophilisate for the resuspension.

The injection canule must have a lumen of 1.0–1.2 (needle No. 1 or 20); for connective tissue and placenta, a lumen of 1.2–1.4, for cartilage and fetal, skin one of 1.4–1.8 should be selected.

One-ware equipments for every tissue are avaiable 1983 (fig. 219–226).

Site of injection

Implantations of cell material can be injected
a) subcutaneously,
b) intramuscularly,
c) intraperitoneally.

(Text continue page 197)

Fig. 210–218:
Implantation technique

Fig. 210:

Owing to the high dryness of the lyophilisates, with a residual humidity of less than 0.4%, it is not easy to resuspend them in the ampoules; the surface of the lyophilisates is moistened with water, which inhibits the penetration of the suspension liquid into the lyophilisate powder. It is therefore advisable to fill the cylinder of a 10–20 ml syringe with 3–5 ml of the suspension liquid after closing the nozzle of the cannula with a sterile small-calibre cannula broken off at a right angle.

Moreover, the lyophilisate can be brought into the cylinder of the syringe with the cannula put on and provided with a protective cap (see fig. 214) direct i. e. without a solvent in the cylinder.

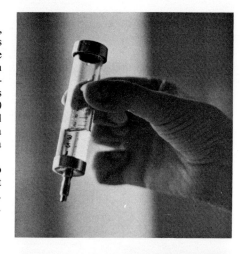

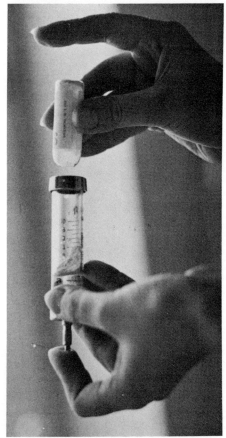

Fig. 211:

After loosening the contents of the ampoule by knocking on a hard bottom, the lyophilisate is strewn into the cylinder of the syringe from above.

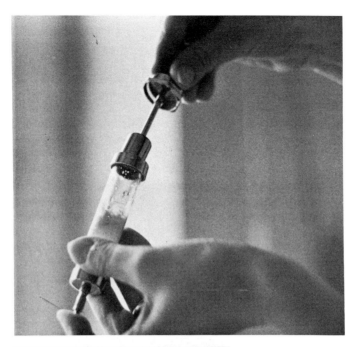

Fig. 212:
After emptying the complete contents of the lyophilisate ampoules into the cylinder, the piston is put on and screwed.

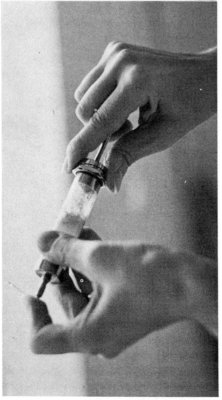

Fig. 213:
The use of sterile disposable syringes spares the screwing. In contrast to this advantage, there is a disadvantage: more tissue remains in the nozzle of the cannula.

192

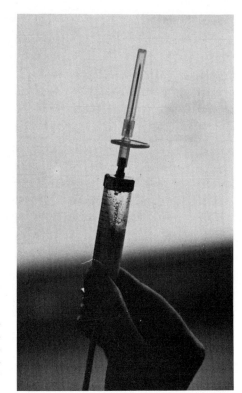

Fig. 214:
The lyophilisate and suspension liquid are mixed in the cylinder by shaking till the dry substance has disappeared completely. The contents of 2–3 ampoules of lyophilisate can be suspended in a cylinder at the proportion of 100 mg of lyophilisate: 4–5 ml of suspension liquid.

Fig. 215:
With the syringe held in a vertical position, the air needed for mixing is evacuated till the first drop of the suspension appears at the needle top. The filling of the needle with suspension avoids the closing of the orifice with a cylinder of skin when the needle is pricked. For most of the tissues, cannulae with a calibre of 1.0–1.2 will suffice, for placenta and connective tissue 1.4, for cartilage and bone-marrow a diameter of 1.8 mm is recommended. Not more than 10 min should pass between the resuspension and the injection or else the swelling would impede the injection and the preservation of the biochemical substance after the rehydration could no longer be controlled.

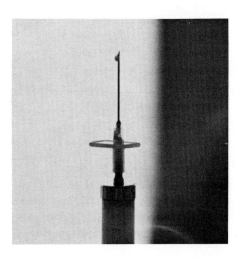

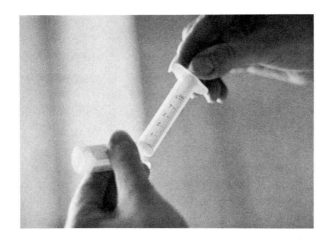

Fig. 216:
To empty the cannula and the puncture channel it is advisable to inject some more suspension liquid. This suspension liquid can be used for the complete cleaning of the lyophilisate ampoules.

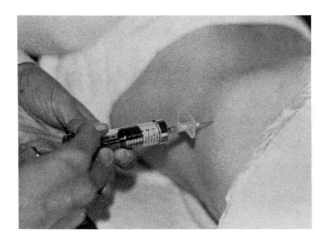

Fig. 217:
The injections (implantations by injection) are applied by deep subcutaneous (epifascial) punctures; there should not be any resistance, which would indicate an improper position of the needle-point. Lumbar regions (i.e. above and outside the gluteal region) and abdominal walls are the most suitable sites for the absorption.

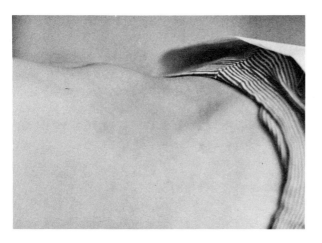

Fig. 218:
The injection lifts off skin and subcutaneous tissue, which causes tenderness on pressure and tension for about 2–3 min. The protuberance will disappear after a professionally applied epifascial injection within 10–15 min. Injuries to blood vessels and bleedings into the area of injection may evoke inflammatory processes (same as with injections of own blood). The puncture-channel should be covered for 2–3 days with an adhesive tape against infections.

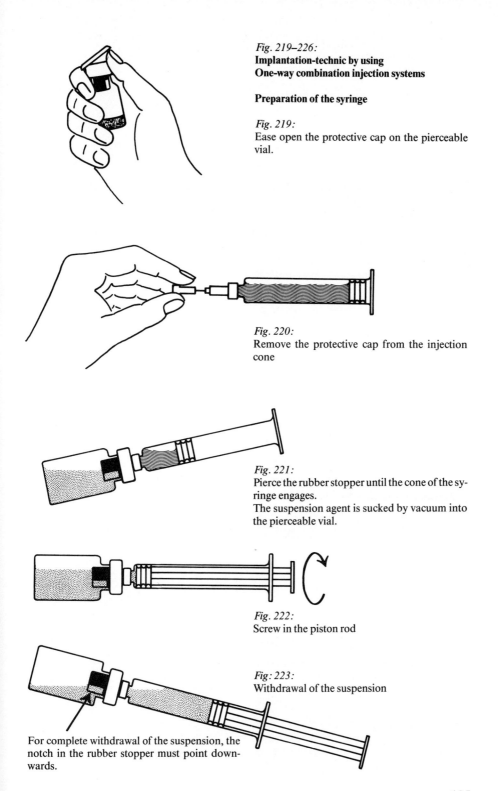

Fig. 219–226:
**Implantation-technic by using
One-way combination injection systems**

Preparation of the syringe

Fig. 219:
Ease open the protective cap on the pierceable vial.

Fig. 220:
Remove the protective cap from the injection cone

Fig. 221:
Pierce the rubber stopper until the cone of the syringe engages.
The suspension agent is sucked by vacuum into the pierceable vial.

Fig. 222:
Screw in the piston rod

Fig: 223:
Withdrawal of the suspension

For complete withdrawal of the suspension, the notch in the rubber stopper must point downwards.

195

The implantation must be carried out immediately after withdrawal of the suspension by deep subcutaneous injection.

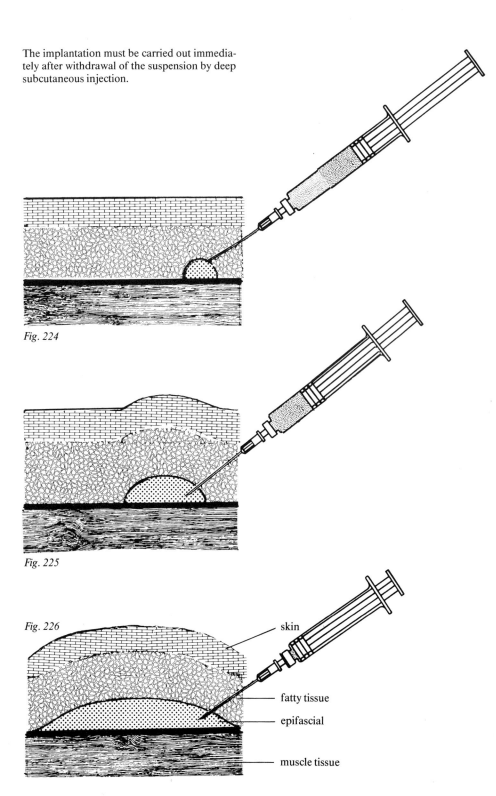

Fig. 224

Fig. 225

Fig. 226

skin

fatty tissue

epifascial

muscle tissue

The *deep-subcutaneous (epifascial) injection* is the most gentle and most physiological application. The space of implantation is dilated by a small injection volume (0.2–0.5 ml) so that the subsequent injection is effected by lifting the subcutis with the liquid, without traumatizing the tissue with the top of the needle. Proper sites for the implantation are areas with fluffy subcutaneous cellular tissue and sufficient elasticity. Best suited are dorsal-lateral areas between the lumbar and gluteal regions (i.e. higher and more lateral than the intragluteal intramuscular sites) as well as the skin of the abdomen; exceptionally, the skin of the back or the thigh may come into question. The most suitable surfaces for absorption are under the skin of the abdomen and under the lumbar region (fig. 217, 218).

The *intramuscular injection* was preferred formerly; for intramuscular injections it must be considered that the comparatively large volume causes spreads and traumatization of the muscles and, possibly, bleedings. Restricted functions of muscles, pain and hematoma are remarkable consequences if more than 2 injections are administered. Rest in bed for several days may be necessary in such cases.

The *intraperitoneal injection* is optimal with respect to the absorption but too risky regarding complications; this application, therefore, should be reserved to special situations, which may occur in cases of cachexia with atrophy of the subcutaneous tissue, further in generalized oedema with doubtful conditions of absorption.

Concomitant phenomena

From the above remarks that the effect depends on the primary disorder, on the requirements of the organism, on the implanted tissues and on the patient's age, it follows how very individual the effect and its extent may be. However, the variety of clinical treatments, subtile casuistics in certain areas and of experiments on animals can be divided chronologically into characteristic phenomena.

The phase of stress

follows the implantation immediately.

The implantation causes pain by the pressure of the volume as the skin is lifted, usually for 2–3 minutes, but also up to 5–10 minutes.

Parallel to the disintegration and transportation goes the phase of stress, properly. It may, in the minority of the cases, be accompanied by slight rises in temperature of 0.5–1.0°C (i.e. about 37.8–38.5°C of body temperature) for some hours or a day. The blood-count shows a rise in leukocytes while the polynuclear multiply (fight of leukocytes). Adults describe a pleasant desire for rest, some a feeling as after a heavy meal, others speak of lassitude for several days.

Children may show two contrary aspects in the phase of stress, namely desire for sleep for several hours up to 2 days, on the one hand, and hypermotility to restlessness, on the other. Most of the children do not change their behaviour at all during the phase of stress.

Whereas young babies respond only seldom with rises in temperature, such rises can be observed more frequently in older babies and infants, practically never in children between 3–15 years of age.

The slight leukocytosis with multiplication of the polynuclears subsides after a few days and results in a monocytic-eosinophilous «overcoming phase» though the qualitative changes are not very impressive.

Inconsistent though it may sound: the stronger the symptoms of the phase of stress the better the therapeutic outcome may be anticipated.

Phase of effect

The positive effect of a «cell therapy» appears usually from the 3rd to 4th week after the injection. This has been registered most convincingly by observations of thousands of parents of disabled children, who speak of *«developmental outburst»* or *«developmental leap»*, sometimes of a *«developmental explosion»*, which may receive expression in motor, linguistic and mental criteria or criteria of conduct. This phase lasts about 3 months, then subsides and falls below the threshold of what can be registered, after 5–6 months.

Besides this general *«time-table»*, there are impressive examples of earlier or later effects. From animal tests we know that according to the effective tissues (spleen, liver) the normalizing deviations of the blood-count are fully developed in leukemic mice already after 3 days. A mongoloid baby who owing to complex immaturity of the liver, sepsis and uncontrollable diarrhea was unable to gain in weight in spite of 3 months of parenteral feeding and moribund got peritoneal injections of 150 mg of liver, 150 mg of placenta and 100 mg of cerebrum, improved within an hour though his condition had lasted for months. After a second series of implantations, the improvement was definitive.

A boy of eight suffering from familial congenital nephrosis was carried to the clinic with a hydrops on a hard plank because his body looked like a jelly-fish. All conventional measures (prednisolon, infusions of protein) failed. Diuresis set in after peritoneal injection of 150 mg of kidney and 150 mg of placenta already on the following day and swept out the edemata completely.

A latency-period

of 1–2 weeks follows the phase of stress till the registrable onset of the action. It is the period in which, after disintegration and removal of the implanted material, the dispersion in the body and the incorporation in the homologous organs (structures) take place. Not until the functions of the organ (tissues) have improved at the site of incorporation, the effect can be registered biologically or clinically. In contrast to the above extremely short intervals pending the onset of the effect, latent periods of several months have been reported for older persons. STÜHLINGER (1979) collected 20 impressive examples showing the different onsets and durations of effect.

The repetition

of the implantations depends on the duration of the effect. As a rule, repetitions should not be initiated earlier than after a time-interval of 5 months. In favour of this minimal interval speak immunological considerations and reasons of effect. In adults and especially old persons, the duration of the therapeutic result is decisive for the indication and time of a repeated treatment. Generally, the intervals will come to 1–2 years.

An exception to this recommendation is the concomitant tumour therapy with a fetal mesenchyme; intervals of several weeks are usual and necessary here.

The frequent question how often a cell therapy should or must be repeated, can be answered very simply: as long as concrete success is obtained.

Compatibility

Lyophilised tissues in physiological solutions are well tolerated, there is no toxicity. As however a xenogenous tissue injected subcutaneously by comparatively large volumes (6–15 ml per injection) is in question, physical irritations at the site of injection are caused, on the one hand, and immunological concomitant symptoms may be caused by repeated injections, on the other hand. The long interval between the injections of implantations, from 5–6 months up to 2 years, is medically justified and provides moreover some safety from an anaphylactic reaction after sensitization.

The side-effects are astonishingly slight even under the forced therapeutic conditions of the frequent implantations in the tumour-immunotherapy. The following picture results from an extensive study by H. RENNER (1979):

71 patients got 324 injections of fetal mesenchyme (Resistocell®), several injections (2–22) were administered to 55 patients at intervals of 4–6 weeks. Even those 324 injections intended for the immunization against fetal antigens showed no threatening allergo-anaphylactic reactions; in one case, a patient developed urticaria but tolerated several equal injections without reaction later.

The evaluation by H. RENNER provided the following outcome:

Of those 324 immunizations, 254 were specified under the following parameters: fever, local pain and local reactions at the point of puncture such as erythema, swelling, overwarming. The reactions were rated by an arbitrary scale from 0–4:

0 = no reaction
1 = slight
2 = distinct
3 = intense
4 = very intense.

No reaction whatever was observed in 57.8% of the immunizations, the rest showed: fever in 6.7% (scale 1 and 2), local pain in 29.9% (among them only 3.2% scale 3) and local reactions in 19.3% (among them only 2.3% in scale 3). These side-effects were partly combined.

But once more it must be made plain: most of these reactions were slight to moderate (scale 1 and 2), only very few were distinct (scale 3). Excessive reactions were not observed (scale 4).

Especially it must be emphasized: all side-effects (100%) were entirely regredient within a short time; there were never any lasting ulcerations, fistulae or fever.

The several immunizations were applied to a group of women with metastasising mamma carcinoma as part of a combined treatment with cytostatic interval-polychemotherapy and local palliative radiation during the first chemotherapeutic courses. The immunization was performed at intervals of 4–6 weeks when the therapy had been interrupted. RENNER treated a woman who by now has got already 31 regular immunizations in the therapy-free intervals within about 2¾ years. Also these several immunizations at short intervals were just as well tolerated as single immunizations or such repeated at longer intervals.

N. WOLF (1966, 1969) obtained similar *time-accelerated results* when treating 65 patients suffering from brain-atrophic processes. The implantations were lyophilisates of placenta and fetal frontal brain, sometimes combined with hypothalamus and ovary; 2–6 treatments at intervals of 4 weeks constitute also an unusual, immunologically provocatory accumulation of implantations at short intervals. Even under these conditions

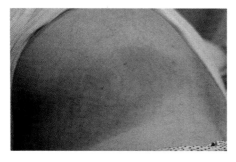

Fig. 227:
Repeated injections at the same site may cause a local reaction round the point of puncture in the form of reddening and swelling. – Intense local reaction in adipositas (striae). Girl of 16.

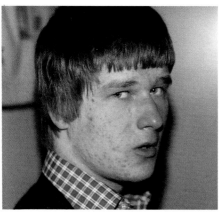

Fig. 228:
High IgE titres may evoke general reactions in the form of a rush or a Quincke edema. Catecholamins (adrenalin derivatives) applied orally or parenterally (specially suprarenin) work faster and more causally than cortison derivatives.

«no complications or remarkable side-effects whatever occurred».

From his own experience based on 74,000 implantations of lyophilised tissues of various organs applied in the course of 25 years, the author can derive the following conclusions: if intervals between implantations of 5–6 months and the precautionary measures described are observed, the percentage of side-effects and complications is much inferior to the rate anticipated for xenogenous tissue.

In particular, the following circumstances must be taken into account:

1. *Local reactions (erythema, swellings)* on the first 2–3 days after the injection; they depend on the injection technique, injected quantity and number of the preceding implantations applied at the same site. Such local reactions must be expected in about 5–10% of the cases if injections are repeated.

2. Irrespective of this, extended non-allergic erythema is often seen immediately after injections of *placental tissue;* in question is a circulatory reaction, which subsides untreated or with only physical measures (cooling, gel).

3. One *abscess* caused by the injection must be taken into account for every 5,000 implantations, according to all serial observations made so far. It should be realized that the cleanliness at the site of injection cannot be assured especially with disabled and young children. The cases observed so far are without exception pyogenous infections from inside the body or infections of the puncture channel.

4. *Hypersensitivity reactions* of the immediate type must be expected for repeated injections – more than three preceeding injections – in 8‰, especially if no freedom from infection is guaranteed. Immediate reactions usually occur through IgE via the complement system and do not constitute a hypersensitivity for the xenogenous tissues.

5. *Infections* of animal epidemics frequently feared specially in the beginning years have so far not been observed. Substantiated reports are available neither for the original fresh-cell method nor for the dry-cell doses.

The general risks and the problems of the complications are treated in papers written mostly in the fresh-cell era. Most of them analyse the matter generally and theoretically. Here is a survey of the more important authors:

BÖSCH 1958;
BOMS 1956;
CAMERER 1961;
CASTENS 1957;
DAHMEN 1953;
DÖDERLEIN G. FANCONI G.
and NONNENBRUCH W. 1955;
HUPFELD 1980;
GRIFFEL A. 1957

IVERSEN 1956, 1959;
JORES 1955;
JUSSEK 1970;
SCHULTEN 1957;
VORLÄNDER 1958;
KANZOW 1960;
KLEIN 1967;
KNÜCHEL 1956;
PISCHINGER 1955;

RAPPOLD 1959;
RIETSCHEL 1955, 1956;
RÜMELIN 1969;
RUPP 1955;
SCHMID F. 1955,
    1978, 1980;
SPRADO 1955, 1958;
SCHÜTZE 1956.

Much more useful than the above figures is the statement that in only 40 of more than 74,000 implantations, suprarenin or cortison had to be applied parenterally (subcutaneously) owing to the dimensions of the urticarial reaction, which is a rate of less than 1‰. Even these situations could have been avoided for the most part if infections of the respiratory tract and pyogenous focuses (otitis, mastoiditis, suppurative sinusitis) had been respected as strict contraindications and no compromises e. g. for excessive travelling distances and economy of time had been agreed to.

Of all postulated incompatibilities and complications for which a temporal coincidence seemed to indicate a causality with cell therapy, the casuistically reported cases of *encephalomyelitis* and *polyradiculitis* deserve special notice. Most of the published cases (GSELL 1975; HUPFELD and WENZEL 1980; BENNHOLD 1954; SEITELBERGER et al. 1957; BRAUCH 1956) are so-called «fresh-cell treatments», for which the quantity and kind of the used material were not known and there was no safety from the conveyance of microbes. As the declarations of the materials used and of their doses were insufficient, the conditions of these complications extremely rare in proportion to the number of the treatments have not been found out.

The fact that, in contrast thereto, more than 40 series of implantations of lyophilised cerebral tissues were applied to mentally ill children in the course of development without a case of neuroallergic reactions becoming known so far, shows that the possible causalities depend on special conditions.

If any substantial quantities of cells are implanted, it is necessary to avoid any excessive physical overexertion, exposure to intensive sunlight and X-ray radiation, further the use of cytostatic drugs within the first 10 days following the implantation.

Cell therapy is a highly specific method, which must be learned. Indications, contraindications, methods of application and, above all, the use of standardized, bacteriologically controlled products declared as to quantity and contents, are prerequisites for an adequately riskless and promising therapy.

Forms of the cell therapy

The publicity for various forms of cell therapy has helped to confuse the public. The «fresh-cell therapy» (tissues of freshly slaughtered animals are dissolved and injected) was wrongly believed to use fresh cells, living to continue life in the organism of the recipient. Decisive for the effect, however, is not the «freshness» but the composition and quantity of the biochemical contents (substrates and enzymes). The faster the tissue is implanted and preserved, the more active ingredients remain intact. Lyophilisation (freeze drying) is the method of choice because all chemical disintegrating processes of the donor's tissue are stopped at once when the water is withdrawn. This is the safest method of guaranteeing the native form of the biochemical outfit of fetal tissues.

A therapy largely applied by the doctors must assure that

a) the quantity of the used «pharmacon» can be declared,

b) the contents are generally known,

c) freedom from microorganisms can be anticipated.

The way of meeting these requirements is not equal for the 3 variations usual nowadays (tab.). Applied by well versed experts and if a team collaborates smoothly, the «fresh-cell method» guarantees a great deal of efficiency and safety provided that not more than 30 minutes elapse between the taking of the donor's tissue and the implantation. Roughly, the lyophilisates offer the highest degree of safety and effect. The entire elementary research has been done with lyophilisates because only these provide the prerequisites for experimental work.

Safety conditions	«Fresh-cell method»	Lyophilisates (freeze drying)	Freeze-cell method
Quantity	not determinable, roughly estimable for experienced	declared by mg of liquid-free tissues	roughly determinable
Biochemical composition	undefined	about 20 cellular substances cytochemically demonstrated Content on minerals and trace elements is analysized	undefined
Sterility	sought to obtain by asepsis, cannot be guaranteed	released for use only after bacterial control	freezing and thawing reduce bacteriological safety usually controlled

Instructions for the production of sterile cell-therapeutic preparations and for the health control of the donor animals

The German Federal Health Gazette 13, pages 116–117 (1970) contains the instructions for the production of cell-therapeutic preparations. These instructions comprise 4 chapters:

I the importance of using healthy donor animals;

II provenance of the donor animals;

III slaughtering hygiene and meat inspection;

IV taking of organs and further treatment.

Here is the wording of the instructions for a safe production and application.

Conditions of production
I The importance of using healthy donor animals

a) Necessity of additional examinations and measures

The cellular therapy in the meaning of these directions is a technique by which material of animal tissue or native animal fluids are incorporated into the body of a patient. Under § 1 paragr. 1, in connection with § 2 No. 3 of the Drugs Act of May 16th, 1961 (Fed. Gaz. I p. 533) – version now valid – such substances become medicaments. Their circulation, however, is prohibited under § 6 No. 1 of said Act if their use as prescribed implies a risk of harmful effects exceeding a degree acceptable in the understanding of medical science. The harmful effects include the transmission of the morbific agents of zooanthroponosis, to which the fresh-cell therapy may give rise. To avoid such a risk, certain precautionary measures must be observed when the donor animals are selected and the preparations are extracted. Some of these measures are already part of the provisions on vaccines and sera (ordinance of the Pr. min. of public welfare and agriculture of July 15th, 1929 (LMBL. p. 447) – still valid). As a matter of principle, only animals healthy in every respect can be used. It is the veterinarian's concern to select and to examine them. Irrespective of this, the doctor is responsible for the application and its consequences.

Slaughter cattle is tested alive and after killing for pathologico-anatomical processes under the Act on meat inspection (FLBG). However, the findings relying usually just on a rough examination allow only to decide on the edibility of meat. These findings therefore do not indicate that certain tissues are suited to be used for the cell therapy. A painstaking bacteriological examination is carried out only in suspicious cases and if animals are ill; they do not come into question to serve for cell donors anyway. The examination under the Act of meat inspection, consequently, is not sufficient to detect all diseases transmissible to man by parenteral application because many infectious diseases and stages of diseases proceed without clinical symptoms or pathological changes. If in cell therapy cells are transmitted immediately from the animal to the patient, the time available between the taking of cells and the application is too short for relevant additional examinations.

203

b) Zoonosis

As chiefly horned cattle, sheep and pig, and the rabbit of the small animals, come into question to serve for donors, especially the diseases of these animals that can be transmitted to man are of interest, namely:

blue-tongue disease (sheep)	brucellosis
enzootic sheep abortion	gas edema
influenza	leptospirosis
looping ill	listeriosis anthrax

lyssa (rabies)
foot-and-mouth disease (aphthous fever)
animal small pox
Rift-Valley fever (sheep)

Wesselbron fever (sheep)
ornithosis

pneumococcosis
erysipelas

salmonellosis
tuberculosis,
psittacosis,
piroplasmosis,
rickettsiosis,
toxoplasmosis
tularaemia (e. g.
Q-fever)
vibriosis

II Descent of the donor animals

a) Selection

To judge of whether an animal is suited to be used as a donor of cells, a time of observation as long as possible is necessary in order to submit it to thorough repeated clinical and additional tests in the laboratory. Best suitable are SPF animals, in special cases gnotobiotic, at least animals kept for the particular purpose of extracting cells and supervised by a veterinarian. If, exceptionally, this requirement cannot be met, the animals used must have lasting distinctive marks, be of a known descent and have been examined thoroughly by veterinarians at regular intervals.

Obligatory are veterinary certificates of health, from which it appears that repeated examinations of the stock of animals in question have not revealed any symptoms indicating an epidemic (e. g. foot-and-mouth disease, erysipelas, myxomatosis), especially one of the diseases mentioned under Ib), and that an animal shows no clinical signs of a disease. These certificates of health should state moreover that the animals have not been submitted to a therapy likely to exert an unfavourable influence on the results of the examinations (e. g. certain inoculations with destroyed or living cultures – possibility of eliminating morbific agents or influence on the results of serological examinations – or treatments with sulphonamides and antibiotics – possible influence on the results of bacteriological examinations -). Sterility, abnormalities of the cycle, miscarriages or abortions and mastitis must not be there. If possible, artificial insemination ought to be used in the original stock of animals; a natural mating can be accepted if the father animal is submitted to the same supervision as the donors. If there was an epidemic in the immediate environment of the original stock and the donors are free from the epidemic though susceptible to infection, the animals of this stock cannot be used unless passing first a quarantine, the duration of which must be fixed by an official veterinarian according to the kind of the epidemic.

The veterinarian and official veterinarian should collaborate closely when a proper stock of animals is selected.

b) Species of animals

Donors of cells are chiefly horned cattle, calf, pig and sheep. The sheep seems to be preferred as it is easy to keep and supervise. Further, small laboratory animals as guinea-pigs and rabbits are used.

c) Quarantine

If animals are to be included in a supervised stock, they must be put under quarantine. This is indispensable unless the animal comes from a known stock looked after by a veterinarian, which must be certified by a veterinarian. The quarantine should last 3 weeks at the least. The stall must be built in such a way as to keep the animals strictly separated from other animals. It must be easy to clean and disinfect and allow clinical inspection of the animals any time. Contacts with wild animals or rodents must be avoided and stinging insects, ticks and flies be kept away.

d) Examinations

The animals selected for donors of cells must be subjected to repeated clinical, bacteriologico-virological, serological and allergological examinations. If parasitical diseases are suspected, supplementary tests (faeces, skin) must be made. In case, the animal experiment must be included. These tests ought to be made also during the quarantine or time of observation.

III Slaughtering hygiene and meat inspection

a) Conditions expected from the slaughter rooms

The room used for slaughtering cell donors ought to be reserved exclusively for this purpose. All necessary structural requirements for hygienic equipment must be met. If such a room is not available, slaughtering must be done in a slaughter-house, with strict separation from the normal slaughtering. The place where the slaughtering is done and its equipment must meet the minimum requirements for slaughtering under the provisions for meat inspection.

b) Qualities expected from the animals

Animals qualified as malnourished by the veterinarian or very excited before slaughtering, unfed for some time or not sufficiently reposed, do not come into question to be used as cell donors. The animals must be cleaned thoroughly before slaughtering. The hygiene of cutting up is very important. Any contaminations of the meat and organs must be avoided (minimum requirements for slaughter-houses under the provisions of meat inspection). Pigs should be brothed preferably in a hanging position. It is advisable to slaughter only one donor animal at a time. Slaughtering several animals simultaneously may impair the hygienic conditions.

c) Examinations under the meat inspection Act

Whilst the meat inspection Act allows, in certain cases, persons other than veterinarians to examine meat, only a veterinarian is authorized to do so if the extraction of cells comes into question. As a rule, it is advisable to release the cell material only after the examination according to § 21 and the foll. of the regulatory statutes A of the meat inspection Act i. e. as soon as the inspection has proved the perfect quality of the meat for human consumption. The parts of the body (genitals, fetuses, etc.) declared unsuitable for human consumption (§ 35 sentence 1 of the regulatory statutes A of the meat inspection Act) can be used for the extraction of cells if the meat and the part of the body in question have been found to be in order and a permission under § 7 of the meat inspection Act has been issued. Animals not subject to the provisions of meat inspection (e. g. rabbits) must be examined in analogy to these instructions. This means that a veterinary examination is obligatory also if an animal is killed only for the production of cells and not used for human consumption.

d) Additional examinations

When tissues are produced for the so-called fresh-cell method (immediate transmission from the donor to the patient), additional laboratory tests on the extracted cell material will usually not be feasible as time is short. The health control ought to be concentrated above all on the living animal. If however parts of tissue are taken for the production of quick-frozen and lyophilised cellular preparations, these additional examinations must be made. They help to reduce still more the risk of infection.

IV The taking of organs and further treatment

a) Qualifications expected from the personnel

The personnel occupied with the extraction and production must, respecting the state of health, come up to the requirements for persons working in the food trade. The provisions of the Federal Epidemic Act apply. The persons entrusted with the taking of tissue must be thoroughly familiar with the special technique of dissection for the various species of animals and, above all, with anatomy.

b) The taking of the organs

The tissue must be taken under aseptic conditions. The unintentional opening of non-sterile organs (oesophagus, trachea, stomach, intestine, etc.) must be avoided.

c) Additional laboratory examinations

For reasons of time, bacteriological examinations can come into question only for tissues that are to be quick-frozen or lyophilised before use (see IIId). If only fetal tissue is taken, these examinations may be restricted to the foeti. Recommended is a bacteriological test

more thorough than that provided by annex 1 to § 20 par. 3 of the regulatory statutes A of the meat inspection Act. Quick-frozen and lyophilised tissues require moreover sufficient bacteriological after-controls of the preparations ready for injection.

d) Further treatment up to the processing or injection

The cell material must be put into sterile containers immediately after taking. Fresh cell material intended for the application must be transported and preserved at low temperatures ($+3°$ to $+6°$C). When cells are quick-frozen, a temperature of about $-70°$C is necessary. The material for quick-frozen and lyophilised preparations must also be treated in such a way as to avoid an unfavourable influence during the subsequent processing. Gradual bacteriological tests should be made during the various steps of production. The methods of production must guarantee the manufacture of sterile injection preparations. The compatibility ought to be tested on small experimental animals before the injection.

Congenital aberrations of functions and structure

Aberrations in the prenatal development of a living being may relate to the structure (form, substrate), the function (enzymes, metabolism, movement) or to both. Innate abnormalities are charged with the myth of the irrevocable, fatal. This mostly because the underlying elementary processes take place on a level partly below the threshold of our recognition but certainly beyond our imaginative power.

In fact, it is really paradoxical that most of the non-hereditary «chromosome abnormalities» show morphological aberrations on the hereditary substrates, the chromosomes, whereas on the other hand no morphological equivalent can be found on the hereditary substance in the recessive or dominant «hereditary diseases».

The two therapeutic ways used so far of *substituting lacking substances* (e.g. insulin substitution in diabetes) or the *elimination of non-processable metabolites* (e.g. reduction of phenylalanin in phenylketonuria) are symptomatic measures. Experimental biology has used the sinister term «gene manipulation» to point to a causal influence on structural and functional aberrations of the genes. A serious question-mark, however, stands before the consequences in medicine.

The cell therapy proved the possibility of influencing innate abnormalities practically already when theory flatly denied such possibilities. The appearance of clinical changes is often called into question if there is no theoretical or logical explanation of what has become visible. Then reference is made to the «present state of science», the relativity and insufficiency of which is disclosed by every following new recognition.

This situation must be borne in mind when «cell therapy for chromosome aberrations» ist the subject of a treatise. The «present state of science» relies on the idea that a chromosome abnormality is *«the cause»* of a mosaic of clinical symptoms. In fact, a morphological ascertainment on chromosomes is not more than an abnormality of the form in other dimensions i. e. those of the subcellular structures. The functional disharmony brought into a phylogenetic and ontogenetic harmony by such an abnormal form uses to be much more important than the aberration of the form proper.

Chromosomal abnormalities

The structural aberrations of chromosomes use to be subdivided by groups into abnormalities of the autosomes and gonosomes (sex-chromosomes), on the one hand, and by disorders of distribution, on the other hand. One speaks of monosomies (1 chromosome instead of 2), trisomies (3 instead of 2), translocations (displacements of chromosome mass) and deletions (injuries to chromosome constituents without numerical aberration or displacement of material). Tab. 23 contains a survey of the clinically most important forms.

Sufficient therapeutic experience with this group of disorders is available only for Down's syndrome and Turner's syndrome. For all other chromosome abnormalities, sporadic cases make, at best, rough outlines for a consistent therapy. The treatment has to rely on the symptoms of clinical results rather than on the findings as to chromosomes, and must be conceived for the entire medicine (fig. 229, 230, 231). Some succerr promises aberrations of the chromosomes Nr. 9, 10, 11; in trisomy 13 und 18 we have no celltherapeutic experience till now.

Tab. 23: **Aberrations of chromosomes**

1. Translocation on chromosome 1	**Abnormalities of the sex chromosomes**
2. Wolf-Hirschhorn-Syndrom (Deletion chrom. 4)	1. monosomy X (45,X)
3. Syndrome of deficiency on the short arms of chromosome 4	2. polysomias a) triple-X-syndrome
4. Cat's-cry syndrome (abnormality of chromosome 5)	b) tetrasomy X c) pentasomy X
5. Monosomy 9	3. XY-polysomias
6. Partial Trisomy 10 q	a) Klinefelter-syndrome (XXY-type,
7. Trisomy 13–15 (Patau's syndrome)	47,XXY
8. Trisomy 18 (Edwards' syndrome)	b)XX-type (46, XX)
9. Deletion chromosom 18 (DE GROUCHY-S.)	c) XXXY-type (48, XXXY) d) XXXXY-type (49, XXXXY);
10. Trisomy 21 (Down's syndrome)	Fraccaro-type
a) free trisomy 21	e) 49, XXXYY und 49 XXYYY
b) mosaic mongolism	f) XXYY-type (Double male)
c) translocation mongolism	4. gonosomal mosaics
d) double-trisomy (48 chromosomes)	
11. Rare aberrations	

Down's syndrome

Down's syndrome (= mongolism, mongolism-syndrome, mongoloidism, trisomy 21, trisomy G) is the most frequent and most important innate disorder accompanied by chromosomal abnormalities. From the correlation of the clinical symptoms to certain (not uniform) chromosomal aberrations (trisomy 21, translocations, mosaicisms) it is often concluded that the symptoms occurring in the course of development are fatal and inevitable. This resignative interpretation

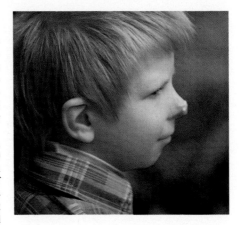

Fig. 229:

Translocation on chromosome 1

A boy of 5 years is admitted for considerable retardation of his development. He used only fragments of syllables, is little concentrated, cannot be brought to work, appears inconstant. Microcephaly, head of 47.5 cm (−4 cm) in circumference, with hypoplastic frontal and temporal parts of the forebrain. Dysmorphy in the upper head-somite including ears and eyes.

After the first implantation already (Apr. 26, 1977: 100 mg of diencephalic lyophilisate, 100 mg of cerebral hemisphere, 150 mg of placenta male fetus), distinct improvements of speech, of sociability and initiative were obtained. After 4 series of implantations at the age of 6 10/12 years (May 1979), the rough movements and sociability nearly correspond to the age and vocabulary of the 2-year-old with certain achievements adequate to the 3rd and 4th years. Circumference of head: 48.6 cm.

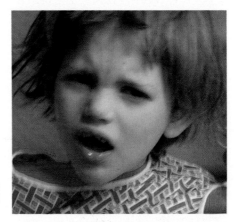

Fig. 230:

Cat's-cry syndrome

Even repeated implantations of fet. brain tissues improve just slightly the general condition and microcephaly.

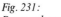

Fig. 231:

Dysmorphy syndrome in monosomia 9.

As a new-born many signs of dysmorphy: hypertelorism, small eyes, deep ears, shield-breast, defect of diaphragm, displacements of body-proportions, nail-hypoplasia and contractures of all joints, only the hands were opened.

At the age of 8/12 years muscular hypotony, no static functions. Learns to be seated at age of 10 months, six weeks after first implantation of 100 mg of diencephalon and 100 mg of cerebrum, learns to walk freely at 2 years, uses 10 words.

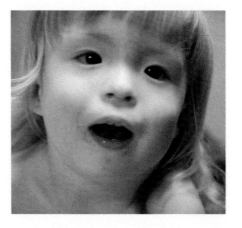

of morphological findings on a subcellular level has done immense damage to generations of afflicted children and parents.

In contrast to this nihilism palliated with the term «present state of science» there have been for 30 years a medical practice and experience proving not only scientifically but also biologically on a generation of mongoloids that Down's syndrome can be influenced. Among the pioneers of this evolutions are HAUBOLD H. (1954–1967); GOLDSTEIN H. (1956, 1959); FAHLISCH K. (1961); MOMMSEN H. (1955–1959); FELDMANN H. (1959, 1979, 1982); SCHUBERT E. V. (1957); SCHOLZ K. (1973, 1974); HALLER B. (1970–1980); ZELLER W. (1957).

The author's own experience covering more than 25 years relies on 1780 long-term observations documented and evaluated under various biometrical, metabolic and therapeutic parameters. The plan of therapy adjusted to all sections of medicine based on these extensive studies and fixed in individual publications between 1953 and 1983 will be explained more at length as example of other innate syndromes in order to work out the interplay of the various treatments (see fig. 232).

Conception of treatment

In contrast to the present conformistic conception that trisomy is the cause of Down's syndrome, the following representations are based on other fundamental ideas and biologico-clinical facts. They relate to the biological central question whether the function makes the structure or whether the structure determines the function. Applied to the processes of germ-cell fusion and to the first processes of division, the following questions arise:

● Is there a primary lower functional valence of the germ-cells leading to abnormal processes of division and fusion in the chromosomes, which provoke a secondary influence on the abnormal forms?

● Is the morphological aberration of the chromosomes really the primary noxa from which all other symptoms can be derived?

The abnormalities of chromosomes confirm the correlation with the clinical symptoms of Down's syndrome, not however their causal importance. The aberrations of chromosomes are probably the consequence of an additional pathogenous principle in the function of the germ-cells, which come into question to be the cause only because they can be identified optically and morphologically. Clinically, this alternative implies the question whether the metabolic aberrations in children suffering from Down's syndrome are the result or the cause of the chromosomal abnormalities.

Important facts speak for the conception that Down's syndrome is a disease correctible in essential partial symptoms rather than a fatal consequence of chromosomal-morphological aberrations.

Therapeutic requirements

Down's syndrome is a disorder affecting the form and function of the entire or ganism, and therefore its symptoms consist of pathological abnormalities (form variants) and functional aberrations. The progredient retardation in untreated mongoloids is the outcome of the dysfunctions, the common denominator of which seems to be a metabolic disturbance in all cellular membranes. This disturbance influences metabolic, rapidly growing tissues (brain, glands of the internal secretion, cartilage, liver, immunocytes) more than metabolic less active tissues.

210

Table 24: **Response to therapy of important symptoms seen in Down's Syndrome**

Removable	Improvable	No Response
Saddle Nose	Hypertelorism	Brushfield Spots
Narrow Palpebral Fissures	Epicanthic Folds	Milk Dentition
Eye axis	Mongolian Eye Axis	Anomalies
Squint	Nystagmus	Broad Upper Part of
Conjunctivitis	Abnormal Ear Formation	Ilium
Blepharitis	Secondary Dentition	Pseudoepiphysis
Macroglossia	Anomalies	Synostosis
Brittle Hair	Abnormal Behaviour	Chromosomal
Obstipation	Flat Acetabulum	Abnormalities
Microcephalia	Coxa valga	Pterygium
Hypognathism	Brachymelia	Ape Furrow
Weakness of Ligaments	Brachycarpia	«Sandal» Furrow
Muscular Hypoplasia	Clinodactylia	Dermatoglyphics
Muscular Hypotonia	Cheilosis	Non-Operable Heart
Umbilical Hernia	Hypogenitalismus	Diseases
Inguinal Hernia	Social Development	
Retarded Ossification	Motor/Kinesthetic	
Osteoporosis	Development	
Lowered Resistance to	Speech	
Infection	Mental Development	
Thickened Skin	Physiognomy	
Cervical Lipomatosis	Stature	
Operable Heart Diseases	Abstract Process of Thought	

The Down syndrome is a multiple handicap which concerns both the

Physical development
a) anthropometrically (insufficient growth, dislocation of proportionate ratios, microcephaly, physiognomy);
b) statomotorically (delay of the statomotoric development, disorders of the fine motorial and coordination systems)
and the

Mental development
a) in the psychic and social areas;
b) in the intellectual sphere.

In addition, there is a general weakness of the defense system against infections.

Inevitably a «multiple handicap» results in the need for multidimensional care.

Numerous experiments made in the past failed because they were structured in terms of too narrow a concept; they did damage to the Down children – not on account of the method of treatment applied but by the fact that further therapeutic requirements were neglected.

Not only a 3-decade experience and the success obtained in this field speak for considering Down's syndrome a treatable disease needing a therapy, but also a number of exact facts:

211

1. *The somatic, stato-motoric, intellectual and psychic developments* decline with the advancing age gradually in relation to the norm of age. Many symptoms distinctive of the fate and position of these children in the society are not original but develop *secondarily* in the course of growth.

2. Many symptoms, primarily not marked but manifesting in the course of growth, are possible only with a participation of the *endocrine system* (nanism, hypothyreosis, symptoms of adrenal insufficiency).

3. The *aberrations of proportions and growth of the brain skull and facial bones* are little marked at birth and in the first months of life, in part they do not exist. The objective measurements are mostly still within the norm, about the mean value. With advancing age, the growth of the cranium lags behind the norm; the brain is not equal afflicted because the occipital and parietal regions stay behind

most. The first anatomic changes are found in the cerebellum.

4. While the growth of the brain is retarded, the *mongoloid physiognomy* becomes more evident as the deformation of the cranium and facial bones continues with the advancing age unless a therapeutic intervention is initiated.

5. Owing to the general *underdevelopment of the mesenchyme*, the weakness of the defense against infection adds much to impair the children's development.

6. There is no direct relation between the findings of chromosomes, the clinical symptoms and the intellectual development. This lack of correlation is most evident in mosaic-like mongolism as a varying percentage of body-cells and tissues show a normal structure of chromosomes.

7. The *nanism* of mongoloid children begins during infancy and reaches the peak in the last puberal stage of

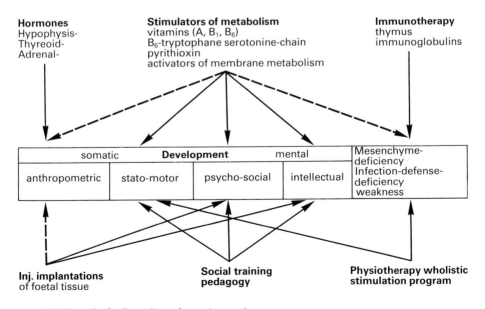

Fig. 232: Therapies for Down's syndrome (see text)

growth. The regularities relying on a long-term observation of mongoloid children seem to suggest a continued *deficit of the puberal phase of growth,* which consequently determines much the dimensions of reduced body length.

Therapeutic postulations

If the practical assessment of the mongoloid syndrome is considered to rely on the fact that here a disease with a progressive retardation of the development is in question, the following therapeutic postulations result:

1. To *regulate the balance of the endocrine glands* in such a way as to reduce or to stop the endocrine deficits.

2. To reduce or to stop the progressive deficit of the *brain growth.*

3. To treat the lowered *resistance to infection.*

4. To remedy the *weakness of the connective and supporting tissues.*

5. To *prevent the deprivation* elicited by therapeutic resignation as an additonal injury to the children.

6. To develop and to use consistently a *pedagogy* adjusted to the outcome obtained.

Consequently, the therapy must aim at all symptoms and groups of symptoms to influence. The following methods are available:

a) hormones
b) stimulators of metabolism
c) immunotherapy
d) implantations by injection
e) social training and pedagogy
f) medico-gymnastic treatment of the whole body (stimulation program)
g) speech therapy.

Therapeutic principles

An analysis of the situation will show first that all developmental sectors are afflicted, most however the intellectual development. Nanism, microcephaly, disturbed proportions of the body stature, timely and formal abnormalities of ripening are distinctive of the anthropometric component of the somatic development whereas the retarded stato-motor development characterizes its functional component. Within the mental sphere, the social development (including the retarded learning of social functions up to antisocialism) is affected just as well as the intellect, which shows the most serious deficiencies in the area of abstract thinking. The therapies are illustrated synoptically in fig. 232.

Metabolic therapy

The literature on metabolic aberrations in Down's syndrome provide only in certain areas binding conclusions on therapeutic consequences. Among them are:

a) disturbed absorption caused by reduced enzyme activities in the intestinal secretion;

b) demand for vitamin A as an expression of reduced protection of surfaces;

c) disturbed metabolism of vitamin B1 and vitamin B6 in connection with the restricted metabolism of tryptophane;

d) abnormalities of the tryptophane metabolism, which entail a lowered serotonin level;

e) cytochemical indications to transport disturbances in the cytomembranes;

f) progressive hyperuricaemia;

g) low taurin levels;

h) aberrations of the calcium-magnesium levels;

i) high phosphate values;

213

j) low intracellular zinc values, potassium-, manganese-selen-values (hair);
k) high transferrin values;
l) low to reduced serum-iron values;
m) enzymatic aberrations;
n) disorders (insufficiencies) in the immunglobulin-synthesis.

Of importance for the therapy are medicaments of metabolic intermediate stages, vitamins and diet recommendations.

Vitamins A, B1 and B6 need continuous substitution; the minimum dose must come up to the daily requirement. If there are symptoms of lacking vitamin B (perléche, cheilosis, lingua scrotalis, chron. conjunctivitis, branny skin, seborrhoic hair-bed), vitamin B1 ought to be increased to 50–150 mg/die. Vitamin C should not be administered by quantities above average, vitamin D by as far as possible small doses; several multivitamin products cover these requirements.

The vitamins of the B-group – which occupy a central position in the entire pathological process of Down's syndrome (SCHMID, REHM and CHRISTOFFER, 1974; READING CH. M., MCLEAY, A. a. NOBILE S., 1979) – intervene in the tryptophane metabolism at six sites. Here is also the point of attack for the pyrithioxin (Encephabol®), a vitamin B6 derivative without the character of a vitamin, which influences specially the development of speech in infancy. The tolerance of pyrithioxin is comparatively low in eretic children; sometimes they do not even tolerate a teaspoonful daily of it. B-vitamins are to raise above all the serotonin level lowered in the mongoloids.

Nutrition

Food may replace many of the mentioned medications. It is easier to make this statement in theory than realizing it in practice, because extensive preservation of basic food items creates a situation in which even an interested doctor is no longer able to clearly recognize the nutritional implications.

The basis for the nutrition of Down children should be a full-value normal diet cutting down on the amount of carbohydrates. The majority of Down children instinctively rejects merchandise containing sugar (candies). This diet should include adequate bread – rye bread, leavened bread, whole-wheat bread – an anbundant amount of salads, raw vegetables and fruit. Salads which are in the stage of transition from the yellow to the green colour, contain particularly many B vitamins.

The daily amount of milk should not exceed the equivalent of 500 ml whole milk because of the calcium supply connected with it. To support the maturation of the medulla a weekly amount of 2–3 beaten eggs or egg yolk is recommended. As far as feasible the addition of small amounts (2–3 tablespoonfuls) of raw brain of young animals, mixed in a Starmix blender, for soups, vegetables, puddings or milk drinks has proven advantageous. From the second half-year on, the objective should be 1 to 2 meals of sea fish weekly.

With selective deficiencies in individual elements and trace elements the following recommendations may provide some help:

Potassium deficiencies can be corrected through diet by giving the child food which is rich in potassium, such as potatoes, carrots, peaches, apricots. For cases of selenium deficiency the best source of selenium is brewer's yeast or other kinds of yeast.

Manganese deficiency is widespread due to the consumption of bleached flour and baked goods; the best substi-

Tab. 25: **Basic therapy for Down's syndrome**
Ground schemes

A. Babies up to 3rd month of age

Rp. *Astrumin*
S. Mo., Wed., Fr. 1 tabl.
2. *Multibionta drops*
S. 20 drops daily
3. *Membravit*
S. 1 tabl. daily
4. *Encephabol juice*
S. 1/2 meas-spoon daily
5. *Pancreon*
S. 1 tabl. daily

Rp. *Thyreoid dispert 0,1*
S. Mo., Fr. 1/2 (till 1) tabl.
2. *Astrumin*
S. Wed., Sat. 1 tabl.
3. *Multibionta-Tropfen*
S. 30 drops daily
4. *Membravit*
S. 1 tabl. daily
5. *Nootrop (or Normabrain) 800*
S. 1/4 tabl. daily

B. Babies from 4–12 months

Rp. *Thyreoid dispert 0,1*
S. Mo., Wed., Fr. 1 tabl.
2. *Multibionta*
S. 30 drops daily
3. *Membravit*
S. 1 tabl. daily
4. *Encephabol juice*
S. 1 tea-spoon daily
5. *Normabrain juice*
S. 1/2 meas-spoon daily

Rp. *Thyreoid dispert 0,1*
S. Mo., Fr. 1 tabl.
2. *Astrumin*
S. Tu., Th., Sat. 1 tabl.
3. *Membravit*
S. 1 tabl. daily
4. *Mulgatol-Gelee*
S. 2 teespoon full daily
5. *Indovert-Juice*
S. 2 teespoon full daily

C. Infants 2–5 years

Rp. *Thyreoid dispert 0,1*
S. Mo., Wed., Fr. Sat. 1 tabl.
2. *Mulgatol jelly*
S. 2 tea-spoons
3. *Membravit*
S. 2 tabl. daily
4. *Neurotrat*
S. 1 bean daily

Rp. *Thyreoid dispert 0,3*
S. Mo., Wed., Fr. 1/2 tabl.
2. *Astrumin*
S. Tu., Sat. 1 tabl.
3. *Membravit*
S. 1 tabl. daily
4. *Indovert-Juice*
S. 2 teespoon full daily
5. *Vitafestal*
S. 1 tabl. daily in the evening

D. Children 6–12 years

Rp. *Thyreoid dispert 0,3*
S. Mo., Wed., Fr. 1/2 dr.
2. *Vitafestal-Drag.*
S. 1 dr. daily with dinner
3. *Membravit*
S. 2 tabl. daily
4. *Neurotrat forte*
S. 1 bean every 2nd day

Rp. *Thyreoid dispert 0,3*
S. Mo., Wed., Fr. 1/2 (till 1) tabl.
2. *Astrumin*
S. Tu., Th., Sa. 1 tabl.
3. *Membravit*
S. 1 tabl. daily
4. *Eunova*
S. 1 drop daily
5. *Neurotrat forte*
S. Mo., We., Fr. 1 tabl.

Suite of table page 216

E. Older school-children and adolescents	
Rp. *Thyreoid dispert 0,3* S. Mo., Wed., Fr. Sat. 1/2 dr. 2. *Eunova* S. 1 dr. daily with dinner 3. *Membravit* S. 2 tabl. daily 4. *Neurotrat forte* S. 1 bean every 2nd day	*The substitution of thyroid preparations must be increased or reduced individually, according to the clinical symptoms. Integral preparations are better than single components T₃ or T₄. If available, a combined preparation of hypophysis and thyroid tissue should be preferred during the first 6 years. the demand for vitamin B₁ is very high i. e. between 100–150 mg per day.*

tute in the food is whole-meal flour and the corresponding kinds of bread.

Stays on the sea-shore of three to six weeks exert a favourable influence on mongoloid children; this is true especially for the inclination to infection but also for the statomotoric development in infancy. The spontaneous development of the mongoloid children growing up on the seashore proceeds usually more favourably than that of the children living in inland or montainous regions, according to the author's experience. The worst spontaneous development is seen in mongoloids of the chalky mountains (Swabian and Swiss Jura Mountains); they must be treated with more tracerelements and hormones.

Enzyme therapy

Malfunction on the part of the digestive tracts (refusal to take food, diarrhea episodes, disposition for obstipation, abnormal gas formation, inflated belly) sometimes requires a substituting treatment with digestive ferments. With the exception of Pankreon® problems are created by a large volume of sugarcoated pills. For later childhood «Vitafestal» offers a suitable combination of digestive ferments and vitamins.

«*Coliacron*» , an injectable enzyme preparation, which may also be applied via the oral mucosa, provides unique help in serious muscular hypoplasias,

muscular hypotonias and general weakness of the connective tissue. It is applied in series of 18–24 injections (2–3 injections weekly).

Up to the present the experience gained with Wobe-Mugos, Wobenzym, and *Ocolucidon* (mucopolysaccharide metabolism) are not sufficient. This sector of therapy has not been developed very much in the face of the numerous known anomalies of the enzyme metabolism of the Down syndrome. Also the relative high enzyme content of fetal tissue provided through injection-type implantations probably has a shorttime effect only.

Endocrine substitution

With the Down syndrome the endocrine system is affected at different levels: diencephalon, hypothalamus, hypophysis, thyroid gland, suprarenal gland; gonades.

The neurocrine sphere is responsible for insufficient growth of the first years of life and probably also for acromicry.

The hypophysis commanding the glands of internal secretion is not an autonomous «control station» but depends, on its part, on the neurosecretory processes, especially on the «releasing factors» of the diencephalo-hypothalamic system (fig. 272–274).

A great deal has been written on the disturbances of the thyroid gland functions, and there have been controversial discussions of the problem. None of the laboratory methods including the auto-antibody determination meets the requirement to provide guidance for a need of treatment. Relying on and waiting for positive reactions obtained with laboratory methods among young people and adults suffering from Down syndromes is not recommended; rather, guidance should be obtained from the chief clinical symptoms from the very beginning such as macroglossia, obstipation, hyperkeratosis, adynamia.

To simplify matters, the endocrine insufficiencies of Down's syndrome can be divided into two types i. e. the thyroid type and the diencephalic type. Hypothyroid symptoms prevail in the former, diencephalic symptoms in the latter (Tab. 24), and the symptoms become evident during the development in untreated mongoloids i. e. they do not exist primarily. These symptoms do not or just slightly develop in treated children.

The Function of the Gonades vitally influences the puberty features among Down children, its onset is early, among girls often as early as between the 8th and the 10th years; it is shortened in terms of time, and abortive as to the functional result. The «puberal growth thrust» effected through gonade hormones fails to develop or remains below the threshold values. In this growth stage the growth deficit is increased considerably.

Meantime the menarche age of mongoloid girls has come closer to the average population due to the multidimensional treatment described. Alone by including suprarenal glands and ovarium between the 5th and 8th years of life it was possible to increase the final height average of Down girls in the last five years to 151 cm (average height of un-treated girls 142 cm); the height of those treated until 1975 was 146 cm.

The elimination of numerous organ preparations from the stock of medications is disadvantageous to the endocrine substituting therapy.

Complex correlations exist between Down's syndrome and the thyroid function. The therapeutic measures must conform to the clinical symptoms. Biochemical data are not reliable as a secondary dysfunction is in question. The doses will have to depend on the response of the symptoms (macroglossia, obstipation, husky voice, thickened skin, dry hair).

Ground schemes for the fundamental therapy with medicaments are contained in Tab. 25. The general rules should be adjusted to the individual requirements.

Mesenchyme insufficiency

The organismic weakness of the connective tissue (mesenchyme insufficiency) is of importance for the development of mongoloid children especially with respect to the following 2 points:

a) the stato-motoric development is inhibited purely mechanically by the hypoplasia of the supporting tissue (hypoplasia of the muscles, ligaments, tendans, vessels and skeleton);

b) the inadequate efficiency of the reticular and loose connective tissue impairs obviously the immunity against infection.

The inferiority of the supporting tissue can be influenced by gymnastic treatments of the whole body and by massage of the connective tissue; the parents should be given a program of physical exercises to carry out for ten to fifteen minutes twice or three times every day, in conformity with the actual state of the stato-motoric development. The gymnastics favour also the socialisation of the children.

Deficient immunity and defense against infection, biochemically identified by low rates of immunoglobulins, manifest themselves clinically by chronic and relapsing infections of the upper respiratory passages, enterocolitis during infancy, chronic rhinitis, tonsillitis, sinusitis, hypertrophy of adenoids, bronchitis and bronchopneumonia.

The defense against infection on the epithelial interface and the lymphatic zone of resistance can be improved by doses of thymus and multi-vitamins (vitamin A!). Moreover, antibiotics as well as inhalations and phytotherapeutics should be administered for short periods, further in certain cases tonsillectomy and adenotomy be performed to fight the chronic infections of the respiratory passages.

Besides the large and thick tongue, voluminous tonsils are an additional factor preventing the children from overcoming babbling and stammering because, mechanically alone, no articulation is possible.

Training therapy

The duty of training methods is to improve the functions of underdeveloped or damaged organs, organ systems or limbs by way of an increased stimulation with a specific objective. Passive stimulation aims at an active response to stimulation. In the case of multiple handicaps this training will cover both physical and mental activities. Transposed to the nerve system this means a stimulation at the periphery of the neuropils – that is at the motoric end-plates, axons, peripheral nerves – in order thereby to prepare the performance of functions up to the centre, the cell body of the neuron. Therefore, all methods of training are peripheral stimulation techniques with the aid of which the performance of the functions of the neurons shall be increased or established.

Methods of training are symptomatic treatment which should not be isolated in the therapeutic concept; rather, they must be embedded in a wholistic biological concept applied to the personality of the patient concerned. A maximum result will only be achieved within this framework.

The Down syndrome is a multiple handicap; under its therapeutic schedule numerous methods of training which start at the peripheral neuron will be applied in the course of development:

a) remedial gymnastics;
b) therapeutic gymnastics;
c) sports for the handicapped;
d) therapeutic swimming;
e) therapeutic horse riding;
f) motion therapy;
g) occupational therapy;
h) speech therapy (preparation of speech; training of speech motoricity);
i) optical training;
k) acoustic training;
l) music therapy;
m) behavioural therapy;
n) psychotherapy;
o) pedagogy.

It is not the purpose of the present analysis to give a valuation of these methods, which, indicated individually, may all have their advantages in specific stages of development. What should be avoided, is any monomaniac concentration.

Implantations by injection

Fetal tissue is implanted mainly to activate brain growth. This method, often incorrectly referred to as «fresh-cell therapy» is the most effective as it helps to remove certain symptoms resisting

Tab. 26: **Injection-implantations in Down's syndrome**

The succession and combination of organs given hereafter are based on statistical information on the growth of the size of the brain. They therefore relate, primarily, to the growth of the skull, the physiognomical changes and, connected therewith, to the social and intellectual development. This succession may be neglected in particular cases, according to individual symptoms or disorders.

As Down's syndrome affects also other organs (thymus, thyroid gland, adrenal gland, gonads, liver, kidney, etc.) and a general metabolic disturbance of cytomembranes is in question, it is advisable to include more tissues in the long-term plan of injection implantations.

For growth of the skull (brain)		Alternative or addition implants	
1. *Fet. mesencephalon*	100 mg	a) *weak resistance to infection*	
Fet. cerebral cortex	100 mg	thymus	100 mg
		adrenal gland	100 mg
2. *Fet. spinal medulla*	75 mg	b) *achondroplastic type (deep, broad root*	
Fet. cerebellum	100 mg	*of nose, micromelia)*	
		cartilage	100 mg
		placenta	150 mg
3. *hypothalamus*	100 mg	c) *in considerable nanism, unless osteal*	
Fet. occipital brain	100 mg	*(see b)*	
		comb. endocrine tissues	
		(hypothalmus, thyroid, adrenal gland	
		sex-spec. ovary, testes).	
4. *Fet. diencephalon*	100 mg	d) *6–10 years*	
Fet. cerebral hemisphere	100 mg	thyroid gland	100 mg
		fet. liver	150 mg
5. *Hypophysis sex. spec.*	80 mg	e) *in girls 6–10 years*	
Fet. temporal brain	100 mg	adrenal gland	100 mg
		ovary	120 mg
6. *Thalamus*	100 mg	f) *in boys 8–10 years*	
Fet. frontal brain	100 mg	diencephalon	100 mg
		adrenal gland male	100 mg
7. *Fet. basal ganglia*	50 mg	g) *in hyperuricaemia*	
Fet. parietal brain	100 mg	placenta	150 mg
		fet. kidney	100 mg
		h) *opacity of lens, vitreous body (early)*	
		placenta	150 mg
		lens	25 mg
		vitr. body	25 mg
		i) *in alopecia*	
		fet. diencephalon	100 mg
		adrenal gland	100 mg
		fet. liver	150 mg

This succession is repeated at intervals of 5–6 months in the first 6 years, of 6–9 months beyond the first 6 years of treatment unless the clinical symptomatology suggests other succession combinations or quantities.

medication and pedagogical measures. Authors sceptical about this method usually have no experience in this field or work with theoretically inadequate preparations (extracts chemically split up cellular derivatives, orally applied dilutions). The concept is to supply the body parenterally in a native biological form with the high outfit of substrates and enzymes of the rapidly growing fetal tissues.

If implantations by injection are made before the age of three years i. e. during the period of the most intense skull growth (= brain growth), progressive microcephalia with its concomitant physiognomical symptoms can much be prevented but merely be lessened beyond the age of three (Abb. 233, 234). After the fourteenth year of life, this method influences microcephalia just exceptionally, and hardly any effects can be expected for the physiognomy.

The implantations are performed by deep subcutaneous (epifascial) injection at five-month (four to six) intervals. If these specific implants are not chosen after the individual symptoms, the following succession is recommended (Tab. 26).

The results obtained so far relate to the given succession of implantations and quantities, and can probably be improved by augmenting the implants and including other tissues.

The mongoloid dyscephalia

The following remarks on the rules of growth in treated mongoloid children rely on the findings in untreated mongoloid children as defined in 1969. The 100 untreated mongoloid children statistically evaluated at that time are contained in the 200 cases of the present survey. The rules of the mongoloid dyscephalia will be treated concisely hereafter (SCHMID et al., 1969, 1972, 1982).

The abnormal development of the head as part of Down's syndrome comprises the formation of the cranium and facial bones as well as the changes of size, form and proportions. Whereas the abnormal development of the cranium is the outcome of the disturbed growth of the brain, the deformations of the facial bones result partly from mesenchymalossary and mechanical factors. The primary hypoplasia of the maxilla, which increases in the course of growth, combines with the consequences of macroglossy and of the adenoid vegetations.

The most important findings resulting from a biometrically founded craniometry shown on X-ray pictures of children suffering from Down's syndrome are:

1. The mongoloid dyscephalia is characterized by a brachymicrophalia increasing with the growth and a hypognatism of the superior maxilla.
2. The cranium, which represents the growth of the size of the brain, lies in the new-born mongoloid child usually within the tolerance of the norm; the microcephalia, therefore, is not innate in the majority of cases.
3. The growth of the cranium lags measurably behind the normal growth from the second trimenon of life; the deficit augments rapidly till the fourth year of life, later slows down gradually. The variation is essentially wider in girls than in boys.
4. The growth of the cranium (identical with the growth of the brain-size unless a hydrocephalus is in question) is not uniformly affected. The growth of the occipital, posterior parietal and temporal regions is much more retarded than the anterior parts of the skull.
5. Untreated, the mongolism develops at the end of the growth of brachysteno-microcephalia with a varying,

220

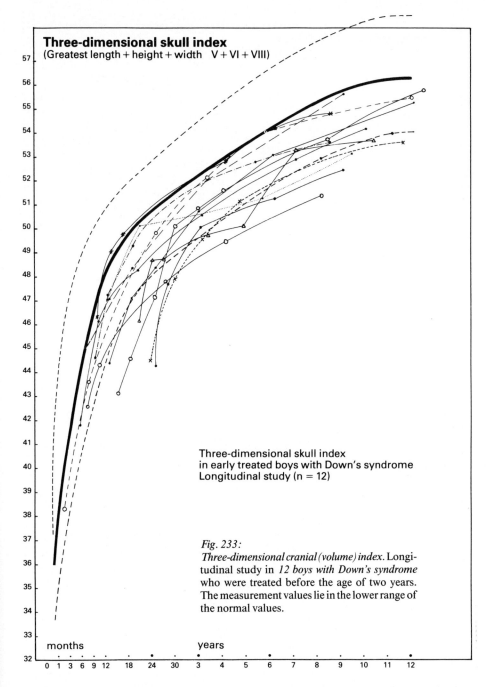

Three-dimensional skull index
(Greatest length + height + width   V + VI + VIII)

Three-dimensional skull index
in early treated boys with Down's syndrome
Longitudinal study (n = 12)

Fig. 233:
Three-dimensional cranial (volume) index. Longitudinal study in *12 boys with Down's syndrome* who were treated before the age of two years. The measurement values lie in the lower range of the normal values.

months   years

though, considerable in the majority of the cases, deficit in comparison with the normal average (fig. 235).

6. Further, the physiognomy is influenced by the changes of the facial bones. These are primary mesenchymal and not caused by the malformation of the brain. The reduced depth of

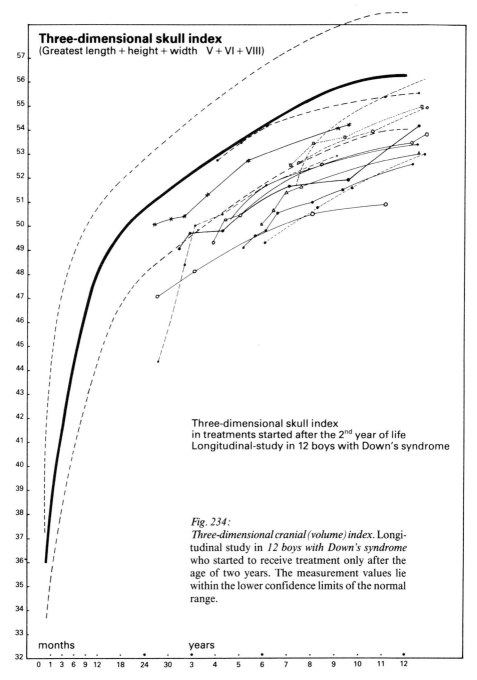

Three-dimensional skull index
(Greatest length + height + width V + VI + VIII)

Three-dimensional skull index
in treatments started after the 2nd year of life
Longitudinal-study in 12 boys with Down's syndrome

Fig. 234:
Three-dimensional cranial (volume) index. Longitudinal study in *12 boys with Down's syndrome* who started to receive treatment only after the age of two years. The measurement values lie within the lower confidence limits of the normal range.

months   years

0 1 3 6 9 12   18   24   30   3   4   5   6   7   8   9   10   11   12

the superior maxilla is there at birth and, together with the steep anterior cranial fossa, constitutes the typical mongoloid face. The central third of

the face is flat to sunken and thus looks broad; these disproportions are still accentuated by the relatively normal growth of the inferior maxilla during the period of puberty and by the absence of the occipital vault (fig. 235, 236).

Material and methods

The following biostatistical analyses rely on craniometric evaluations obtained from 200 mongoloid children under the conditions mentioned below:

1. The cases were not selected i.e. they relate to mongoloid children treated in 2 years, without regard to the gravity, age and sex;
2. the measurements must be available before the treatment is initiated;
3. the therapy must last 2 years;
4. apart from the biometrical initial values, at least two groups of measured patients determined during the treatment must be available.

As part of the radiological cephalometry, 10 distances and 6 angles are measured on cranial radiograms of all mongoloid children. Of importance for the growth of the cranium size are mainly 3 distances namely the largest length (V), the largest width (VII) and the largest height (VI) of the skull. These 3 distances make an index of the cranium size, which reflects correctly the growth of the cranium under physiological and pathological conditions and provides a metric scheme.

The initial values before the initiation of the treatment and cases, in which only a so-called basic therapy was performed, have shown that without a treatment and with basic therapy an influence worth mentioning on the growth of the cranium size cannot be obtained. In the 200 analysed cases, therefore, implants of heterologous fetal cerebral tissues (sheep, calf) were injected.

These implantations are applied by subcutaneous (epifascial) injections. As a rule, 2 × 100 mg of various parts of the

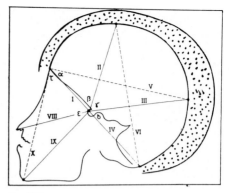

Fig. 235:
Skull-size deficit in untreated mongoloids at the end of growth.

brain, exceptionally minor quantities of 50–80 mg (hypophysis, basal ganglia, medulla oblongata) are used. After a re-suspension in a Pannett-Compton solution, the volume of the implant is 7 ml, and another 3–4 ml of Pannett-Comptom solution are injected subsequently through the lying needle into the implantation depot. Used were only original packs of lyophilised tissues of the siccacell series. The analysis includes 1400 implantations administered to 200 mongoloid children as described.

Results of the implantation therapy

The most serious symptom to Down's syndrome is the mongoloid dyscephalia, a combination of brachy-steno microcephalia with a flattened central third of the face. The initial values of the index of 3-dimensional size of the skull – at birth mostly within the tolerance of the normal average – decline strikingly in the course of growth in untreated mongoloid children, with decisive deficits in the 2nd–4th years.

Implantations by injections of heterologous fetal cerebral tissues in doses of 2 × 100 mg and at intervals of 4–6 months normalize much the configuration of the cranium and improve the physiognomical conditions (fig. 235–243).

223

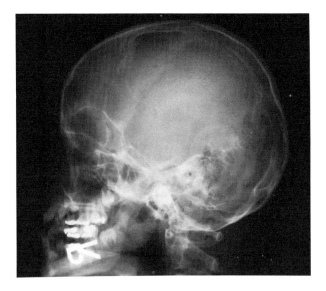

Fig. 236:
Brachymicrocephaly in a $9\frac{1}{2}$ year-old girl untreated so far. Flattening and asymmetry of occipital skull-vault, rough sella, hypoplasia of the middle face, high density of the cranial bone.

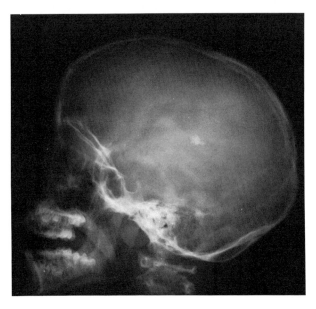

Fig. 237:
Cranial proportions in a 9-year-old mongol girl treated since early childhood. The cranial dimensions are slightly inferior to the normal figures, good relief of the cranium vault. Calcification of the plexus.
The children were compared because they came for the (first, repeated) examinations on the same day immediately one after the other.

The following principles result from the biostatistical evaluation of a prospective study on 200 non-selected mongoloid children before the treatment and after 2–3 implantations:

1. An increase of the cranial-size index can be obtained in about 2/3 of the cases treated.

2. The increase is not restricted to infancy and babyhood, as supposed formerly, but can be brought about also in the early years of school time.

3. The increase of the cranial-size index depends gradually on the initial situation; in other words: the greater the deficit of the size of the cranium at the

Tab. 27: **Effect of various tissular combinations on the growth of the skull size in 761 implantations**

Sex, age, initial situation and succession of implantations are not taken into consideration in this summation (with negative values subtracted).

Combinations of tissues		increase of volume index
cerebral hemisphere	+ mesencephalon	54,3 %
	+ diencephalon	54,3 %
	+ hypothalamus	54,3 %
	+ hypophysis	36,1 %
	+ frontal brain	36,1 %
cerebral cortex	+ hypophysis	49 %
	+ diencephalon	41,8 %
	+ hypothalamus	41,8 %
	+ mesencephalon	41,8 %
Occipital brain	+ diencephalon	36 %
	+ hypothalamus	36 %
	+ mesencephalon	30 %
parietal brain	+ diencephalon	12,8 %
	+ hypothalamus	12,8 %
	+ mesencephalon	15,6 %

beginning of the treatment, the more the size of the cranium increases after the implantations.

4. The essential effect is seen after the first implantation; after the second implantation, the indices reach a distribution pattern corresponding to Gauss's bell i. e. they range within the normal tolerance.

5. Gradually the best effects are attained by combinations of 100 mg of an deeper cerebral area (diencephalon, hypothalamus, mesencephalon) with a hemisphere- or cortical preparation (cerebral cortex, cerebral hemisphere); Tab. 27.

6. The biostatistical remarks relate only to anthropometric measures, which show no strict correlation with the function of the brain i. e. mental efficiency.

Efficiency of the therapy

Assessing and proving the success and shortcomings of a therapy require special factors if a clinical aspect with more than 200 possible individual symptoms is in question. Among them are:

a) a great number of observations;
b) a steady observation over several years;
c) differentiated, provable criteria (parameters).

The first two conditions are fulfilled by treatments of 1780 mongoloid children over 1–25 years. Criteria for assessments were there by hundreds and thousands but could not be evaluated until the «spontaneous development» of untreated mongoloids had been cleared biostatistically. Most of the supporting data had to be established because the medical science had until then been satisfied with global, non-founded, data in this field.

Tab. 28: **Average ages of mothers and fathers of mong. children by the years of the age classes of the children**

Age class	Number of cases	Average ages of mothers	fathers
1953–1961	30	35,0	36,6
1962–1965	54	33,85	35,9
1966	32	32,9	34,0
1967	29	33,5	36,0
1968	54	32,8	34,5
1969	71	33,5	35,5
1970	67	34,2	36,7
1971	61	33,5	36,5
1972	70	32,6	35,3
1973	70	33,7	36,8
1974	51	33,7	36,5
1975	29	31,9	33,9
1979	56	32,1	
1980	64	28,3	
1981	47	30,9	35,1
total	785		

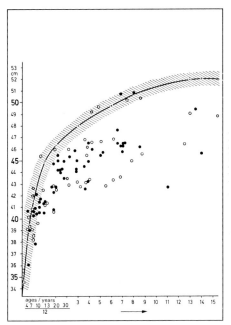

Fig. 238:
Three-dimensional brain-skull quotient

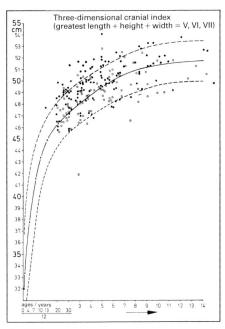

Fig. 239:
Three-dimensional brain-skull quotient

Three-dimensional cranial index (greatest
length + height + width = V, VI, VII)

in medically untreated Downs-children:
(n = 100 mongoloids;
● = boys
○ = girls)

(n = 200 mongoloids, including the 100 cases
of fig. 238
● = boys
○ = girls)

Most measurements are clearly below to normal
variations.

After the second inj. implantation of fet. cerebral tissue, the brain-skull-index is mostly normal.

The efficiency of the therapeutic
measures was largely proved to a degree
seldom possible in medical treatment.
The most important results have been
outlined hereafter:

1. Stature

Untreated mongoloids are of short to
dwarfed stature, boys averaging 148 cm,
girls 142. However, it must be stated that
also untreated children show considerable variations (plus/minus).

Conclusive information about the influence of the treatment on the stature
was not possible prior to an observation

period of 6 years and compiling some
1500 values measured. This surveyable
space of time shows clearly that the treatment influences the stature without
using growth hormones. As in the case of
other anthropometric values, the effect
differs according to sex. Long treated
males reach a final stature of some
161 cm (fig. 234), females 146 cm (1975
study; 1981: 151 cm). The influence of
the treatment has been demonstrated for
both sexes, especially so by the T-test
comparing the ages, and was up to 1976
slighter in girls than in boys.

The measured values remain constant

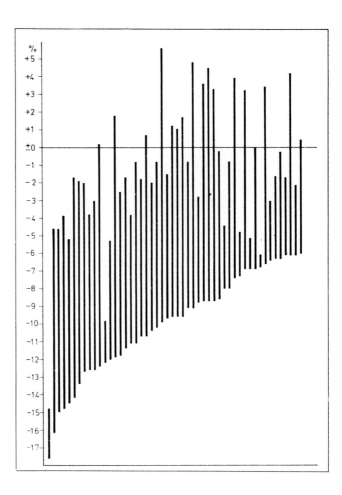

Fig. 240:
Increase of 3-dimensional skull-index in extremely microcephalic mongoloid children (initial values below −6% of normal; n = 50) after the first implantation of lyophilised fetal cerebral tissues. Chiefly considerably increased volumes.

if the therapy is continued. The final stature was about 161 cm for boys when a prospective examination was made in 1979. A changed succession of implantations by including adrenal and ovarian tissues in prepuberty improved the growth of the girls to an average final stature of 151 cm.

Circumference of the skull

Brachy-microcephaly is one of the most constant symptoms of Down's syndrome and is recorded in about 92% of all cases. At the first measurement in the first trimester of life the greatest fronto-occipital skull circumference is just below the normal values (39 cm compared with 41 cm in boys; 38,5 cm compared with 40 cm in girls). Up to the third year the deficiency increases (46.6 cm against 50 cm in boys and 46.2 cm against 48.6 cm in girls). While in mongoloid boys the deficiency becomes somewhat less up to puberty, in girls it remains constant. At the age of 18 years, untreated mongoloid boys have an average skull circumference of 52.7 cm and girls 50.9 cm.

In the 1979/1980 random group of treated children the average values were 53 cm (against 54.5 cm) in 14-year-old boys and 51.8 cm (against 54.0 cm) in girls. At the age of $17\frac{3}{12}$ years the corresponding comparative average values are

227

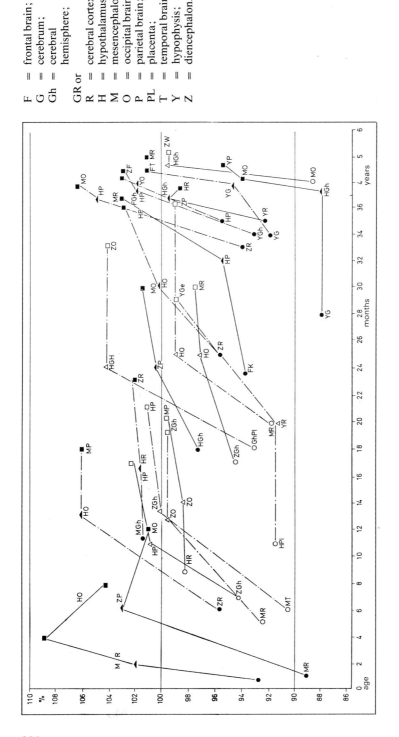

F = frontal brain;
G = cerebrum;
Gh = cerebral hemisphere;

GR or
R = cerebral cortex;
H = hypothalamus;
M = mesencephalon;
O = occipital brain;
P = parietal brain;
PL = placenta;
T = temporal brain;
Y = hypophysis;
Z = diencephalon.

Fig. 241:
Individual courses of the three-dimensional skull-index in 20 mongoloid children (● = boys, ○ = girls). Taking the average age as 100% mean value, the curves show the specific response of the skull growth to the various combinations of implants.
Circle = first implantation, triangle = second implantation, square = third implantation.

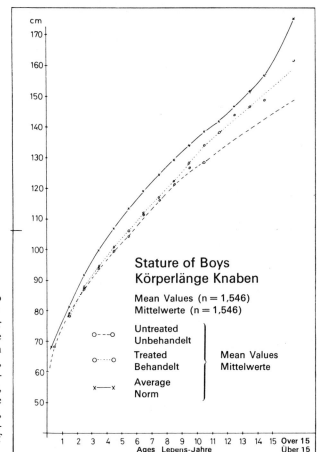

Fig. 242:
Average statures
Boys (n = 1546). The group of treated mongoloids (n = 981) is just slightly superior up to the 10th year to the group of untreated children (n = 565). For the untreated, a final tallness between 148–150 cm may be anticipated, the averages of the treated are about 161 cm and, therefore, in the middle between the untreated and the average of healthy boys (174).

53.4 cm (54.9 cm) in boys and 52 cm (54.4 cm) in girls. The skull circumference of boys reaches 97.3 % and that of girls 95.4 % of that of healthy comparative groups.

To improve the circumference of the head still more, a more specific (with medicaments or implantations) effect on the growth of the cartilaginous preformed base of the skull is necessary. Cartilage, osteoblasts and life as lyophilisates or hydrolysates should be used in the first three years of life (fig. 243).

3. Brain-volume index

Whereas the brain-size of untreated mongoloids retards gradually behind the normal average in the course of growth (with the main deficit evolving in the first three years of age), a treatment initiated in early infancy will normalize the index values much or completely. This follows from three-dimensional index measurements on radiographs. This effect can be achieved only with implantations by injections of fetal brain-tissue; an approximation of the skull-size index to the normal average is reached usually after 2–3 implantations (Tab. 27) (fig. 235, 237, 240, 241).

4. Analysis of development

In the course of a programmed analysis, the therapeutic effect on the motoric

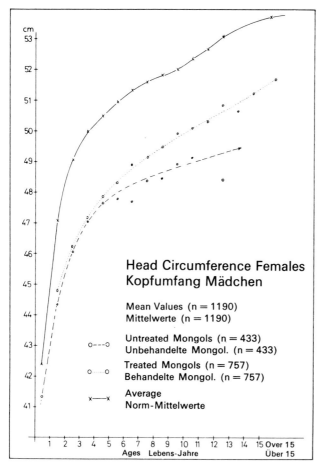

cm
53
52
51
50
49
48
47
46
45
44
43
42
41

Head Circumference Females
Kopfumfang Mädchen

Mean Values (n = 1190)
Mittelwerte (n = 1190)

o---o Untreated Mongols (n = 433)
       Unbehandelte Mongol. (n = 433)

o...o Treated Mongols (n = 757)
       Behandelte Mongol. (n = 757)

x—x   Average
       Norm-Mittelwerte

1 2 3 4 5 6 7 8 9 10 11 12 13 14 15 Over 15
      Ages Lebens-Jahre   Über 15

Fig. 243:
Averaged head circumferences
Girls (n = 1190). The treated
mongoloids (n = 757) show
from the fifth year a slight
plus over the untreated girls.
This difference increases with
the growing age; the considerable variations of the mean
values among the untreated.
At the end of the body
growth, the mean head circumferences of untreated
mongoloid girls are about
49.5 cm, and 51.5 cm in
treated mongoloid girls as
against 54.5 cm in healthy
girls.

development, fine motoric and coordi-nation, speech, social behaviour and mental development was studied in more than 4000 findings. Whereas un-treated children reach usually a state of development corresponding to that of a 4–6 year-old patient, the results achieved by the treatment came up to the criteria of 8–12-year-old children. This creates important conditions for social integra-tion and for learning the elementary cultivation of mind.

5. Intelligence quotient

The retardation of mongoloid chil-dren affects above all their instellectual capacity. The findings on the intelli-gence quotient outside the author's clin-ic showed a considerably higher average of the intelligence age of treated mongo-loid children. The intelligence quotient found in infants range from 60–90, and an average increase of the intelligence quotient by 20 points effected by treat-ment can be ascertained at all ages.

6. Cultivation of the mind

Whereas formerly mongoloid chil-dren were considered listless and non-educable, and educational efforts cen-tred on practical training, it has become increasingly obvious that treatment can certainly make the majority of these chil-dren learn to read, to write and to speak.

Curves of growth

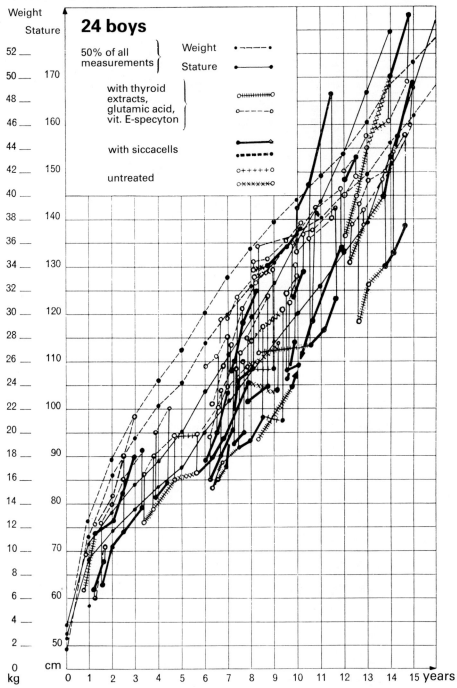

Fig. 244: Courses of the growth of statures in 24 mongoloid boys treated by various methods (H. S. Feldmann, 1979).

Fig. 245–247:
Scenic representations by mongoloid children

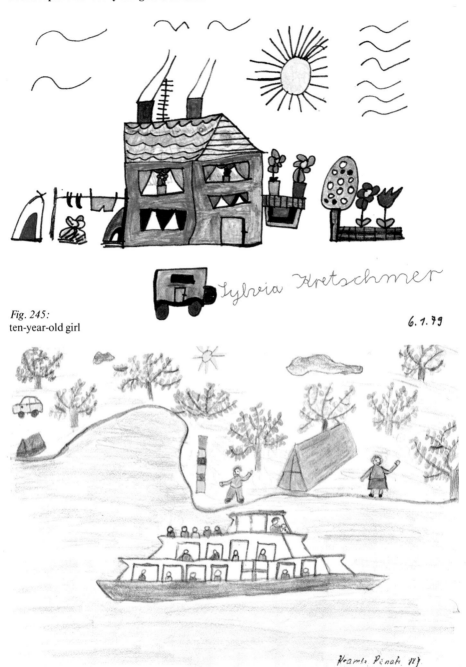

Fig. 245:
ten-year-old girl

Fig. 246:
twelve-year-old girl

232

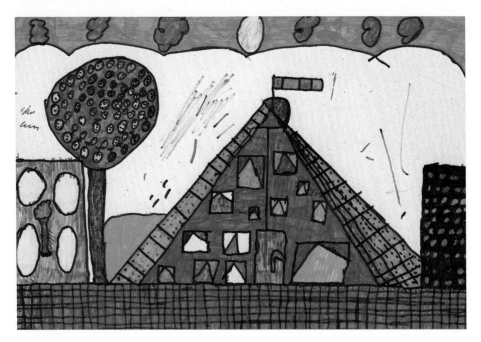

Fig. 247:
fourteen-year-old boy

The important thing is to begin early with the pedagogical work. In most cases, the possibilities of pedagogical training made available by modern medical methods are not utilized sufficiently.

7. Creative capacities

If mongoloid children are early, i. e. in late infancy, encouraged to learn techniques of elementary cultivation of the mind and through play are acquainted with creative activities (handwork, painting), they may sometimes achieve remarkable creative results, especially in the field of descriptive drawing and handicraft. Everything will depend on a good encouragement within the family and at school (fig. 244–247).

8. Morbidity

According to the latest extensive statistical findings (OSTER, 1953); RECORD and SMITH, 1955; CARTER, 1958),

50–60% of untreated mongoloid children die during the first five years of infection of the respiratory passages (pneumonia, stenosing laryngotracheobronchitis), hyperpyretic infections, infections of the gastrointestinal tract and of heart-failure.

In contrast to these statistical data, which have probably improved somewhat during the last few years, 1780 patients observed by the author have shown that the predisposition of mongoloid children to illness under long-term treatment is not greater than that in normal children of the same age. The risk of illness is much reduced by the treatment and comes close to the normal average. Adequate basic medication is a prerequisite.

9. Mortality

In contrast to earlier data (see above), the mortality of the mongoloid children

233

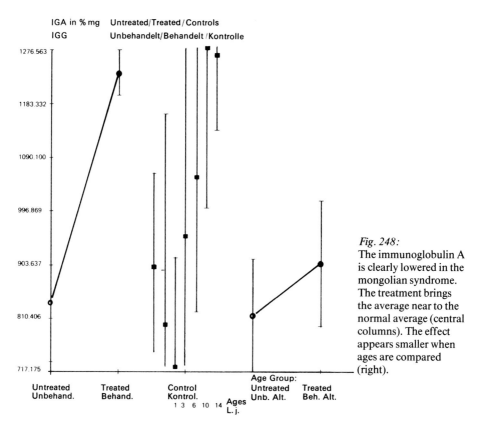

IGA in % mg   Untreated/Treated/Controls
IGG   Unbehandelt/Behandelt/Kontrolle

Untreated   Treated   Control   Age Group: Untreated   Treated
Unbehand.   Behand.   Kontrol. Unb. Alt.   Beh. Alt.
                      1 3 6 10 14 Ages
                                  L. j.

Fig. 248:
The immunoglobulin A is clearly lowered in the mongolian syndrome. The treatment brings the average near to the normal average (central columns). The effect appears smaller when ages are compared (right).

and youngsters is below 3 per cent among the author's patients. The latest statistics established between 1950 and 1960 confirmed for mongoloids a death rate exceeding about 20 times that of the normal average. The reduction of the death rate of children to the level of the normal population may be looked upon as one of the greatest results of the long-term treatment. The rest of the deaths within the first ten years of age were chiefly caused by congenital heart-failure serious enough to influence the children's fate alone. The second important cause of death among the treated cases was traffic accidents.

Life expectancy of mongoloid children cannot yet be indicated definitely because this would require observations of at least 2–3 decades. The long-term treatments conducted so far cover 1–20 years. Life expectancy of mongoloid children is nearly the same compared with the age-groups of a «normal» population.

10. Immunological functions

The shift within the pattern of immunoglobulins helps much to reduce the resistance to infection in untreated mongoloid children. Whilst the recurrent infections usually augment the immunoglobulins G, there is a lack of immunoglobulins A and M. Comparative studies on 142 cases showed that the treatment brings the deficient immunoglobulins clearly to a point approximating the normal average (fig. 248, 249) though that average is not attained. Moreover, the resistance to infection is improved. Only children which already suffered from

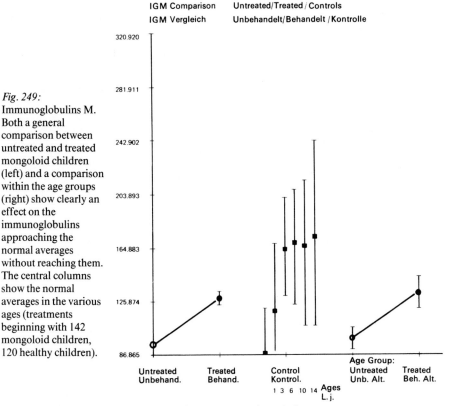

IGM Comparison   Untreated/Treated / Controls
IGM Vergleich   Unbehandelt/Behandelt /Kontrolle

Fig. 249:
Immunoglobulins M.
Both a general
comparison between
untreated and treated
mongoloid children
(left) and a comparison
within the age groups
(right) show clearly an
effect on the
immunoglobulins
approaching the
normal averages
without reaching them.
The central columns
show the normal
averages in the various
ages (treatments
beginning with 142
mongoloid children,
120 healthy children).

Untreated   Treated   Control   Untreated   Treated
Unbehand.   Behand.   Kontrol.   Unb. Alt.   Beh. Alt.

Age Group:

1 3 6 10 14 Ages
L. j.

chronic infections in the upper respiratory tract (sinusitis, chronic rhinitis, adenoids) before the treatment will react less favourably for a short while.

11. Biochemical parameters

Of the biochemical changes occurring with the mongolism syndrome, the following are of major consequence for retardation:

low serotonin level;

disturbed tryptophane metabolism;

disturbed metabolisms of the vitamins B1, B2 and B6;

disturbed taurin metabolism;

values of uric acid increasing progressively with age;

increase of certain intracellular enzymes;

reduced serum iron;

elevated transferrin;

reduced zinc;

low extracellular calcium levels caused by early calcinosis; comparatively high intracellular aluminium levels, low levels of potassium, manganese and selenium.

It is not yet possible to describe definitely the effect of general treatment on the biochemical aberrations; whilst certain factors (e. g. iron vitamin B2, vitamin B6, uric acid) may well be influenced, the therapeutic concept has still not yet been elaborated to obtain regular patterns. Specially in this field, the therapeutic goals are still too new.

12. Physiognomy

The facies of an untreated mongoloid is characterized by the distorted proportions of the head and the resulting changed physiognomy: slanting palpebral fissures; epicanthus; hypertelorism; short, flat nose; drooping corners of the mouth; flat middle part of the face; small skull, flat occiput; short, fat neck.

The chance of influencing the physiognomy depends on the time when the treatment is initiated and on how consistently it is conducted. If the therapy is started in early infancy and at the age of three at the latest, the generally unaesthetic appearance can largely be modified. Photographs from long-term studies in individual cases and comparisons between consistently treated children of different age have shown great differences between treated and untreated mongoloids (fig. 250–252).

13. Socialisation

As also untreated mongoloids may spontaneously show a favourable development, most of the mongoloids were considered as unsuited for integration into society, a view frequently leading to the suggestion that the children should be sent to an asylum. Life in an asylum, therefore, was a predestinate fate for untreated mongoloid children.

Treated mongoloid children, particularly those treated at an early age, are definitely enabled to reach a condition assuring their full integration into their families and environment. A poll on the social situation in 220 cases has revealed that the parent – child relation and the children's reaction to their environment are not problematic in most cases.

14. Motor ability

Untreated mongoloid children show a deficient motoric and kinetic ability. The physical appearance is usually limp, with stooping shoulders, dropped lower jaw with mouth open, gawky and straddling gait.

This condition, too, can largely be remedied by treatment, with major impor-

tance attributed to systematic physiotherapy in early infancy. The improvements include kinetic reactions, handling of musical instruments (even the piano), working materials and mechanical toys, weaving and gymnastics.

15. Clinical symptoms

For the most important symptoms of more than 200, findings have revealed that long-term treatments can repair well over one third, another third can provide improvement and less than a third cannot be influenced (Tab. 24).

The list of clinical manifestations responding to treatment is not complete. Yet, comprehensive clinical and biostatistical data for the above-mentioned fields are available whereas other fields, as metabolism, lack sufficient investigation. Considering the great numbers of tested and proved measurements and the exceptionally many cases observed, the remark uttered frequently by certain institutions and persons that «no therapeutic success has been demonstrated so far for mongolism» can be denoted only as anachronistic cynism for the parents of retarded children or, possibly as an excuse for own failure.

Development

If in development (= unfolding of the biological powers inherent in the living organism) one sees a complex system of characteristics (present or missing), then it is in principle wrong to try to express this complexity in the abstract figures of an IQ (Intelligence Quotient) or a DQ (Development Quotient). An analysis of development which does justice to the overall biological situation of humans has to consider the following components separately:
a) Coarse motoricity statics
b) Fine motoricity coordination
c) Speech

Fig. 250–252:
Physiognomical changes
in the course of an early
consistent therapy

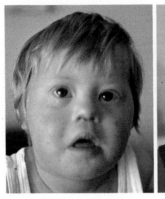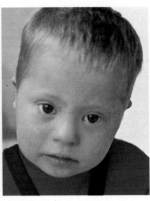

Fig. 250:
Mongol. boy with chronic
infections of the upper
respiratory passages
a)   before treatment
b)   5 months later

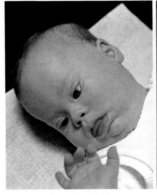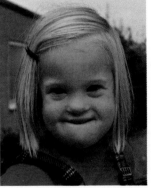

Fig. 251:
Mongol. girl with typical
physiognomical changes
a) at the age of 4 months
b) with aesthetical
    physiognomy after a
    5-year treatment

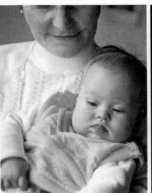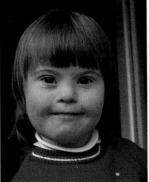

Fig. 252:
Mongol. girl, whose
treatment began when she
was 7 months old (a), $4\frac{1}{2}$
years later (b).

d) Social development
e) Intellectual development

With a development analysis which has been in use for over ten years, 200 criteria (parameters) can be checked. The individual function must be easy to check and the questions must be answerable by the parents, without any question of doubt. The development tempo is symbolized in a pseudologarithmic, vertically oriented system. At the annual follow-up examinations it does not matter when a function was learned, but rather whether it is (or was) mastered or not. In this way one gains a comprehensive visual overview of the capacities and the failures, the latter at the same time indicating an immediate need for treatment. This analysis is in direct contrast to an IQ

Longitudinal course development.

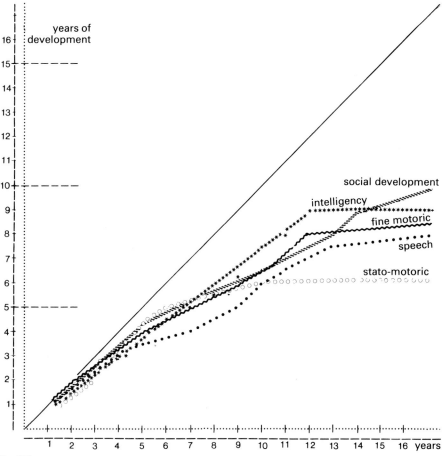

Fig. 253:
Longitudinal course of development in 374 children with Down's syndrome from a prospective investigation carried out in 1980. While in infancy the development almost corresponds to that is retarded. The highest average values which are children with Down's syndrome, of school age, of the average normal child, the development of reached are in intellectual development and social development, which at the age of 14 years correspond to those of normal children aged $9\frac{1}{2}$ years and $10\frac{1}{2}$ years, respectively (for details, see text).

238

test, which only results in classification into a particular category and has certain advantages but only for official purposes.

If one today (1981) analyses a random sample of children with Down's syndrome who have been treated with drugs on a relatively uniform basis, but whose education and social care has been very different, the development status is as set out below. «Random sample» means children and adolescents with Down's syndrome, with and without other anomalies (e.g. heart defects, gastrointestinal abnormalities etc.), studied over a prospectively defined period. This analysis gives the following average state of development in 14-year-old children with Down's syndrome (Fig. 253):

a) Coarse motoricity statics: average equivalent age 7 years
b) Fine motoricity coordination: average equivalent age 8 years
c) Speech: average equivalent age 9 years
d) Social development: average equivalent age $10\frac{1}{2}$ years
e) Intellectual development: average equivalent age $9\frac{1}{2}$ years

These retardation values have a range of variation of ± 2 years. Surprising at first was the considerable retardation in motoricity. When one takes into account, however, that after early infancy almost nothing is done as far as motor training is concerned, then this result is understandable, but it does demonstrate the need for therapy during a neglected phase of development.

Of far-reaching significance, however, are the average values in speech, social and intellectual development. If for these, which are very important as far as scholastic advancement is concerned, one takes as a basis an average equivalent age of $9\frac{1}{2}$ years (with a maximum of 12 years), then this means that

the school programm of the first three primary-school classes can and must be made available to children with Down's syndrome.

It is a tragedy that in many «special schools» syllabuses are used in the first three years which are at a lower level than that of the last year in the normal kindergarten. At the age of 8 of 9 years a child with Down's syndrome is generally no longer capable of meeting the normal demands of school to the desired extent, if he has not already acquired a consciousness of achievement and learned to concentrate and persevere at the age of 6 and 7 years. The syllabus of the first three primary school classes, taken at a slower pace than normal, covers, to the limited extent to be expected in these children, reading, writing and arithmetic.

This basic schooling, combined with a good social structure and a mostly above average memory capacity, is the prerequisite for taking up an occupation, under guidance and supervision. The «intellectualization» of most forms of occupational training have certainly made it difficult for those with only average gifts to take up most occupations. These training and apprenticeship regulations have made it completely impossible for the handicapped to complete an occupational training adapted to their practical abilities. It is laws and regulations which present the greatest obstacles to the advancement of the handicapped in their schooling and their working life. Wherever it has been possible to overcome these obstacles adolescents with Down's syndrome have proved themselves to be conscientious, friendly, polite, clean and in most cases also responsible helpers. Social occupations (e.g.

239

hospital orderlies or assistants) suit them best.

How has the fate of mongoloids changed?

In contrast to the situation existing between 1866 and 1970 it is today no longer disputed that children with Down's syndrome should be treated, nor do people in fact warn against treating them any longer, but the argument still goes on about how to treat them. While a minority of authors, who seem to be totally uninfluenced by the knowledge of the efforts being made in this field worldwide, still propagate «affection» as their main advice, the principal line of attack today in fact ranges between «cytotherapy» and the other methods of treatment. «Whether» has been replaced by «How?». As a result, the sociological and medical situation of patients with Down's syndrome has changed decisively.

The majority of mongoloid children today attend a normal kindergarten without integration problems. The learning effect of the «normal» environment cannot be estimated too highly. Almost all mongoloid children go to school, 5 % to primary and elementary schools, 22 % to special schools for learning handicapped children and the remainder to special schools for the mentally handicapped. With a few exceptions, such children born in the last 12 years grow up within their families and are hardly ever felt to be «handicapped» by those around them. Whereas up until a few years ago children with Down's syndrome were still excluded from all social insurance schemes, here too there has been a clear change, although a really satisfactory solution still has to be found.

If all the therapeutic possibilities are used, then the overall biological situation of children with Down's syndrome today approaches more closely the average for the normal population than the previous classification under the designation «mongolism». In contrast to the irresponsible claim that therapeutic successes «have not been proven», extensive comparative studies of many different parameters are now available which provide evidence of the effects of therapy. Table 29 gives an overview of this, which will be discussed in detail in the following chapters.

The argument between the theorists about which method of treatment provides the decisive therapeutic effect is futile, because it is with the wholistic therapy that one strives to promote and develop the personality of the patient – assessments on the value of the individual therapeutic steps are not the important thing.

Table 29: **Comparative investigations between untreated and treated children with Down's syndrome are available in the following parameters:**

1. Height
2. Body weight
3. Circumference of the skull
4. Cranial volume index
5. Physiognomy
6. Motor development
7. Fine motoricity coordination
8. Speech development
9. Social development
10. Intellectual development
11. Morbidity
12. Mortality
13. Immunglobulins
14. Metabolic investigations:
    a) Vitamins B_1, B_2, B_6
    b) Na, Cl, K, Fe, Cu, Mn, Zn, Mg, Ca
    c) Ferroxidase I
    d) Transferrin
15. Scholastic situation
16. Creative capacities

The therapy of Down's syndrome as adopted nowadays is one of the most convincing and satisfactory fields of pediatrics. Development during recent years has shown that improved basic knowledge of the biochemical processes has helped to perfect increasingly the therapeutic concept. This therapy is probably the best possible now available but still far from being optimal. Further developments based on present knowledge may necessarily be anticipated for the next years.

Gonosome aberrations

The female determination is localized in the X-chromosome, the male determination in the Y-chromosome. The female sex is homogametic XX, the male is heterogametic XY. There are gonosome aberrations in the structure, in the number and in mosaic combinations.

Turner's syndrome

is the most frequent numeric aberration of the gonosomes. A monosomy X (caryotype: 45, X) is characterized by a number of obligatory and facultative somatic symptoms:

nanism with sexual infantilism; dysgenetic of hypoplastic ovaries; hypoplasy of the genitals, lack of mammae; primary amenorrhoea; increased secretion of gonadotropin in the urine.

After the first description by ULLRICH (1930), the aspect has been augmented by multiple facultative abnormalities, referred to as *Ullrich-Turner's syndrome* or as *Status Bonnevie-Ullrich.*

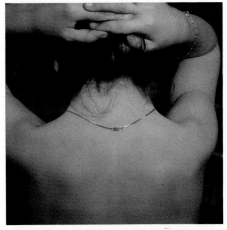 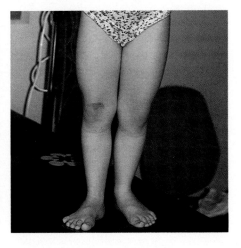

Fig. 254 a, b: Turner's syndrome (45 X)
Carried to term, weighing 2250 g and having a stature of 47 cm when born, nanism ascertained at age of 1 year. (79 cm, − 16 cm), 10.3 kg at three years. Typical symptoms: disproportionate nanism, pterygium, small ears, deep limit of hair, shield thorax, atypical finger furrow, male physical appearance (a, b).

To these symptoms belong:
poker face;
deep limit of the cervical hair (fig. 254 a);
pterygium colli;
carp's mouth;

multiple pigmented naevi;
hypoplastic mamillae deficient in pigment,
cubitus valgus;
shortened metacarpal IV;
stenosed aortic isthmus.

Besides these two nosological conditions, there is moreover the *pure gonad dysgenesia (Swyer's syndrome)*, a defective development of the gonads and of the secondary sex characteristics without any further corporal stigmata.

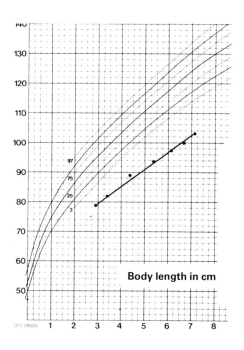

Body length in cm

Fig. 254c, Turner's syndrome (45 X)
Regular implantations of adrenal gland, ovary, diencephalon (every dose: 200 mg of lyophilisate) at intervals of 6 months, ovibion, later combined with cortiron, brought the growth rate to about 6 cm per year so that the deficit of stature has not much increased since the treatment began (c).

Male Turner's syndrome

Cytogenetically determined by the chromatin-negative karyotype 46, XY, this aspect is also called *«testicular germinal dysgenesis»*, *«male gonad dysgenesis»* or *«Noonan syndrome»*. The symptoms are the same as those of Turner's syndrome, with infantilism, hypoplasy of the testicles and nanism as the most important. Lymphangiectatic oedemata and skeletal abnormalities especially on the hands (brachycarpy, brachydactylia) are more frequent, pigmented naevi rarer than in female Turner's syndrome. The testicles are hypoplastic, dystoptic and secondarily injured with advancing age. There are less 17-ketosteroids in the urine. The gonadotropin level is low also after puberty (hypoganadotropic hypoganadism). There is no or little secondary hairiness on the body, the development of bone is evidently retarded (fig. 255); adults develop osteoporosis and premature regression (HIENZ). X-

monosomy has not yet been detected in male Turner's syndrome.

Fig. 255 a, b, c:
Male Turner's syndrome ▶
A boy of 8 years, who moreover suffers from a valvular pulmonary stenosis, is presented for the first time with a nanism of minus 18 cm. Dystrophy, mild ptosis bilaterally, deep ears, shield thorax; breeches-like thighs, the testicles are small and soft, palpable in the inguinal canal. An extremely loud, high-frequent, long-drawn-out noise due to the valvular pulmonary stenosis can be heard. The ossification at this time corresponds to that of a $4\frac{1}{2}$-year-old boy and thus conforms much to the real stature (a).
Beginning of treatment by implantation of 100 mg of male adrenal gland, 100 mg of hypothalamus and 120 mg of testis.
Basic treatment: cortiron and primogonyl.
With implantations at half-year intervals, the boy grows 14.5 cm within $2\frac{1}{2}$ years, shows a growth rate (c) somewhat above average during that time and recovers much of the deficit also with respect to the ossification. The testes have grown, but still palpable in the inguinal canal.

242

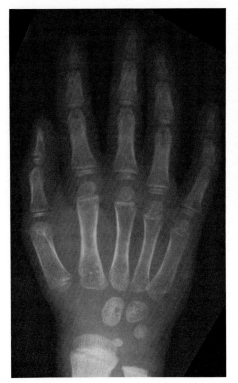

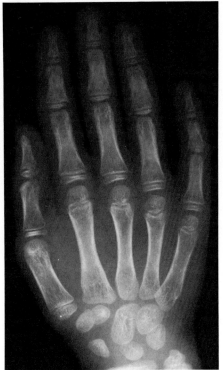

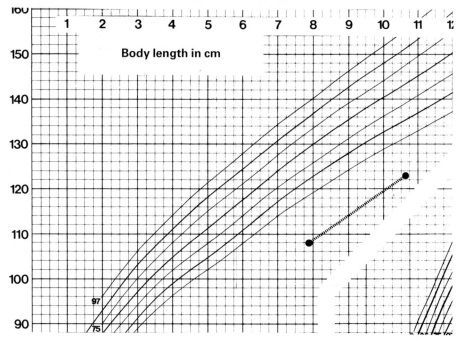

Fig. 255 a, b, c

is based on the constellation XXY of the sex-chromosomes. As the picture varies much with the central symptoms hypogonadism plus high-growth, Klinefelter's syndrome is referred to as classical (XXY) and atypical; numerical, structural aberrations and sex-chromosome mosaics are found in various constellations. The nucleo-morphological findings are chromatin-positive. The testicles are hypoplastic due to tubular sclerosis and hyperplasy of interstitional cells.

The facultative symptoms comprise:

partial baldness;
scanty or lacking beard,
gynecomastia,
hairiness of female pubes,
osteoporosis.

The structural build includes the following types: eunuchoid, dysplastic, somatically normal and pyknic-feminine-matronlike.

Celltherapeutic approaches

Sufficient experience on cell treatments of chromosome abnormalities is not available. Nevertheless, observations justify the postulation to treat with cell therapy these gonosome abnormalities, which cannot be influenced otherwise. Of the 9 Turner's syndromes (7 of them observed for several years), the female syndromes have shown different courses, the male syndromes astonishing results. During the first ten years, especially the effects on the growth of the build indicate success or failure, and no respective results can be anticipated for the female Turner's syndrome after the 10th year of age.

For the male Turner's syndrome, however, the effects on the growth of the body, the ossification, the social behaviour and the impulse are convincing (fig. 255 a–c); not only the growth rate is normalized but also the lacking ossification is largely completed (fig. 255 b, c).

For female Turner's syndrome,

female adrenal gland	100 mg
ovary	120 mg
hypothalamus	100 mg
alternating with:	
placenta	150 mg
ovary	120 mg
female adrenal gland	100 mg

are used at intervals of 5–6 months.

A substitutive basic therapy with $2-3 \times \frac{1}{2}$ tabl. of cortiron per week and ovibion dosed according to age daily is recommended even if an objective outcome cannot be proved.

For male Turner's syndrome, the following doses are applied alternately at intervals of 5–6 months:

hypothalamus	100 mg
male adrenal gland	100 mg
testicles	120 mg
and diencephalon	100 mg
placenta of male fetus	150 mg
male adrenal	100 mg.

The basic therapy should use $3 \times \frac{1}{2}$ – 3×1 tabl. of cortiron per week, according to age.

Experience with Klinefelter's syndrome is not yet available, a therapy is certainly promising here, too.

Genetic aberrations

The genetic i.e. hereditary illnesses and abnormalities comprise nosological units under the mode of inheritance. According to this individual criterium, dominant, recessive and sex-linked hereditary diseases are comprised. The cellular primary defect and the clinical symptoms give heterogeneous and heteromorphous pictures.

On principle, *enzymes or substrates* or both metabolic components can be affected. The connection between these biochemical constituents is outlined in fig. 256 a, b. Enzymes are pilots catalyzing the transformation of biochemical substances without being part of the balance of this process. Normally, a substrate (1) is conveyed into another substrate (2) by an enzyme (alpha) (fig. 256 a).

The damming up overcharges the cell with undigested metabolites, disturbances of the cellular metabolism, inflation of the cytoplasm, storage.

The absence or want of substrate 2 causes the interruption of the metabolic chain at this point, from which disturbances of growth and development, dystrophy, skeletal abnormalities result.

These then are the two cardinal processes in innate metabolic disturbances, and the important clinical aspects have been compiled in Tab. 22, 30, 31. This survey of a group of more than 400 known metabolic abnormalities, seen from the genetic and the clinical point of view, shows that the enzymopathies prevail, followed by the metabolic tissular systems mesenchyme (skeleton) and the central nervous system.

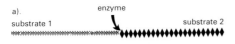 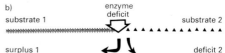

Fig. 256 a, b:
Principle of the metabolic disorders. A chemical substrate is changed into a substrate 2 by the pilot-function of an enzyme (a). The enzyme does not go into the bilance of the process. If the (b) enzyme is insufficient or lacks, a surplus of substrate 1 (= storage, intracellular poisoning), on the one hand, and a lack of substrate 2 (= interruption of the metabolic chain, dysfunction or failure, disturbed development) will take place.

So if this enzyme lacks or is reduced, the substrate 2 cannot or not sufficiently be formed. The two resulting biological consequences are

a) excess (damming up, storage) of substrate 1 because it cannot be metabolisized further;
b) lack of the substrate 2 because it is not synthetized, which means metabolic insufficiency on this level.

More important for clinic and therapy than the adjectives «dominant» and «recessive» is knowledge of the subcellular localisation of the disorder and the affected biochemical substances: enzymes, substrates or both. Sticking to the hereditary adjectives favours the therapeutic nihilism, the knowledge of the origin and of the substances in question provokes action.

Tab. 30: **Genetic development disorders**

A. Dominant	B. Sex-linked – hereditary
tuberous cerebral sclerosis (Bourneville-Pringle's syndrome) H.-Lindau's syndrome neurofibromatosis chorea huntington dystrophia myotonica Moebius's syndrome (diplegia facialis cong.) Sturge-Weber's syndrome Oxycephaly (due premature suture-synostosis) dysostosis craniofacialis (Crouzon) Apert's syndrome (acrocephalo-syndactyly, type I, II) Goldenhar's syndrome (oculo-auriculo-vertebral dysplasia) Treacher-Collins's syndrome (dysostosis mandibulo-facialis) Franceschetti's syndrome Noonan's syndrome Christ-Siemens-Tourraine's syndrome (hypohidrotical ectodermal dysplasia maxillary hypoplasia) Engelmann's disease (progressive diaphysical dysplasia)	Mucopolysaccharidosis (Pf.-Hurler's syndr.) gangliosidosis progressive muscular dystrophy Lowe's syndrome (oculo-cerebro-renal syndrome) Lesch-Nyhan's syndrome incontinentia pigmenti (Bloch-Sulzberger's syndrome) Norrie-Warburg's syndrome resistance to vasopressin familial hyperuricalmia **C. Recessive-hereditary (significant or probable)** Amaurotic idiocy (gangliosidosis) phenylketonuria galactosaemia endemic struma maple-sirup disease homocystinuria hyperhistidinaemia

Therapeutic methods

The so far scarce therapeutic methods rely on two principles, namely the elimination of the dammed up substances by withdrawal (e. g. food poor in phenylalanin in cases of phenylketonuria) or the substitution of the lacking enzyme (e. g. digestive enzymes in cystic pancreatic fibrosis). A reasonable treatment of the innate metabolic diseases, therefore, is restricted to a few forms because the pathological chain is virtually not changed.

It would be more promising to try and influence the subcellular source of the aberrations by cellular organelles (mitochondria, lysosomes, membranes) but the necessary preparations are not available in an adequate concentration. Only tissues and cellular suspensions can be supplied for practical use so that the proportion between the active ingredients and ballast substances for cellular injections is not favourable.

Reproduceable effects were meanwhile demonstrated for a considerable number of metabolic diseases but the therapeutic action is limited as to time and quality. Observations have been made for:

mucopolysaccharidosis (fig. 310);
gangliosidosis;
Noonan's syndrome;
hyperammonaemia;
cystinosis;

Familial dysautonomy
 (Riley-Day-syndrome)
alkaptonuria
albinism
Hartnup's syndrome
cystathionurie
arginin-succinic-acid imbecility
citrullinuria
hyperammonemia
cystinosis
gluco-amino-phosphat-diabetes
hyperglycemia
histidinemia
imidazolaciduria
hyperprolinemia
hydroxyprolinemia
Joseph's syndrome
Oasthouse-urine syndrome
familial genetic microcephaly
Grigler-Najjar syndrome
porphyria erythropoetica
hypophosphatasia

Neuro-ectodermal symptom prevalence

Ataxia teleangiektatica
 (Louis-Bar's syndrome)
Sjörgen-Larson's syndrome

Cockayne-Neil's syndrome (nanism)
pigmentxerodermia
Rothmund's syndrome (congen.
 poikilodermia)
Friedreichs-ataxia
Canavan's disease (spongy
 degeneration of the central nervous
 system)
Alexander's disease (megencephalia
 and hyaline panneuropathia)

Mesenchymal or polytope symptoms

Craniostenoses
 (premature suture-synostosis)
acrocephalo-syndactyly
osteopetrosis (infantile form)
pyknodysostosis
Laurence-Moon-Biedl-Bardet's
 syndrome
Conradi-Huenermann's syndrome
 (chondroangiopathia calc.)
Ellis-van-Creveld's syndrome
 (chondroektodermal dysplasia)
Smith-Lemli-Opitz's syndrome
Zellweger's syndrome
 (cerebro-hepatorenal syndrome)
Meckel's syndrome (splanchnocystic
 dysencephaly)
Fanconi's syndrome (anaemia)

gluco-amino-phosphate diabetes;
Grigler-Najjar's syndrome (fig. 257);
tuberous cerebral sclerosis (fig. 275);
Christ-Siemens-Tourraine's syndrome (fig. 290);
progressive muscular dystrophy;
Louis-Bar's syndrome (fig. 206);
Rothmund's syndrome (fig. 289);
Friedreichs's ataxia (fig. 275);
Ellis-van-Creveld's syndrome;
Fanconi's syndrome (fig. 322).

In cellular therapy, one should rely on the clinical guiding symptoms, the supposed or statistically established locali-sation in the organs, cells or cellular organelles. Irrespective of these special requirements as appearing from the synoptic Tab. 30, the doses of fetal liver (150 mg of the lyophilisate) and sex-specific placenta (150 mg of lyophilisate) seem to exert generally the most favourable effect of innate metabolic diseases. Examples are shown in the fig. 206, 257, 274, 275, 276, 277, 278, 289, 290, 310. Special attention should be paid to a reasonable medication and dietetic concomitant therapy for innate metabolic disorders.

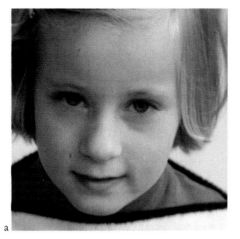
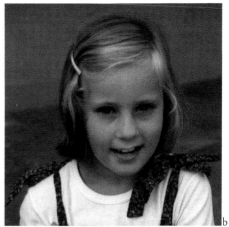

a

b

Fig. 257:
Grigler-Najjar's syndrome. At 6 years (a) icterus, serum-bilirubin values between 25–35 mg%, reduction of speech, increasing ataxia; at 10 years (b) bilirubin about 25 mg%, scanning and distinct speech, ataxia remedied.

As far as multiple disabilities with symptoms centred in the central nervous system are in question, the synoptic concept of an integral medical treatment will be discussed in detail hereafter.

Tab. 31: **Metabolic disorders**

Of the more than 400 known metabolic disorders, those of importance have been listed in a synopsis by R. G. SCHMID (1979). It has been divided into classes of matter in metabolic disturbances of carbohydrates, fat, amino-acids, porphyrin, plasma-protein, metals, vitamins and purin. The table, intended to be used as a guide in the practice, comprises definitions of the basic disturbances, clinical guiding symptoms, frequency and age-disposition and diagnostic proofs. The data have been taken from: H. OPITZ and F. SCHMID, 1965; U. STEININGER and H. THEILE, 1974; H. MEHNERT, 1975; K. SCHREIER, 1979. ▶

Carbohydrate metabolism disorders

A. Enteral			
1. Disaccharidmalabsorption: Lactose/Saccharose/Isomaltose Primary/secondary forms	Diarrhea, dehydratation, dystrophia. In time of first milk meals, but various forms also at higher age.	H: dependent on type A: from birth	test for lactose tolerance test f. sacch. tol. biopsy of small intestine
2. Monosaccharidmalabsorption: glucose/galactose	Diarrhea – dehydratation when supplies of milk are initiated.	H: rare A: from birth	test for glucose tolerance test for galactose tolerance
B. Intermediary metabolism Metabolic disturbances of galactose: galactosaemia lack of galactokinase	Hyperbilirubinaemia, non appetite for drinking, vomiting, dystrophia, hepatomegalia, cataracts, spasm	H: 2–10 A: 0–18 M.	reduction samples + clinistix – enzymes in erythrocytes
2. Metabolic disturbances of fructose: intolerance to fructose Benign fructosuria Fructose 1,6 diphosphatase	vomiting, hypoglycaemia, hepatomegalia, laktatacidose, spasm. After beginning of fruit feeding.	H: 1–5 A: fruit feeding	reduction samples + clinistix – test for fructose tolerance
3. Glycogen storage disease: type I–X (Gierke, Pompe, Cori, Forbes)	Diabetes mellitus with frequent hypoglycaemia, hyperlipaemia, laktatacidose, cardiomegalia, hepatosplenomegalia	H: up to 0.5	sugar after fasting – fat values + test for glucagon + test for adrenalin +
C. Diabetes mellitus **1. Diabetes mellitus:**	acetonaemic vomiting, dyspepsia loss of weight, hypo/hyperglycaemia	H: 3000 A: old age	acetone-glucosuria blood sugar daily prof. test for fructose tolerance

H = frequency on 100.000; A = age in days, months (M) years (J.) any age (old age)

249

Disorders of complex carbohydrates

1. Mucopolysaccharidoses: type I–VII, Pfaundler-Hurler. Hunter. Sanfilippo, Morquio. Lamy.	facial dysmorphie, progressive dementia, nanism, convulsions, dysostosis multiplex, corneal disorders, hepatosplenomegalia	H: 1 A: 1–2–6 Y.	test for toluidin + urine of heparansulfat urine of keratansulfat urine of dermatansulfat
2. Mucosulfatidosis	like mucopolysaccharidosis + leukodystrophia	A: 1–3 Y.	prove in leukocytes
3. Mucolipidoses type I–III (I also sialidose)	like mucopolysaccharidosis	A: 0–4 Y.	prove in leukocytes
4. Fucosidosis I + II:	like mucopolysaccharidosis	A: 4–12 M	prove in fibroblasts
5. Mannosidosis:	like mucopolysaccharidosis	A: 1–3 Y.	prove in serum
6. Aspartylglucosaminuria:	like mucopolysaccharidosis, speech-disorder	A: 1–5 Y.	prove in urine

Fat-metabolism-disorders

A. Enteral **1. Cöliakia:**	Anorexia, vomiting, period. diarrhea, fatty stools, dystrophia, blown-out belly, steathorrhea	H: 100 A: 5 M–3 Y.	test for xylose 80 % + (blood) fats test for gluten-tolerance sucking biopsy small intestine
2. Mucoviscidosis	Mekoniumileus, pancr. insuff., offensive fatty stools, diarrhea and obstipation in menopause, dystrophia, chronic emphysembronchitis	A: 10–100 A: 0–2 Y.	test for sweat steathorrhoea + trypsin activity – iontophoresis
3. Enteritis: Gastroenteritis, colitis. Morbus Crohn, enterocolitis	gripes, nausea, muco-bleeding diarrhoea, obstipation possible, vomiting	H: 100 000 A: 0–old	test for morbific agents in stools fats in serum protein in serum – BSG + stom. – intest. – passage
B. Changed lipoprotein **1. Hyperlipoproteinaemia:** type I–V	nausea, vomiting, atherosclerosis, xanthoma hepatosplenomegalia, colic in the upper abdomen	H: up to 3000 A: 0 – old	blood fats unchanged lipidelectrophoresis
2. Hypolipoproteinaemia: blood fats lipidelectrophoresis unchanged	ataxia neuropathia, avitaminosis	H: rare A: 0 – old	

250

C. lipidosis **1. Niemann-pick:** type A – E	refusal of food, vomiting, hepatosplenomegaly, psychomotor retardation, red retina spot, hypotonic – ICP, idiocy	H: rare A: 6 m – 50 y	hypertriglyceriaemia hypercholesterinaemia osteomalacia thrombocytopenia
2. Morbus Gaucher: type I (adults) type II (infantile) type III (juvenile)	indigestion, (Hepato-)splenomegalia, hypertone ICP (type I), kachexie, idiocy night-blindness	H: till 50 A: 3 m – 20 y	Acid phosphatase pelvic osteolysis bone-marrow: Gaucher cells
3. Refsum's disease	night-blindness, paraesthesia, ataxia, paresis, attacks of pain	H: rare A: 2 – 20 y	Triglycerides + (in liver, kidney, muscle) liver biopsy protein + – liquor
4. Glycosphingolipidosis: Fabry	teleangiectasia, diarrhea, leg oedema, burning in fingers and toes	H: rare A: 10–20–30	proteinuria, haematuria opacity of the cornea
5. gangliosidosis (amaurotic idiocy) GM – 1 (type O, A, B) GM – 2 (type I, II, III) GM – 3	psychomotor- regression, amaurosis, nystagm, decerebration rigidity, idiocy, megalencephaly with «hydrocephalus» paroxysm	H: 0,25 A: 6 m – 6 y type 15 y	fovea centralis red EEG leukocyte enzymes biopsy of the rectal mucosa
6. leukodystrophies: metachromatic leukodystrophy Pelizaeus-Merzbacher's syndrome Schilder's disease, spongy degeneration, morbus Krabbe	muscular hypotony, weakness, psychomotoric retardation, spasm, tetraplegia, paroxysm, opticus atrophy	H: rare A: 0–1–19 y	liquor protein + EEG arylsulfatase urine + histology

Disorders of amino-acid metabolism

Disease	Clinical features	Frequency (H/A)	Diagnostic tests
1. Alcaptonuria	Black-brown staining of napkins, skin pigmentation in old age	H: 0,1 A: from 0	FeCl 3 green, Fehling +, urine deposit black osteoarthrosis paperchromatography
2. Albinism: yellow, black, white, ocular	White (in case with black spots) pigmented skin, red iris, photophobia	H: 0,3 A: from 0	Ophthalmology
3. Phenylketonuria:	Smell of mouse urine, dermatosis (eczema) paroxysm, psychointellectual retardation	H: 10–15 A: 0–5 M	FeCl 3 deep greenish-blue phenistix-test, guthrie-test, EEG
4. Disturbed tyrosin metabolism tyrosinaemia (three arts)	Vomiting, diarrhea, dyspnea, cataracts, hepatosplenomegaly, hypophosphataemic rachitis, retardation, blisters on feet and fingers	H: rare A: 1 W – 8 M	hypophosphataemia, glucosuria, proteinuric/leuko/thrombocytopenia, aminoacid-chromatogram, hypoglyaemia
5. Histidiaemia:	Disturbed articulation, reduced hearing	H: 6–8 A: 0–5 J	FeCl 3 green (from 2. week)
6. Maple-syrup disease:	Refuse of food, apathy, moro + apnoe, paroxysm, Maggi-like smell from 6th day)	H: 1 A: 3–4 T	FeCl 3 greyish-green chromatography, EEG
7. Homocystinuria:	Tallness, longfingers, lens ectopy, suited to thrombosis, reduced intelligence, changes of vertebral column, paroxysm	H: 0,3–1 A: 2–30 Y.	nitroprusside test + chromatography
8. Cystinosis:	Polydipsia, polyuria, anorexia, obstipation, vomiting, photophobia, rachitoid osteopathy	H: 1 A: 6–12 M	glucosuria, erythrocyturia, slit-lamp examination
9. Hyperammonaemia I + II	vomiting, spasm, lethargy	H: rare A: from 0	serum-ammoniak +
10. Citrullinuria:	cerebral lesions with fits	H: rare A: 0–30 Y.	serum-ammoniak + Ehrlich Reganz yellow chromatogram-blood
11. Argininsuccinicacid disease	paroxysm, ataxia, reduced intelligence	H: 0,25 A: 0–old	Ammoniak in the serum + GOT Arg. succ. acid-secretion

Porphyrin metabolism disorders

1. Porphyria several types and courses	Red urine, blisters in irradiated skin, photomatosis, polyneuritis, psychoneurological syndrome	H: rare-D A: 0–20 years	test for aldehyde + uroporphyrin + koproporphyrin +

Anomalies of plasmaproteins

1. Plasmaproteinemia: group of diseases	Bleedings at intervals, relapsing fever, emphysembronchitis, diarrhea, vomiting, dystrophy, neuropathy, oedema, hypotonia, hepatosplenomegaly with cholostasis up to hepatic coma. Accord. to disease very different courses	H: accord. type A: 0 – old	electrophoresis path. lipidelectrophoresis path. tranferrin path. alpha 1 antitrypsin path. fibrinogen + HLA system

Disturbed metallic metabolism

1. Haemosiderosis primary/secondary form	loss of weight and thirst, weakness, hepatosplenomegaly, diabetes mellitus, bronced skin	H: pri-sec! A: 0 – old	serum iron exceed. 200 μg Desferal test path.
2. Wilson's disease	hepatosplenomegaly, ascites, «parkinsonism»	H: 1 A: 11 – 25 years	proteinuria, Kaiser-Fleischer's corneal ring (ophthalm.)

Hereditary disturbances of vitamin metabolism

1. Disturbances of pyridoxin	Shrieking, tonic-clonic spasm, restlessness, tremor anaemia	H: rare A: 0–2 M	B 6 i. v. under EEG B 6 substitution
2. Vitamin B-12 malabsorption: familial/primary-secondary	anorexia, megaloblastanaemia, inflammations, pernicious anaemia	H: rare-p. A: 2 – 5 M	proteinuria blood-count
3. pseudo-vit. D defiency rachitis:	rachitis	H: rare	alkaline phosph. parathormone + calcium

Purine metabolism disorders

1. gout	Podagra, pellagra, painful inflammatory articular swellings	H: 2500 A: 20 – 40 years	BSG + , leukocytosis urea exceeding 6 mg %

Mental and multiple disabilities

Concept of a therapy system

Remarkable progress has been made in the last 30 years by medical therapy for mentally handicapped – in comparison with a stagnation that had lasted for centuries. The impulses came from various marginal areas of medicine and pedagogy but to a lesser extent from principal areas such as neurology and psychiatry. Physiology, biochemistry and - morphology created a better understanding of the structure and functions of the nervous system; pediatricians, physiotherapists and pedagogues worked out practical techniques for treatment.

Let us again summarize the contrast between present and past. In the past, people were helpless when faced with the manifestations of mentally handicapped persons or diseases of the central nervous system. This helplessness was reflected by isolating and tranquilising the patient; that is, the central nervous system was not trained and depressed. But in our days the active principle of encouragement and training has basically found general acceptance though not everywhere in practice. In terms of historical development, we should have overcome the periods of eliminating the handicapped (in antiquity and remnants of that age in modern times), of isolating the patient (behind big walls in medieval times). The main duty of medicine in our times is the integration of handicapped people into the environment. Despite basic progress and positive trends, individual cases still nowadays point out the limitations of these possibilities – but also the limitations of quite a few erroneous developments in terms of organization. Long years of my own experience on more than 5000 cases of handicapped

children have shown that the potential offered by therapy is in most instances utilized only in a unilateral and thus incomplete manner; barriers erected in terms of organization often obstruct rather than favour the development of these children. A few medical and educational examples are intended to clarify this statement.

The Drawbacks of Specialization

Certainly, *medical gymnastics, physiotherapy, stimulation-programms* have been and still are one of the most important elements of therapeutic progress. In the course of the change of designation from «infantile cerebral paresis» to «cerebral motor disturbance» remedial gymnastics – primarily through specialized methods breathing sectarian intolerance – are emphasized to such an extent – both in the projecting line of thought and in terms of time – that other methods of treatment are neglected or can no longer be accommodated in terms of time.

The *introduction of anticonvulsive agents* was a step forward which took the notion of unavoidable fate from the seizure conditions. Wherever such progress became an end in itself, where the symptom of the «convulsive cerebral attack» was made the centre of the condition and the sole target on which therapy should focused, the usefulness of symptomatical treatment may be perverted to damage to the personality of the patient; this may happen due to a neglect of other ways of treatment and the suppression of the central nerve functions. The gamut of the disadvantages of a one-sided therapy ranges from serious damage to the skeleton (Rachitis anticonvulsiva) to «Morbus anticonvulsivus» where the consequences of a high-dosage and unsuitable anticonvulsive medication are of a more serious pathological nature than the seizure condition proper.

The system of our *specialized pedagogy* may be compared with an excellent network of roads where, unfortunately, there are no cross-connections. The patient who, due to geographical location, is put on such a road (i.e. a special school G for Mentally handicapped, special school L for Learning handicapped, school for physically handicapped), will as a rule have to keep on that road since he is given the result of an intelligence test as a starting position to serve as an identification card.

The *field of testing* (psychological, behavioural, intelligence tests and others) is highly diversified with its more than 1000 test methods. However, practical experience shows that the result often testifies more to the abilities of the tester than to the abilities of the tested patients. A handicapped child who lives in contact with one or a few reference persons in his environment, will never show the same performance which he is able to show when confronted with strangers; often any cooperation is refused during the test. An intelligence quotient (IQ) labelled from such test situations is an unsurmountable obstacle for many children who are to be given adequate supportin their development.

Handicap as an Integral Concept

The development of the child, that is the evolution of the biological potentials contained in the genotype in accordance with the laws of nature, is a complex process composed of a somatic and an intellectual (mental) group of factors; the physical area includes anthropometric data (length of body, weight, circumference of head, growth), and statomotoric functions. The mental area consists of psychic, social and intellectual components. In handicapped patients the individual components are usually not affected in uniform manner; the assessment (often identical with diagnosis) is formed in most instances, according to the most serious deficiency (spastics, debility, numbness, speech disorder, ataxia). Here it is often overlooked that the patient is a personality who, besides his shortcomings, has also positive (and in this case often above-average) qualities (for example social attitudes, willingness to give help, tidiness, a good instinct).

An optimized therapeutic concept must be based on the integrality of the patient who is handicapped, primarily recognize the mosaic of symptoms, evaluate it and work out an individual scheme for treatment and guidance from the individual possibilities and shortcomings. The supreme therapeutic target must be the encouragement of personal development, not the elimination of a symptom.

Diagnostic Requirements

Looking at the changes that have occurred in the judgment and classification of mental handicaps in the last 50 years by referring to the diagnoses used, which ranged from

«Vitium cerebri»
over
«Oligophrenia» (debility, imbecility, idiocy)
to

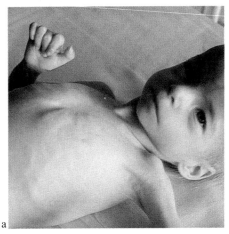

a

«Cerebral palsy»
(infantile cerebral paresis),
«cerebral motoric disorders»
and finally to
«brain damage in early childhood»,

two things are evident:

As against the general organ-related diagnosis, individual symptoms (such as the degree of intelligence, motoric handicap, seizure conditions) were given predominant attention in the course of time and promoted to « Diagnosis» status. The provisional end of this trend, the «brain damage of early childhood» is to be assigned to the period where, about 150 years ago, developments started:

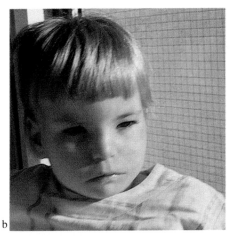

b

Fig. 258:
Progeria series of development 710812-780523

a)
The boy of $3\frac{5}{12}$ years was admitted with 75 cm stature (-24 cm $= -25\%$), 5.56 kg bodyweight (-4.5 kg related to stature = about -75%(!) -9 kg corresponding to age = about -150%) because he was unable to ingest food. Dystrophic, senile appearance, frontal vessels as thick as pencils. No reaction to optic, acoustic stimuli, no sounds, little spontaneous movement. On polyvitamins, digestive ferments, primobolan gains in weight up to 12.9 kg, increase of stature to 80 cm in 7 months, but no static and mental progress.
At $4\frac{3}{12}$ years, implantation of 100 mg of cerebral lyophilisate. Slowly beginning, then rapidly visible motor and mental development; at $5\frac{4}{12}$ years 92 cm (-19 cm), 17.2 kg, according to age.

b)
At $5\frac{8}{12}$ years 98 cm (-16 cm), 18.4 kg. Implantation: 100 mg diencephalon, 100 mg frontal brain; grows 3 cm in 40 days; reacts to environment, sits, stands, walks, utters first sounds.

c)
At $10\frac{6}{12}$ years, the boy attends special school, speaks indistinctly owing to Moebius's syndrome, fully integrated in social respect, 126 cm (-12 cm), 30.5 kg. At 12 years, 4th class of special school, reads, writes, counts up to 20, is interested in everything; 133 cm, 31.8 kg.

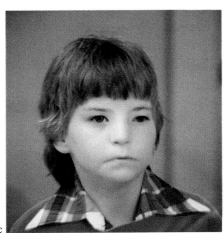

c

256

Tab. 32: **Important diagnostic partial symptoms of mental retardation and multiple physical disability**

somatic		mental		Sens-organs	Peculinities
anthropo-metric	stato-motoric	psycho-social	intellectual		
general growth anomalies nanism microsomia high stature giantism dystrophy adiposis **partial growth anomalies** microcephalia macrocephalia dyscephalia hypognathia hypergnatia hypogeny hypergeny brachymelia brachycarpia brachydactylia brachy-mesophalangy acromicria dolichomelia dolichocarpia dolichodactyly acromegalia cranial hypoplasia (bird's head) caudal hypoplasia dysraphia dysmelia	**muscular hypertony** monoplegia diplegia triplegia tetraplegia (Little-S.) hemiplegia **muscular hypotonie** Foerster-S. puppet phenomenon «Floppy infant» **muscular dystony** **Dyskynesia** athetosis chorea chorea-athetosis **ataxia**	apathie hyperkinesis erethism aggressivity listlessness helplessness tyrant uncleanliness autism	debility imbecillity idiocy partially disturbed performance no abstract thinking no discrimination absent-mindedness echolalia perseveration cortical blindness cortical deafness loss of initiative	**skin** analgesia hypalgesia trophic disturbances disturbed circulation anomalous pigmentation **speech** lacking understanding of speech motoric speech disturbance (dyslalia) **hearing** hardness of hearing deficient selective pitch of voice deafness **vision** **strabism** nystagmus microphthalmy macrophthalmy opacity of lense retrolentary fibroplasia glaucoma amblyopia blindness	increased predisposition to infections lacking immunoglobulins **gastro-intestinal disorders** inappetence lack of ferments chronic obstipation chron. gastritis ulcera oesophagitis gastro-oesophageal reflux frequent vomiting **vegetative symptoms** vegetative lability disturbed peripheral circulation acrocyanosis trophic disorders lost or weakened regulation of body-temperature

There is merely a difference in degree compared with «Vitium cerebri», no basic difference. But the most dangerous attribute is the Intelligence Quotient (IQ), a figure computed with sources of error; such figure lends itself to easy processing by government offices but often entails disastrous consequences for the treatment and encouragement of the children because, in many instances, the qualification for being encouraged, the possibility of treatment and the type of schools to be attended are determined with this figure.

Starting with this negative aspect it is pointed out that the mosaic of a handicap is composed of individual symptoms which should also be covered and formulated in each single instance; otherwise we lose sight of them in our therapy. There is a momentous difference as to whether the label of a handicap reads:
a) brain damage in early childhood or
b) motoric and mental retardation;
   athetosis;
   ataxia;
   strabism;
   dyslalia.

Tab. 33: **Multifactorial damages**

anencephaly	arthromyodysplasia (arthrogryposis)
hydrancephaly	Hallervorden-Spatz degeneration
arhinencephaly	Sturge-Weber's syndrome
parencephaly	(trigeminus-angiomatosis)
microcephaly	syndrome with aniridia, cerebellar
hydrocephaly	ataxia
	oligophrenia
clefts of lips, maxilla, palate	Pierre Robin's dysmorphia
rachischisis	bird-face (Seckel's nanism)
lacunar skull	Hallermann Streiff-disease
	(oculomandibulo-dyscephalia with
dysmorphia-syndromes	hypotrichosis)
Cornelia de Lange-syndrome	Many more, mostly rare, syndromes
Rubinstein's syndrome	

Tab. 34: **Environmental Factors which may lead to mental damage or impairment:**

Prenatal Damage	**Natal Dangers**
Maternal Noxae:	Immaturity
Nicotine abuse	Prematurity
Alcoholic abuse	Umbilical-cord strangulation
Drug abuse	Prolonged birth
Antiepileptic therapy	Difficult birth
Cytostatica	Prolonged hypoxia
Radiation damage	Anoxia
Infections:	Artificial aids (forceps, suction cup)
Bacterial sepsis	
E. Coli	**Postnatal Damage**
Pyoceanus	Encephalo-enteritis (toxicosis)
Proteus	Encephalitis
Staphylococcos	Vaccination encephalopathy
Beta-hämol. B-Streptococcos	Meningitis
German measles	Subdural hematome-hygroma
Virus conditions	Anaesthesia accidents
Toxoplasmosis	Cerebral angiographies
Cytomegalia	Traumatic damage of central nerve system
Lues	cardiac arrest
Anemia	Chronic hypoxia
Bleedings (hemorrhages)	Cerebral seizures
Toxicosis	Athyreosis-hypothyreosis
Nidation anomalies of the fetus	Hypocalcemia – hypercalcemia
Blood group incompatibility	Hypoglycemia

Under a) there is a statement not related to any target, it does not lead to a therapeutic consequence;

Under b) there is a comprehensive stock-taking with direct therapeutic demands (see Table 32):

The diagnosis that serves as a premise for a therapy suitable for the individual case, should include the following basic elements:

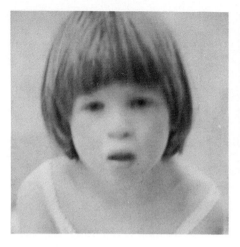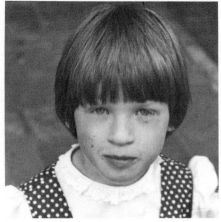

Fig. 259:
Alcoholic-embryo-fetopathy: retarded development, retarded development of speech, mimic expression (a) before and (b) after two treatments with implantations 2 years later; most distinct is the progress in speech development.

Tab. 35: **Infantile cerebral paresis**

Hypertonic Forms Muscle hypertonia Spastic monoplegia diplegia triplegia tetraplegia Spastic hemiplegia	**Dyskinetic Forms** Chorea (motoric restlessness) Athetosis (motoric stiffness) Choreo athetosis (coexistence and change of motoric restlessness and spasm) Fine motor «clumsiness»
Hypotonic Forms Muscle hypotonia Stuffed doll syndrome «Floppy infant»	**Atactic Forms** Cerebellar ataxia Cerebello-spinal ataxia **Mixed Forms** Combinations of the above listed symptoms among each other with sensory
Dystonic Forms Changes of hypertonia and hypotonia	deficiencies, trophic disturbances, reduced intelligence and psychic deviations.

1. Anthropometric data (length of body, body weight, proportions);
2. Size of skull and shape of skull
   a) visual judgment;
   b) circumference of skull (= surface measurement of skull basis);
   c) Radiological skull measurements including the volume index of the skull;
3. Analysis of development (fig. 263)
   a) stato-motoric;
   b) fine-motoric, coordination;
   c) eating, drinking, speaking;
   d) social development, psychic development;
   e) intellectual performance;
4. Neurological symptoms (fig. 264).
5. Anthropological age (bone age).

6. Electroencephalogram (EEG). Additional data can be obtained for special areas, which may be relevant for therapy:
7. Echoencephalogram;
8. Computer Tomogram;
9. Audiometry;
10. Psychological tests;
11. Eye examinations;
12. Analyses of the metabolism;
13. Diaphanoscopy;
14. Cerebral angiography.

Genesis and Types

Most classification principles concerning handicapped conditions are based on the genesis and the clinical symptoms or represent a complex of criteria.

We can distinguish the following main groups based on the genesis:

1. *Hereditary metabolic disorders (Tab. 31);*
2. *Chromosomal aberrations (Tab. 23);*
3. *Environmental handicaps (Tab. 34);*
4. *Multifactorial damages (Tab. 33).*
5. *Types of infantile cerebral paresis (Tab. 35)*
6. *Partial disturbances of performance.*

The summaries in Tab. 29–35 and in the following list give a concise survey of the total field.

Partial disturbances of performance

The probably mildest forms of consequences of brain damage in early childhood are the so-called partial disturbances of performance in various areas of the motoric system, particularly of the learning process. Such partial disturbances may be located within the mosaic of infantile cerebral palsy, but also occur as individual symptoms. The following forms must be distinguished:

1. *Disorders of reading techniques*

a) Incorrect vowels (for example I instead of A);
b) Incorrect consonants;
c) Reversals (e.g. pit/tip);
d) Omission of sounds or added sounds (for example ... un instead of sun; shipi instead of ship);
e) Substitutions (instead of saying «I live in Aschaffenburg»/«my home is in Aschaffenburg»);
f) Repetitions (for example the ca, ca, cat or the cat, cat, cat);
g) New words added or omitted (e. g. instead of saying «a dog» the child says «a vicious dog»; ... was a king instead of there was a king);
h) Refusals (e. g. the sentence «one of the most wonderful experiences...» is spoken as follows: one of the experiences...
i) Inability to articulate unknown words, while the other phonetic structures are degenerate;
j) Deficient differentiation of letters, parts of words and syllables (e. g. between bead and bed);
k) Lack of ability to discover differences between sounds and words;
l) Difficulty in observing lines;
m) Difficulty in proceeding from the right side to the next line below on the left;
n) Poor understanding of the material read;

2. *Writing-disorders*

a) Delayed and slow learning to write;
b) Writing in reverse;
c) Letter size cannot be coordinated;
d) Slipping characters;
e) Strikingly irregular line thickness;

f) Legasthenia;

3. *Speech disorders*

a) Disorders when spelling (e. g. loss of letters, telegraph style words);
b) Inability to spell, that is to differentiate the individual letters contained in a word;
c) Poor understanding of language;

d) Disturbances of language motor system (difficulty in pronouncing);
e) Difficulty in finding words;
f) Poor structure of sentences (difficulty in establishing the right word order);
g) Difficulties in orientation;
h) Stuttering and stammering.

Possibilities and limitations in biological development

The central nervous system of man is the sole organ system the «fetal stage» of which is not completed at the time of birth. Processes of fetal maturation and differentiation extend up to the 4th year of life; they are completed only upon maturation of the medullary sheath. This results in a few essential aspects for vulnerability and therapeutic possibilities and limitations. The following facts should be kept in mind (fig. 260):

1. With a maturely born child the final number of nerve cells is already present; no new ones will be added during his lifetime.

2. Despite the final cell number the weight of the brain of a mature newborn is 350 g on the average; at the end of the somatic growth it is 1250 g on an average, the number of cells being the same.

3. Without increasing the number of neurons the brain volume triples $3\frac{1}{2}$ times by way of formation of secondary structures of the neuron.

4. The main increase in brain volume (= weight) takes place in the first three years of life, that is in the «caught-up» fetal period of the central nervous system. About $\frac{3}{4}$ of the

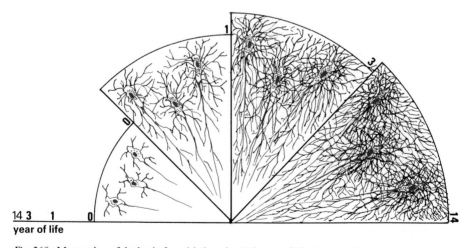

14 3 1   0

year of life

Fig. 260: Maturation of the brain from birth to the 14th year of life. By way of formation of secondary structures the brain volume (= weight) increases $3\frac{1}{2}$ fold; the number of neurons present at the time of birth is not changed.

261

postnatal brain growth takes place in this age period.

These biological laws result in a higher vulnerability of the central nervous system in the first four years of life but also the possibility of acting on it by way of therapy. In particular, the first three years offer chances and potentials for therapy applications with biological «building stones» and a training program from the periphery. These possibilities are no longer available after the fourth year. Possibilities of treatment not utilized in the first three years of life will remain wasted chances throughout life. Even with an increased therapeutic input and effort they can be corrected only in part.

Therapeutical approaches

Looking at the elementary structure of the central nervous system, the neuron, we can see basically three processes:

a) a deficit in neurons;
b) an impairment of maturation and differentiation of the neuropile;
c) destructive (degenerative) processes.

Mental impairment constitutes by far the most important proportion; it goes back to an impairment of maturation of the central nervous system on account of which the functional state of the brain remains in the stages of early childhood. Several points of approach are offered for therapy applicable to this condition, which is known clinically under names such as «brain damage from early childhood», «infantile cerebral palsy» or «cerebral motor disturbance» (fig. 261).

1. *Nonspecific Stimulation of the Metabolism* through increased supply of substrate; in most instances a better supply of blood to the brain is achieved. These agents have so far been used predominantly for elderly people and not sufficiently utilized for children. They include:

euphylin,
heart glycosides,
caffeine,
amphetamines,
complamin,

ephedrine derivatives,
camphor and others.

2. *Specific influences on metabolism* by agents which selectively stimulate individual metabolic processes in the neuron. This field has been neglected by pharmacology and clinics for a long time; it is still in its infancy since sufficient clinical experience can support the theoretical basic concept only in the case of a few substances. The biocatalysts include

a) Pyritinoldihydrochloride monohydrate (Encephatol);
b) Piracetam (Normabrain, Nootrop);
c) Centrophenoxin (Helfergin);
d) Actihaemyl;
e) Nicotinic acid derivates;
f) Membrane activators;
g) Monoamino-oxydase inhibitors;
h) Adrenocorticotropes hormone (ACTH);
i) L-Dopa.

3. *Biological Organ Therapy* (*«Brick-Therapy»*)

Up to the present biological substances of various biochemical dimensions have not been available to a sufficiently great extent for the stimulation of the metabolism of the neurons, for repairing and synthesizing defective and unmatured neuron structures; more-

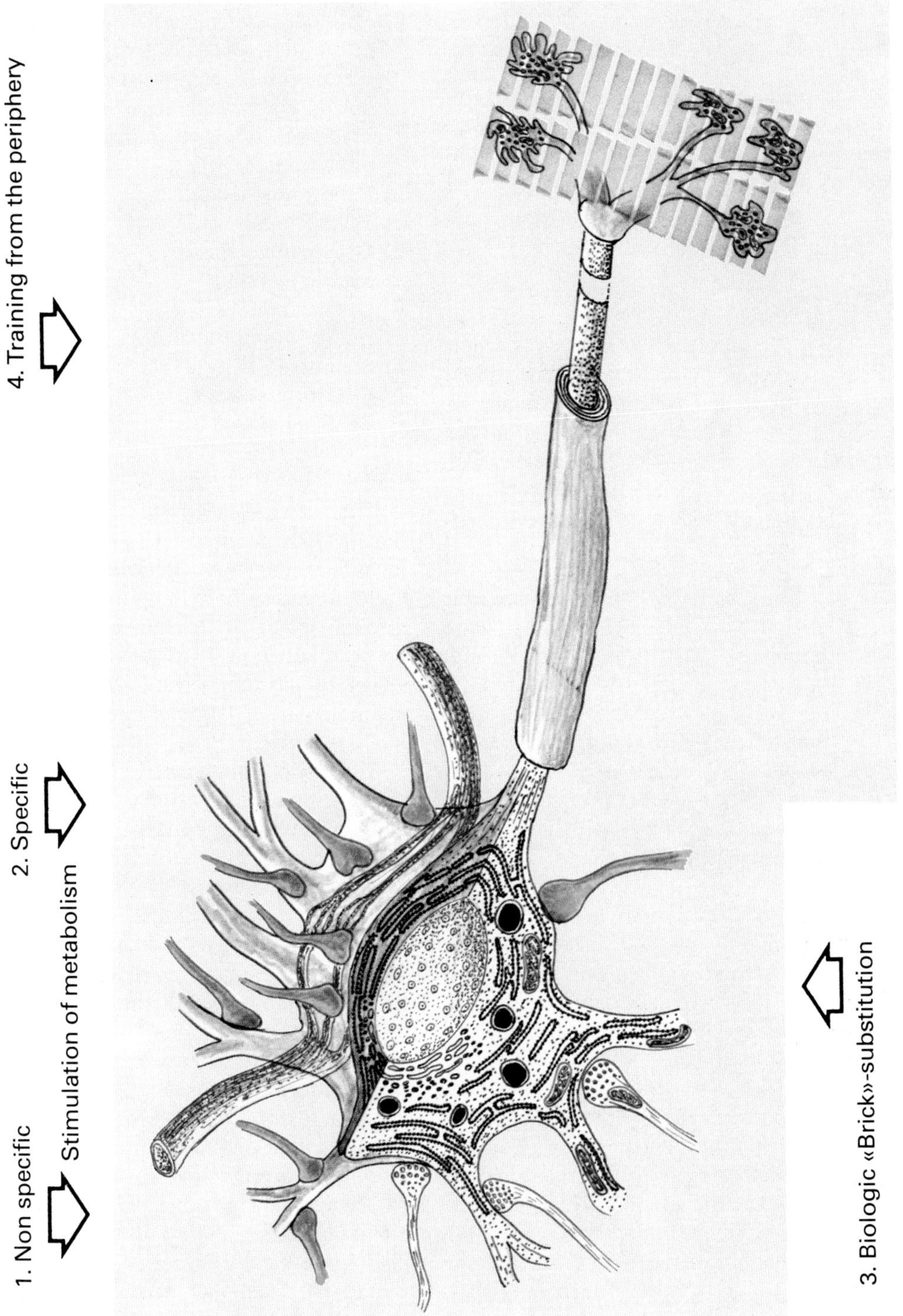

4. Training from the periphery

2. Specific

Stimulation of metabolism

1. Non specific

3. Biologic «Brick»-substitution

Fig. 261: Therapeutic approaches on the neuron

263

over, they have been used without specific targets. The following types are used:

a) Lyophilisates of brain tissue in the form of injection-implantations (so-called cell therapy);
b) Hydrolysates from animal brain in the form of amino acid mixtures (Cerebrolysin);
c) Ultrafiltrates;
d) Enzymes;
e) The supply of constituents is supplemented by enzymatic preparations, where in particular experience has been gained with Coliacron and Wobenzym. With its 3 enzymes Coliacron is suitable for influencing hypotonic and atonic muscles with lasting effect.

These biological substances are causal and not only symptomatic action principles; their fields of application range from disturbances of the brain in the maturing process to the degenerations of the aging and aged brain. The «molecular brick substitution» often forms a first basis for the effectiveness of other methods of treatment, particularly of training methods.

4. Training of Periphery

While the methods listed under 1–3 serve to increase the metabolism and rebuild the nerve cells, another group of methods which is differentiated in itself, avails itself of another principle: the principle of (functional) training of the neuron from the periphery. Sequences of functions, which the neuron is unable to initiate, are released passively in order to prepare the grounds. Thus it is possible to passively initiate processes of differentiation of the central nervous system which, due to functional weaknesses, cannot be realized actively. These methods include:

a) Physiotherapy (remedial gymnastics, gymnastics for special diseases, remedial eurythmics, sports for the disabled, motion therapy, therapeutic horseback riding, therapeutic swimming etc.);
b) Behavioral therapy;
c) Psychotherapy;
d) Occupational therapy;
e) Speech therapy;
f) Optical training;
g) Acoustic training;
h) Stimulating current therapy;
i) Electric impulses;
j) Bioenergetics.

Nonspecific stimulation of Metabolism

The methods of unspecific increase of the metabolism in cerebral affections include an increase of physical activity and influences of the brain metabolism through medicine. Narrow limitations are set for attempts to dilate the cerebral vessels by way of medication, due to the autonomous regulation of the supply of blood to the brain.

The blood-brain barrier is formed by the functional unit of capillary-astroglia-neuron. The astroglia formations envelop the capillaries almost completely. Swelling and edema formation in the central nervous system, on the one hand, and cicatrisations, on the other, lead to a narrowing of the capillary networks and thus to an impairment of the metabolic chain in the capillary area; this is due to increased volume or shrinking of the astroglia. More experience is available in the area of geriatrics than in pediatrics, with agents for circulation and the heart. The use of strophantine, caffeine, fludilat, complamin and other substances leads to short stimulation of the blood supply; however, the counteradjustment should be taken into account, which takes place after the main effect has subsided. For these considerations alone,

264

the methods of unspecific increases of the metabolism serve to treat acute conditions rather than chronic diseases of the central nervous system.

A very important way of nonspecific influences on the brain-metabolism is a disease-orientated-nutrition and diet.

Specific influenser on the metabolism of the Central Nervous System

The intent to increase the performance of the brain goes back to time immemorial; it ranges from the pneuma of GALEN of BERGAMON over the mixture of ether and spirits of Friedrich HOFFMANN (1760, Halle) (in the form of ether drops, used up to the present century) to the «modern» *psychostimulants, psychoenergetica* and *nootropica* (J. KUGLER, 1977). The first specific entry was made by LEVIN (1927) with *amphetamines,* which increase the ability of perception, concentration and reaction. Similar, though shorter improvements of performance of the central nervous system can be achieved with *coramin, ephedrin* and the previously much used *camphor.*

The practical applicability of these substances is limited because, in part, they cause dependence and addiction; without exception, they lead to a counteradjustment, a reduced performance of the central nervous system, after a stimulated stage which may last minutes or hours.

A few substances affecting the brain metabolism do not result in such a counteradjustment; their focus is more specific than the above mentioned substances and the agents that have the general effect of encouraging circulation (cardiac tonics and circulatory stimulants).

In theory and clinical practice certain substance groups, to which specific metabolic stimulation must be ascribed in experiments on animals and humans,

have found general acceptance during the last two decades.

Pyrithioxin, Pyritinol (Encephabol®)

The probably most comprehensive experimental materials and clinical experience with a neurodynamic agent are provided by Pyrithioxin (Encephabol). An increase in glucose utilization and protein synthesis is attributed to this vitamin B6 derivative without vitamin character. Probably this does not do full justice to its complex mechanism of action. Before evaluating the therapeutic importance the experimental data must be analysed. In previous basic pharmacological examinations (HOTOVY, R., ENENKEL, J. H. a. o., 1964), Pyrithixion (150 mg/kg) had a calming effect on cats, increased circulation of A. carotis in dogs, connected with a nitrogen reduction in the urine, a diminishing experimental catalepsy in cats, an improved training of rats for running, and an increase in the psychomotoric efficiency in persons. Circulation and visceral organs remained unaffected. There were no criteria of central stimulation such as an awakening effect, locomotoric action and tremor which are particularly characteristic of amphetamines.

Membrane Effects

In hemolysis experiments on human erythrocytes, MARTIN succeeded in starting, in vitro, a monophasic reversible labilisation of the erythrocyte membrane; the membrane-stabilizing action of benzyl alcohol was antagonized by Pyrithioxin derivatives. The antialcohol effects oberserved in vivo may be bound up with these membrane-influencing properties. The choline transport through the membranes of human erythrocytes and in synaptosome preparations from rat brains is inhibited. The retardation of the c-AMP-synthesis with procaine – checked on brain sections of rats – is antagonized. The last two findings show that the membrane effects of Encephabol are not confined to erythrocyte membranes but can also be demonstrated on neuron membranes. The protective mechanism against alcohol is also assumed with regard to the cholinergic spinal marrow synapsis (BENECKE a. o. 1972).

ENDO assumes that Pyritinol influences the interplay of phospholipid-protein substances; the extractability of firmly bound phophorus lipids increases. Membrane permeability increases; some substrates such as for example sodium, glucose, choline, are transported easier.

Clinical Effects

The short-time memory and the immediate memorization in 48 persons subject to experiment was markedly improved according to investigations by I. M. DEUSINGER and H. HAASE (1972) under 300 mg of Pyrithioxin daily for 4 weeks. Increases in vigilance in school children, 8–13, were substantiated by K. D. STOLL (1973) by way of concentration tests after administration of Pyrithioxin. G. LOGUE and others (1974) reported on further positive action on learning attitudes; Ch. FEHLING-JOSS reported on such effects with dyslexia (1974).

Additional effects were registered with regard to brain contusions (BYSTRICKY a. o. 1977; S. Y. OH 1974; LAHODA), with the appalic syndrome (K. v. WILD and G. DOLCE, 1976), with organic psychosyndromes (MISUREC and others, HAMOUZ, W., 1977), with chronic alcoholism (J. MASARIK and J. DEMEL 1974). The probably most interesting interactions were found with cerebral seizures. The consequences on cerebral seizures were examined by GASTAUT on 48 patients with a double-blind experiment. In

5 cases a reduction of the seizures was noticed, in 5 cases an increase. The electroencephalogram changed in the Encephabol group in 8 cases, among them 5 cases changing toward the positive; in the placebo group the change was noticed in 2 cases. On the whole, interest, language, academic and occupational performance were judged favourably. TASSINARI did not see any influence on the electrocardiogram in 30 seizure conditions, when Encephabol was administered intravenously. A differentiated study of infantile seizure conditions (43 cases of 4–14 years) was made by ROGER, ROBAGLIA and C. DRAVET. In a pyridoxin insufficiency test conducted by means of tryptophane loads, 22 of these children were subjected to pyridoxin insufficiency; a negative test was made with 21 of the children. Administered were 300 mg (600) daily for several weeks. In a group of 21 children who were not free from seizures during the experiment, the seizures were reduced in 7 instances, and increased in 13 instances.

According to DIEMATH pyrithioxin effects can be noticed after 4–6 minutes in the electroencephalogram, but they remain confined to the depth branches and are reversible in a few minutes.

Precisely these seemingly contradictory results in seizure conditions and the effects on the electroencephalogram suggest that pyrithioxin is a substance which acts on the neuron specifically and in a highly efficient manner. The mechanism of action is most probably of complex nature; the increase in membrane permeability is probably only at the beginning of the metabolic chain; only on account of this it is possible to improve the cytoplasm metabolism. Since the initial substance, Vitamin B_6 attacks at 6 different points the tryptophane-serotonine metabolism, the B_6 derivative pyrithioxin could play a similar role. The positive action in hypodynamic disturbances (Down's syndrome, hypotonic cerebral paralysis, impulse insufficiency), on the one hand, and an increased effect in hyperdynamic conditions, on the other, suggest a pharmacodynamic emphasis in this metabolic chain.

Piracetam (Nootrop®, Normabrain®)

This is a derivative of the *gamma aminobutyric acid* to which an improvement of the synapsic function is attributed. In animal experiments it was possible to shorten the hypoxic recovery times, to prevent hypoxy-contingent cancellations of short-time memory, and to improve learning effects. In the clinical field various authors observed impulse increases and depression-reducing effects (KANOWSKI 1975). My own observations among more than 1000 children suffering from cerebral retardation extended over 10 years; they were made in a nonsystematic examination series and gave some enlightenment on the effects and limitations of application. The incorporation of piracetam in the therapy for hypodynamic cerebral paralyses and mongolism is probably advantageous between the second half-year of life and the end of the second year. Symptoms such as slowness, poor initiative, weak power of concentration can also be influenced in a positive way among older children. On the other hand, hyperactive erethitic children can respond already under lower dosages (1/4 measuring spoon, 100–200 mg daily) with increased restlessness and excitement; even with a onetime administration in the morning it may be possible that sleeplessness will occur. With the single individual these oberservations can be reproduced by several starts of administration and dis-continuation, so they have practical significance.

The indicative range of this surely interesting substance deserves to be given a better analysis.

Centrophenoxin (Helfergin®)

This is a synthesis product from an aminoalcohol and p-chlorphenoxy-acetic acid. In animal experiments the influence on cell respiration and glucose metabolism has been established (K. NANDY). Without changing pulse frequency and blood pressure, an increase in spontaneous activity has been achieved in animals. The lipofuscin formation, a morphological expression of the aging process in the cytoplasm of the neurons, seems to be delayed by centrophenoxin. The ability to learn and to remember were increased and the life of C47BL/6-mice was prolonged (K. NANDY, 1977). Lipofuscin is considered a degeneration product of the mitochondriae (P. GLEES 1977), the intracellular digestion of which is more difficult for older cells than young ones. S. RIGA and D. RIGA (1977) attribute even a lipofuscinolytic action to centrophenoxin. RODEMANN and BAYREUTHER (1977) registered, under specific experimental conditions, a significant increase in the metabolism of glial-cells in humans. Contingent upon dosage and duration, centrophenoxin activates the pentosephosphat-cycle (making ribose-5-phosphate available for the nucleotide and nucleic acid synthesis) and influences the transport of specific nucleic acids from the cell nucleus into the cytoplasm (K. KANIG, 1977). S. HOYER and K. KENDEL as well as R. COIRAULT have pointed out the increases in cerebral insufficiency circulation.

In the clinical field influences of centrophenoxin were ascertained on the aging process (J. BÖGER, 1977), by way

267

of flicker-photometric examinations; it had also influence on children with learning difficulties and legasthenia (PERET, WEHRLI and HAFEN, 1977). According to HOYER, a significant increase is achieved by centrophenoxin among children suffering from a pathologically reduced brain circulation. This lets us visualize effects with the organic psychotic syndrome to be within reach. In the treatment of mongolism HAUBOLD included Helfergin in the basic therapy, probably with the idea of delaying a premature aging process and increasing the neuron metabolism.

Actihaemyl

This is a haemodialysate from the blood of young calves; is contains approximately 30% organic compounds and about 40–45 mg/ml dry substance. The organic share contains amino-acids, nucleic acid components, low-molecular peptides and substances of the intermediary metabolism – glucose, acetate, lactate, hormones.

An improvement of transport mechanisms of oxygen and glucose, a stimulation of the cell metabolism and of the cell regeneration are attributed to actihaemyl. In particular, it is said to have the following effects on the cellular metabolism, inclusive of the neurons:

Increase in activity of key enzymes of the respiratory chain.
Increase of the intracellular stock of energy-rich phosphates;
Diminution of pathologically increased lactate and pyruvate values;
Increase of the oxygen transport to the cell;
Increase of the glucose transport.

Actihaemyl is a biological medicine free from side-effects; it may be administered at a dosage of 100–300 mg daily the oral way. Under seriously traumatic and apallic conditions of the brain, the dosage administered may be up to 1000 mg a day parenterally.

Nicotinic-acid derivatives

Nicotinic acid compounds lead to a relatively speedy improvement of the blood circulation at the peripheries. Whereas the improvement in circulation in the central nervous system is problematic, distinctive pharmacological effects on the central nervous system have been secured with regard to nicotinic acid amides.

Niamid® = 1-/2-benzylcarbamylethyl 1/2-isonicotinoylhydrazin is an effective monoamino-oxydase inhibitor with remarkable metabolic and psychotherapeutic effects. As part of the basic therapy of mongoloid children and in other hypodynamic symptoms of mentally retarded children it is possible to improve the psychomotoric activity, social contact and emotional control.

Similar effects can be expected from the following preparations: Hämovanad® (= Inositolnicotinate) and Nicoacid® (= sodium nicotinate), Progresin fortard® (= Mg-nicotinate), Nicoplectal (= 50 mg of nicotinic acid + 200 mg of buckeye extract).

L-Dopa

A favourable effect on certain cases of dyskinetic cerebral paresis, besides an influence on Parkinson's disease, is ascribed to L-Dopa (Nacon®) (SIEVERS, 1980)

Membrane Activators

These are substances and biocatalytic combinations intended to improve the functioning of the cytomembranes. Membrane disturbances play their part in numerous congenital disorders of the metabolism and in the aging process of the tissue. Following are the areas of indication:

a) Physiological and premature aging processes;
b) innate metabolic disturbances caused by the membranes;
c) Down's syndrome (basic treatment);
d) Hypothyreosis-athyreosis.

The function of the membrane activator is not confined to supplying intracellularly lacking or reduced substances; it also creates the premises for transmembral movement. Numerous preparations and combinations of vitamins, trace elements and biocatalysators increasing the blood circulation aim at this effect.

Long years of practical experience with various individual constituents have resulted in a biocatalytic combination which is available as *Membravit®*; it contains 3 magnesium compounds, zinc, iodized common salt of Tölz compound, vitamins B1, B2, B6 and tryptophane. The substitutes magnesium and zinc activate the DNS and membrane metabolism in connection with asparagin and orotic acid. The B-vitamins catalyze numerous enzymatic processes, for which magnesium and zinc are essential co-enzymes. After all, the metabolic chain of tryptophane to serotonin can only function if tryptophane is offered to a sufficiently great extent and is also transported into the cell.

Biological Therapy

Decisive progress in the treatment of mental development disturbances was achieved in the last 20 years by the introduction of the so-called cell- and enzyme therapy into the therapeutic concept. The offer of fetal cell suspensions serves to maturate secondary structures of the central nervous system – dendrites, neurites, medullary sheaths, synapses. Naturally, nonexisting cells cannot be replaced. This «Brick-component» therapy in the form of lyophylised fetal cerebral tissue, i. e. the offer of substrates, is supported by the stimulation of the incorporation, namely enzyme therapy. Whereas substrate preparations are available in sufficient differentiation, the availability of enzyme preparations is still fragmentary. The possibilities and limitations of both therapy methods which complement each other, will be briefly described hereafter.

Injection Implantations (Cell therapy)

The following process is initiated by deeply subcutaneous (epifascial) injection of cell and tissue suspensions of xenogenic fetal cerebral regions, in the organism of the recipient:

1. The fetal heterological donor material contains a high concentration of organ-specific substrates and enzymes which is characteristic of rapidly growing embryonal and fetal tissues.

2. The injected suspended tissue material is dissolved like a net within two hours in an animal experiment intraperitoneally, decomposed and attached to the microphage membranes as tissue particles; a leukocytosis develops in the peripheral blood picture.

3. The complex of microphages (= polynuclear) + tissue particles is subject to a phagocytosis during the following hours, through macrophages (monocytes, histiocytes); in a kind of « microphage battle» the complexes are intracellularly decomposed in the macrophages. The process is completed after 48 hours to such an extent that optically no

Symptom	CENTER OF LESION		recommended cell suspensions for implantation
Intelligence normal			
Debility (iQ 80-50)			cortex, hemisphere, frontal-, temporal-,
Imbecility (iQ 50-20)			parietal-, occipital brain
Idiocy (iQ ander 20)			according to cause and conc. symptoms
normocephalic			
macrocephalic			
microcephalic	CEREBRAL CORTEX		
Monoplegia	CEREBRAL		
Diplegia spast.	HEMISPHERE		cortex, hemisphere, frontal-, temporal-,
Hemiplegia limp.			parietal-, occipital brain
Triplegia			possibly diencephalon spinal medulla
Tetraplegia			according to cause and symptoms
Contractures			
Rigor			
Muscle-Hypertonia			
Muscle-Hypotonia			mesencephalon, occipital brain, Medulla oblong.
Dystonia (alternat. Tonus)			mesencephalon, occipital brain, Diencephalon
Convulsions			Petit-mal: mesencephalon, Medulla oblong., Thalamus, cerebellum
Hyperkinesia			Grand-mal: cortex or sections
Coordination-Disorders			cerebellum, basal ganglis, Diencephalon, cortex
Tremor			basal ganglia, Diencephalon, cortex
Chorea	BASAL GANGLIA		diencephalon, basal ganglia, temporal brain
Athetosis			frontal brain, basal ganglia, temporal brain
Restlessnes	DIENCEPHALON		diencephalon, basal ganglia, temporal brain
Eretism			Thalamus, basal ganglia, temporal brain
Autism	HYPOTHALAMUS		Hypothalamus, diencephalon, frontal brain, hemisphere
extrapyramidal Symptoms			basal ganglia, diencephalon, mesencephalon
Initiative-Disorder			frontal brain, diencephalon
Concentration-Weakness			thalamus, diencephalon, cortical areas
Emotional Incontinentia			Hypothalamus, diencephalon, cortex
Perseveration			diencephalon, cortex
Legasthenia			hypothalamus, diencephalon, cortex
Polydipsia			diencephalon, hypothalamus, hypophysis
Polyphagia			diencephalon, hypothalamus, hypophysis
Hypertrichosis			diencephalon, hypothalamus, mesencephalon
Vegetative Disorders			mesencephalon, Medulla oblong., diencephalon
Trophic disorders			mesencephalon, Medulla oblong., diencephalon
Lability of temperature			mesencephalon, Medulla oblong., diencephalon
Hypersensibity	MESENCEPHALON		mesencephalon, Medulla oblong., parietal brain
Hyposensibility			mesencephalon, Medulla oblong., parietal brain
Hyperhydrosis	MEDULLA OBLONG.		mesencephalon, Medulla oblong., diencephalon
Anhydrosis			mesencephalon, Medulla oblong., diencephalon
Ataxia		CEREBELLUM	Cerebellum, diencephalon, frontal brain, basal ganglia
Strabism			
Eye-Paresis		VISUAL DUCTS	diencephalon, thalamus, occipital brain
Nystagmus			
Reduced Visual-Capacity		OCCIPITAL BRAIN	
Amaurosis		EYE	optic nerve, retina, lens
Reduced Hearing-Capacity	HEARING DUCTS		diencephalon, mesencephalon
Deafness	TEMPORAL BRAIN		temporal brain, occipital brain
Dyslalia	EAR		
Swallow-Discorder			basal ganglia, Medulla oblong., mesencephalon

The most frequent symptoms of cerebral damages in early infancy have been classified roughly according to their o ligin in the central nervous system.

Fig. 262: Symptomatological implantation therapy.

foreign particles are any longer identifiable.

4. The intracellular digestion of the phagocytised complexes of microphages + donor tissue takes place in intracellular digestive cisterns (vacuoles). The main mass of the ingested tissues disappears rapidly from the digestive cisterns; remnants of the complex of microphage membrane + donor tissue particles are identifiable for a relatively long time (48 hours).

5. The bulk of donor material is rapidly moved away and utilized. Vital storage and radioactive taggings concordantly show the removal within the first 6 hours after implantation; the main contingent is moved away within the first hour.

6. Whereas the bulk of the donor material is handed over to the metabolic passages of the recipient (utilization), the smaller remaining complex of microphage membrane + donor tissue particles may have an immunogenic effect. This applies primarily to connective tissue structures (glia, mesenchyme).

7. Two premises are vital for the incorporation:
   a) There must be a need in the corresponding organ of the recipient (defect, illness, insufficiency).
   b) For the incorporation the biochemical components must have the corresponding organ-specific structure.

8. The incorporation can take place in accordance with the needs of the recipient by various dimensions; experimental evidence available ranges from oligopeptides to (heterological) macromolecules (immunoglobulin M).

9. The advantage of implantations by injection as against conventional transplantation techniques is as follows:
   a) the implanted tissues are not dependent on blood supply in the recipient; they do not suffer any structural changes on account of degeneration as a result of a lacking blood supply and anoxaemia.
   b) the implantation technique reaches organs inaccessible to conventional transplantations (e.g. brain, liver, pancreas, endocrine glands, thymus and others).
   c) the implantation technique alone can supply substantial quantities of biochemical substrates and enzymes of fetal tissues.

10. The clinical effect of the implantations by injection sets in during the third week after implantation in measurable way; it extends to 4 months up to two years, depending upon age, organ and basic illness.

In some organs (placenta, liver, suprarenal gland) a short immediate effect can be seen within minutes to hours after implantation.

Selection of implantation-tissue

In the case of disturbances of the central nervous system, the organ (= brain region) is selected by symtoms or symptomatological localisations. Fig. 262 provides a guiding survey for practical application.

The following principles used for implantation treatment have resulted from so far 70000 implantations on handicapped infants, children and youngsters:

A) The therapeutic expectations are the greater the earlier treatment is start-

Age	STATO-MOTORIC	FINE MOTORIC, COORDINATION	DRINKING, EATING, LANGUAGE, COMPREHENSION OF LANGUAGE
14			
13			
12			
11			
10		uses knife for cutting	data learned «auditively» are utilized
		copies geometric figures	repeats sentence of 20 syllables
9		writes skilfully and fast	interprets material which was read or seen
			spontaneous statem. w. compl. sentences
8		catches flying ball	repeats sentence with 16 syllables
		draws variety of people	picture stories are interpreted
7	rides a bicycle		sentence constr. stabilized; future tense
	Jumps at least 3 feet wide, 1 foot high		reads short text
6½	walks backward on toes	ties bows, shoestrings	retelling possible
		throws ball further than 3 y	learns characters
6	Roller-skating	draws 6-part man	
5½		eats with knife and fork	
	goes forward on toes	copies square	
5		uses knife for cutting bread	repeats sentence of 10 syllables
	uses a swing by him(her)self safely	draws 3-part man	learns simple verses
			puns; creates own words
4½	climbs ladder	catches bouncing ball	
			asks for meaning («why»)
4			repeats sentence of 8 syllables
	jumps on one leg	able to button	uses names and surnames
		safe sequence of movements	uses childrens' songs
3½		threads perls on to string	asks «why?», «how?»
	goes down stairs	catches rolling ball	uses «J»-form
		copies round shapes	vocabulary more than 200 words
3	drives on tricycle or quadricycle		repeats sentence of 6 syllables
	jumps with two legs	puts shapes into the proper holes	uses plural
			forms sentences of 3 words
		builds tower with 4 bricks	asks «where?», «who?», «what?»
2½	goes up stairs with-out holding to railing	builds bridge of 3 parts	asks about names and things
			eats by him(her)self
	stable balance		
2		scribbles upon his(her) own initiative	forms «sentences» of 2 words
	pushes ball with foot	uses spoon safely	eats «normal» food
	goes up stairs while holding on to railing	able to decant liquids	points to named parts of the body
			uses 2–8 words
1½	goes also backward	uses spoon, insecure	imitates noises
	walks without help	builds tower from 2 parts	repeats simple words
	walks with support		reacts to simple request
	stands freely	grips with thumb and index finger	chews; takes coarse food
1	stands with support	handles building blocks	says «Mom» specificly to mother
	crawls forward and backward	points with hand or finger	drinks from cup
	creeps forward	reaches for, holds toy; cannot let it go	
9/12	sits without aid for a long time	grabs threads	says «Mom», undirected
	sits for a short while without aid	able to hold two toys	bites off biscuit
	supports him(her)self on hands	changes toys from one hand to the other	
6/12	lets him(her)self be pulled up for sitting	turns toy between hands	forms syllable chains
	turns body from dorsal to abdominal pos.	targeted individual movements	laughs sonantly
	supports him(her)self on arms	tries to grab toys	takes pap from spoon
3/12	holds head upright for at least 30 seconds	holds rattle in hand	squeaks, chatting
	holds head upright for at least 5 seconds	untargeted complex movements	screaming stage
	turns head to side		

Name, Surname: Birth date:

Fig 263: Developmental Analysis.

SOCIAL DEVELOPMENT	INTELLECT. PERFORMANCE; IDENTIFICATION; UTILIZATION; COMBINATION	SPECIAL DATA ON INDIVIDUAL DEVELOPMENT	Age
			14
is able to exercise self-criticism	explains terms		13
criticizes others	repeats 6 figures		12
discovers its own «self»	indicates the opposite		11
	interest in legends, technics		10
ancious to have pals	masters figures up to 100		
team games	recognizes nonsensicalness		9
thinking in terms of rank	explains pictures		
	identifies shapes in the maze of signs		8
	describes a picture		
efforts to perform are identifiable	repeats 4 figures		7
is conscious of his(her) duty	distinguishes between right and left		
ties bows, laces			6½
	interest in fairytales		6
constructive common games	knows all basic colours		
combs his (her) hair	recognizes shortcomings, deficiencies		5½
strong feeling for family	knows meaning of «1–4»		
sex-specific game	has scale for sizes and quantities		5
makes friends	names 3 colours		
cleans teeth	relates experiences		
first signs of competitive feeling	constant memory		4½
observes rules of game	knows meaning of figure 3		4
is dependable, clean and dry			
	brings 3 objects upon request		
	knows 3 basic colours		3½
able to dress and undress	repeats 3 figures		
able to dress of			
goes to the bath-room by him(Her)self	distinguishes between front and back		3
plays with other children	recites simple nursery rhymes		
plays for a long time	assigns the proper colours to each other		
wants to do a lot by him(her)self	recognition stays for months		
plays games with assigned parts	repeats 2 figures		2½
	differentiates between «a lot» and «a little»		
reacts logically to situation	matches simple figures		
dry during the day	differentiates «round», «square»		2
expresses wishes			
is potty trained (stool)	differentiates «top», «bottom»		
	differentiates «large», «small»		
follows simple commands			1½
gives toys up	reacts to names		
rolls ball to the mother	points to familiar objects		
calls, when wet	recognition lasts 2 weeks		
resistance, when mother leaves	understands simple words		1
waves «bye, bye»	reacts to light colors		
fetches toys		The data are so timed, that 90% of children with normal development are capable of these functions. The aproximate logarithmic orientation symbolises rate (tempo) of development. Developmental manquos are immediatly visible. The time of testing will be signed by a (colored) horizontal line. The criteria below this line are noted in the same color in the squares to the right.	9/12
helpes to hold cup	recognition lasts hours		
recognises people as unfamiliar	turns head to sources of noises		
imitates simple movements	differentiates kind and stem voices		6/12
shows contact-pleasure	listens to music		
interest for toys	looks to toys, when removed		
answers smile by smiling	follows light	■ total ability ▣ unsure ☐ inability	
visual contact with mother	reacts to noises		3/12

273

ed, that is the earlier the evident growth phase of the human brain is utilized, (the first 4 years of life).

B) Implantations by injection should always be incorporated into an wholistic medical concept of medicamentous, pedagogical and training methods.

C) Implantations should be continued as long as substantiated progress can be registered.

Special Indications

The effect of «cell therapy» depends on the basic condition, age and the wholistic therapeutic concept. The following possibilities and limitations result for various disturbances of the central nervous system:

Congenital Metabolic Disorders

They represent a highly diversified field of more than hundred, partly very rare, illnesses. As a rule, enzyme defects are at the base of these diseases of the metabolism; before the enzymatic step,

substrates are dammed up and tissues damaged. Tissues with a high degree of metabolic turnover such as liver, brain, cardiac muscle, are affected usually more frequently and more seriously than tissues having a smaller metabolic turnover. Tab. 31 gives a survey of the important innate metabolic disturbances.

Up to this day it has not been possible to make special recommendations for the application of implantations by injection for innate disturbances of the metabolism because only individual observations relating to rather few disturbances of the metabolism have become known.

The following tissues seem to occupy a central position in implantation therapy: liver, mesenchyme, suprarenal gland, placenta.

With innate or acquired immuno-deficiency (antibody deficiency, syndromes) the use of thymus, bone marrow, liver and mesenchyme is recommended.

Infantile Cerebral Paresis

A classification of the types and subdivisions of infantile paresis can be seen from Tab. 35.

The age limit of the 4th year of life is particularly important for the use of cell therapy in the case of a cerebral paresis. The later cell therapy is applied in addition to the other methods in the first 4 years, the lesser the success will be.

The following is worth mentioning with regard to the various types: In spastic types, a spastic condition fixed once and not influenceable to a noteworthy extent by gymnastics, cannot be influenced by cell therapy methods beyond the 4th year of life. What can be done is to improve the biological overall condition of the children and the mental functional capacity. Compared with this rela-

tively small responsiveness in the cases of fixed spastic types, effects can be achieved with the dyskinetic forms (choreoathetosis) and the atactic forms up to the time beyond the first decade of life though they are smaller than in earlier stages of life.

For the *spastic forms* the following materials are used: cerebral cortex preparations, cerebrum hemisphere, thalamus, midbrain, cerebellum, spinal marrow.

For the *dyskinetic forms* the emphasis of therapeutic application is on the diencephalon, basal ganglia, hypothalamus, thalamus, temporal brain, and cerebellum.

For the *hypotonic types* of infantile cerebral paresis, mainly fetal spinal marrow, occipital brain, cerebellum and midbrain should be used.

Atactic types originating, in the cerebellum or in the spinal marrow should primarily be treated with spinal marrow, cerebellum, midbrain and, possibly, occipital brain.

Heredo-degenerative conditions of the central nervous system present a diversified field of rare types of diseases which, up to this day the therapeutic experiences and observation-times are limited (see special chapter).

The application of fetal cerebral tissue in previous years has shown that no effects on a progressive development or even a healing process in these diseases can be achieved; on the contrary, in individual instances fever reactions developed after implantation. This was proof that also fetal tissue is not tolerated well with most of these degenerative conditions, which, in part, are combined with an autoimmunisation process.

Only the administration of fetal liver, placenta, suprarenal glands, in connection with a subsequent specific enzyme therapy, has opened up trends promising for the future, even if a binding judgment of the final value cannot yet be passed. Considering the otherwise usually poor prognoses and the inescapable progressive development it is recommended, however, to try this therapy.

Enzyme Therapy

Enzymes are synthesis products of the cell organelles; as to their action they are catalytically active proteins. Numerous enzymes are made available to the organism of the recipient through the injection implantations of fetal tissues applied to specific organs. Unlike biochemical substrates, however, their action is only short, because they are rapidly utilized and transformed. According to the logical consequence of this reality it is advisable to maintain the introductory catalysis by a prolonged application of enzyme preparations. Parenterally administered enzymes are governed by the same laws of action as substrates; they penetrate into the cells where they are lacking or are present in reduced quantities; a local need, a cellular insufficiency is the premise for effectiveness. The live cell behaves toward enzymes the same way as toward vitamins, minerals, amino-acids, peptides and other substances.

The selection of enzyme preparations that can be used unter the therapy concepts for mental retardation is still in-complete. The application presents problems.

For many degenerative disorders of the central nervous system digestive enzymes are indicated.

What is available in sugar-coated pill form are the following: *Wobe-enzym-Tabl.®*; as enema tablets: *Wobe-Mugos Klistier-Tabletten®*; as soluble preparations administered subcutaneously or as preparations of Enzypharma in ampoules, which can be administered via the mucous membrane of the mouth. The following preparations among them are of importance for the disturbances of the central nervous system:

Aminosäure-Komplex®

contains ligases of the Amino-Acyl-Ribonucleic acid synthesis.

Coliacron®

suitable for diseases of the neurohormonal system and applicable to hypotonic forms and general weakness of connective tissue; it contains the following active substances:

275

Symptom	Age / Years																						
	0	2	4	6	8	10	1	3	6	9	2	3	4	5	6	7	8	9	10	11	12	13	14
Intelligence normal																							
Debility																							
Imbecility																							
Idiocy																							
normocephalic																							
makrocephalic																							
mikrocephalic																							
Monoplegia																							
Diplegia																							
Hemiplegia																							
Triplegia																							
Tetraplegia																							
Contractures																							
Rigor																							
Muscle-Hypertonia																							
Muscle-Hypotonia																							
Dystonia (alternat. Tonus)																							
Convulsions																							
Hyperkinesia																							
Coordination-Disorders																							
Tremor																							
Chorea																							
Athetosis																							
Restlessnes																							
Eretism																							
Autism																							
extrapyramidal Symptoms																							
Initiative-Disorder																							
Concentration-Weakness																							
Emotional Incontinentia																							
Perseveration																							
Legasthenia																							
Polydipsia																							
Polyphagia																							
Hypertrichosis																							
Vegetative Disorders																							
Trophic Disorders																							
Lability of temperature																							
Hypersensibity																							
Hyposensibility																							
Hyperhydrosis																							
Anhydrosis																							
Ataxia																							
Strabism																							
Eye-Paresis																							
Nystagmus																							
Reduced Visual-Capacity																							
Amaurosis																							
Reduced Hearing-Capacity																							
Deafness																							
Dyslalia																							
Swallow-Disorder																							

For use: Symptome complete ■ partial ⊠ abortive ⊡

Fig. 264: Documentation of the neurological symptoms.

276

(i. u. = international units)

Succinate-dehydrogenase	8 i. u.
NAD-kinase	8 i. u.
Acetyl-CoA-synthetase	6 i. u.
Glutamin synthetase	6 i. u.

Rheumajecta®

for mesenchymal metabolic disorders
contains:

Sulfate-adenyl-transferase	2 i. u.
Chondroitin-sulfo-transferase	2 i. u.
Cholinacetyl transferase	$3\frac{1}{2}$ i. u.
Katalyse: hydrogenperoxyde-oxydo-reductase	$6\frac{2}{3}$ i. u.

Oculucidon®

for building up mucopolysaccharides, usable for mucopolysaccharidoses and eye conditions
contains:

Hexokinase	6 i. u.
Glucosamin-kinase	6 i. u.
Glucosamin-acetyl transferase	2 i. u.
Sulfate-adenyl transferase	50 i. u.
Chondroitin sulfo-transferase	50 i. u.

Hydrolysates

The biological components for diseases of the central nervous system are supplemented by hydrolysates. Here the most comprehensive experience pertains to the raising of prematurely born children, the apallic syndrome and psychic diseases treated with the preparation Cerebrolysin®. This preparation may be used for injection and for permanent infusions.

Ultrafiltrates

Cell-free ultrafiltrates as oral preparations are used

as brainfiltrates for brain disorders

as liver-placenta-pancreas-intestine filtrates for degenerative disorders of the central nervous system, muscles and metabolic diseases,

as cartilage-bone filtrates for innate and degenerative bone diseases,

as thymus-spleen filtrates for immundeficiencies.

Documentation and Control of Development

With disease patterns which, as is the case with mental and multiple handicaps, are so diversified in terms of development and symptomatology, a comprehensive documentation on the findings made (examples of neurological symptoms see fig. 264, Tab. 24, 36) is as important as a detailed control of the development of the condition. Suitable for this are the clinical and technical data listed in the section «Diagnostic Requirements», also the development and intelligence tests enumerated there, provided they were conducted with a good knowledge of the subject-matter and interpreted within the limitations of their indicativeness; and the determination of the various development age groups according to HELLBRÜGGE; naturally also a verbal report of oberservations.

Documentation on findings and checks of development have been rendered most comprehensively in the foregoing pages (fig. 263). The vertical half-logarithmic principle symbolizes developmental progress which slows down with increasing age. The criteria selected are taken from steps of development observed in actual practice; they take into account practical capacities and to a great extent avoid abstract areas. Since the formulations are kept intelligible, parents and medical assistants can complete the development analyses and check the course of a disease. This way the observations made in the natural en-

277

Tab. 36: **Speech-Development and progress control.**

Age	Examination criteria	3 months	6 months	9 months	1 year	1½ years	2 years
10 years	Further development of memory span						
	Detailed interpretation of events (of the written / read)						
	Development of the word and script						
9 years	Interprets symbols and their meaning						
	Completion of abstract thought						
	Recognition of illogicalities						
8 years	Grammatical development in both word and script						
	Concentration span: 30 minutes uninterrupted						
	Memory span: repeats four numbers (1–10)						
7 years	Vocabulary and sentence construction with full grammatical structure						
	Development of concentration span						
	Development of memory span						
	Speech comprehension expanded						
6 years	Logical interpretation of a story						
	Stabilisation of sentence construction						
	Visual and acoustic interpretation of the seen and heard						
5 years	Stabilisation of articulation						
	Simple sentence construction (beginning)						
	Names forms – colours reliably						
	Visual interpretation of a picture sequence						
	Comprehension of time						
	Reliable form – colour identification						
4 years	Vocabulary of 190–200 words						
	Sentence construction of 5–6 words						
	Logical formation of statements, use of adjectives						
	Faulty articulation						
	Names three to four colours						
	Names 3–4 forms						
	Memory: Nursery-rhymes and stories						
	Comprehends 3–4 commands						
	Identifies colours						
	Identifies forms						
	Understands quantities						
3½ years	Verbal formulation of plans						
	Comprehends constructive toys						
3 years	Understands 2–3 part commands						
	Articulation faulty						
2½ years	Asks questions «where» and «who»						
	Uses 2–3 word phrases («ball gone», «door shut»)						
2 years	Reacts logically to situation (fetches pegs when M. hangs washing out)						/
1½ years	20 words with meaning					/	
	Completes sentence (pat a . . .)					/	
	Imitates simple words					/	
	Understands simple commands					/	
	Imitates of noises, sounds and games (peek a boo)					/	
1 year	Says mommy and daddy with meaning				/		
	Simple word comprehension (come, no)				/		
	Immitation of movements				/		
	Reaction to own name				/		
9 months	Combination: Sounds and gestures indicating wishes			/			
	Babbles sounds, incorporating high and low intonation			/			
6 months	Localisation of voices and noises		/				
3 months	Babble noises	/					
	Awareness of voices and facial expressions	/					
	Crying and cooing	/					

2½ years	3 years	3½ years	4 years	5 years	6 years	7 years	8 years	9 years	10 years	Specific notes and observations

The full / empty

squares symbolise

■ = Function completed
● = Function partly completed
□ = Function lacking

The diagonal lines symbolise the average norm.
The time of testing is marked by a vertical line appropriate
to the age of the child. A different coloured pencil should be
used for later control tests. The same colour should be used
throughout one test.

Author: Patricia Braun, Sprachtherapeutin,
Prof. Dr. med. F. Schmid, Städt. Kinderklinik,
875 Aschaffenburg, Am Hasenkopf 1.

vironment are governing and there are no shortcomings that are usually found in test situations. The doctor will be left with the job of checking whether the entries are correct. The development criteria are selected in such a manner that, at the time of the age scale, 90% of normally developed children will have a command of this function. Thus the absence of such function indicates a pathological condition, which represents, for therapists and parents alike, a request for a specific therapeutic action.

The time of the test has been marked by a horizontal line, all criteria below this line are checked. It does not matter when a child learned the function but whether and how perfectly he knows the functions necessary for the test age. Later findings in the analyses of development should be entered in other colours so as to get a survey of the development periods.

Revitalization

The endeavour to retard or to repair losses of the somatic and mental functions due to age has been a very old wish dream of medicine. Tales and legends of «the fountain of eternal youth» or of the magic drug, which garantees eternal youth, are expression of this human wish dream.

Since cell therapy entered the public consciousness, it has been labeled with the idea of being a *«rejuvenating cure»*; this is very appropriately expressed by the English term *«rejuvenation»*. In fact, the therapeutic endeavours do not aim at rejuvenation but at the restablishment or improvement of biological functions, the total capacity of which is referred to as «vitality». If vitality is interpreted as optimal performance of the functions (capacities) existing in a living being, «revitalization» means a re-establishment of lost functions.

Vitality is moreover a concept comprising the total organism with its triad «body, soul, spirit». Although the dysfunctions relate mostly to partial spheres (difficulties in findings words, disturbed potency, depressive ill-humour), the term «loss of vitality» means the restricted vital expansion of the entire personality (Tab. 37, 39).

This statement must be realized when the objective character is necessarily restricted to individual parameters whereas the patient expects a subjective treatment in order to feel subjectively better and free from complaints. In other words: a research worker is interested in measurable data of individual factors, the physician and patient hope for an improvement of the general condition to re-establish the well-being.

Losses of vitality can be due to illness or old age. In youth, the progressive

Tab. 37: **Leading symptoms of «devitalisation»**

Lacking initiative
loss of activity
rapid exhaustion
reduced physical achievements
reduced psychological reactivity
reduced tolerance to alcohol
reduced tolerance to nicotin
loss of ambition
reduced self-confidence
unfounded depressive ill-humour
dullness, despair
lack of concentration
impaired memory
insomnia

---

phase of life, a living being develops its biological capacities, uses them during the phase of maturity, and loses them in a reciprocal succession during the regressive phase. Problems of revitalization, therefore, are chiefly problems of old age. «Geriatrics» are offered in large quantities, beginning from the good advice «to take plenty of exercise» to mysterious magic roots from a possibly far-off country.

Cell-therapy, probably, is the only of many «geriatrics» likely to do justice to the two postulates of

a) an experimental establishment of statistical significance –

b) a practically proved effectiveness.

Effects of revitalization demonstrated by experiments

Revitalization has been defined by A. KMENT as follows: «Revitalization is the prolonged maintenance of re-establishment of a vitality level substantiated by several age parameters after transgressing the maximum of vitality, which corresponds to an age biologically younger than suiting to the organism chronologically». KMENT and his co-workers have fulfilled the postulates of this definition in a so far unique manner by experiments conducted from 1960–1983.

Various parameters have been tried on substantial groups of animals by long-term tests, the extent and arrangement of which appear from the representative Tab. 38. Of these series of tests, the following are of importance for the questions of revitalization:

Labyrinthian tests

A multiple T-shaped labyrinth with 7 crossings was used to test the learning capacity and memory of rats. Animals treated with lyophilised cells (testis, placenta) showed a significantly reduced running time and number of errors as against a control group. Especially, the memory of the treated rats was improved (KMENT, 1956).

Tissue respiration

During tissue respiration (biological oxidation), substrates rich in energy are transformed into compounds poor in energy. The energy so released is used for the intracellular processes needing energy. Tissue-respiration and age are interrelated. Direct measurements in the Warburg apparatus have shown that tissue homogenates of heart, liver, kidney and aorta consume less oxygen in old rats. Tissue of 2-year-old rats absorbs about 50% less than tissue of 6-months-old rats. Tissue lyophilisates injected into 12 and 17-month-old animals effected, at ages of 20 to 24 months, rates of consumed oxygen that corresponded to much earlier biological ages (10–12 months) (KMENT 1960).

Mitochondria

The increase of the energetic cellular performances by fetal tissue lyophilisates was proved moreover by the numbers and sizes of the mitochondria (KMENT, 1971). The activity of the enzyme succinic-dehydrogenase was also increased.

Collagen-experiments

The degenerative dysfunctions of the supporting apparatus and connective tissue are caused above all by the aging collagen. The collagenous fibres lose elasticity, grow more rigid, the cross-linked pattern of the thread-molecules increases same as fibrillary structures at the expense of the amorphous gelatin-

281

Tab. 38: **Parameters of age for long-term tests on rats** (by KMENT).
Determinations at 5 points of time (9, 15, 21, 27, 32 months) on 168 animals at a time.

Parameter		measured per animal	measurements/group	
Motor activity	electronic kinematographic	240	40 320	
running		1	168	
ECG		60	10 080	
tail tendon	isometr. contraction	120	20 160	
	therm. solubility	2	336	336
	hexosamin	2		
skin	thermically soluble collagen	1	168	
	hexosamin	1	168	
elasticity of the aorta		40	6 720	
lipofuscin	chemical: heart, brain	4	772	
	histolog: frontalbrain hippocampus cerebellum	150	12 000	
succinodehydrogenasis	heart liver	4	672	
plasmalipids		2	372	
plasmacholesterol		2	372	
minerals trace elements	heart, kidney	10	1 680	
	total total test:		94 324 ca. 472 000 measured values	

ous part of the volume. Tendinous threads of rat tails, which virtually consist only of collagen, were treated with heat to prove with biostatistically established significance that after the use of testicular lyophilisate the contractibility of the collagen in the tendons of rat-tails corresponds to earlier ages (KMENT et al., 1963, 1967).

Elasticity and tensile strength of the skin

According to these results seen on collagenous fibres, the statistical significance of an improved elasticity and tensile strength of the skin was established. KMENT and co-workers (1967) availed themselves of the method described by WENZEL (1950).

Further experimental studies

The authors demonstrated the same rejuvenating effect in another experimental group for the elasticity of the aorta.

– The following tests served for the substantiation of the revitalizing effect on animals:
– Tests on the thyroid activity in guinea-pigs with radio-isotopes (J 131) after siccacell products (KMENT, 1958). Quantitative electron-microscopic studies on cardial mitochondria of rats after injections of placenta or testicular tissue (KMENT, 1966).
– Tests on the revitalizing effect by myocardial cells, myocardial nuclei and myocardial mitochondria in rats (KMENT, 1974).
– Analyses of the spontaneous activity in old and revitalized rats by means of electronic registration (KMENT and HOFECKER, 1972).
– Tracer elements in the heart, liver and brain of rats of various ages and after revitalization by cell injections (KMENT, HOFECKER and NIE-DERMÜLLER, 1973).
– Studies on the effect of the revitalization in rats on the absorption, dispersion and secretion of penicillin V (KMENT and NIEDERMÜLLER, 1973).
– Article on the method of the cinematographical registration of the activity of rats, as part of the research into revitalization (JELENIK 1971).
– Gerontological studies on the revitalization (KMENT, 1977).

Identical are the results obtained by WRBA (1961/62) respecting the influence of organic extracts and sera on the metabolism of organic cultures.

The revitalization in clinic and practice

Whereas, experimentally, success or failure can well be demonstrated and reproduced by means of individual parameters, effect and substantiation on a clinical level are confronted with difficult problems. Success or failure of a treatment are items of objectively conceivable factors and subjective sensations that cannot be defined by analytical-scientific standards.

In the *life profile of man,* three periods can be abstracted:

a) the *progressive period* of ripening in infancy, childhood and adolescence (from 0–20 years);
b) the *maturity-period* between the 3rd and 5th decades of life;
c) the *regressive period*, which begins in the 5th decade and reaches to the end of biological existence.

The biological functions for the maintenance of existence subside in the regressive period of senescence inversely to the succession of acquisitions during the ripening period. At the end of these losses there is a living being unable to guarantee its existence by its own strength. In the extreme case, man at a high age is in the same situation as a newborn: he cannot move on, must be fed, has lost his cleanliness functions and is no longer conscious of what happens around him. The loss of vitality sets in during the (4th) 5th decade and proceeds at an individually different pace, with «logarithmical» progression; it comprises all parts of the biological functions, the rough and fine movements, coordination, speech, social behaviour and the intellectual performances.

These functions fit organismically into each other and sum up the total image of personality. The biological position of man in his environment is defined by the extremes rather than by the average of these capacities. Special achievements in one or several fields or particular shortcomings determine the sociological position more than the average qualities.

Findings on various levels of perception

Development and senescence are processes following biological laws; they are the consequence of permanently changing structures and their functions; both influence each other mutually i.e. changes of structures cause changes of functions, and changes of functions transform the structures. For instance the muscles: they can be augmented and strengthened by increasing the functions (training) and undergo atrophy when the functions are restrained (immobilization, long rest in bed). On the other hand, a defective structure or an inadequate innervation i.e. a structural shortcoming will impair the functional power. One must bear in mind the close connections between function and structure for all evolutionary and involutionary processes, especially for the mental and somatic disintegration caused by senescence.

The findings are individual according to our abilities to perceive and to establish proofs in the various dimensions, and the interpretations of the connections between these dimensions (cell – tissue – organism) is incomplete.

Cellular level

The familial cumulative occurrence of long-lived and short-lived persons, of good or bad natural resistance to illness, early or late senescence in a family suggest a genetic fundament.

Here, the nucleic-acid-protein-synthesis apparatus is of central importance. As a carrier of genetic information, the desoxyribonucleic acid (DNA) transcribes its potential and pattern of infor-

mation to the ribonucleic acid (RNA). This *transcription* is followed in the area of the ribosomes (fig. 32) by the *translation* into the sequence of amino-acid of the (characteristic) protein. STREHLER supposes that the growing «internal disorder» in senescence is due to a gradual loss of genes. Of the about 500 genes available for the formation of protein in the nucleolus (fig. 8) at birth, approximately 50 per cent are functioning in old age so that there is, partly, no organ left to effect a sufficient translation into proteins. Functionally, the genetic information is increasingly reduced as the genes diminish.

A statement of account rendered at the first Viennese symposium on experimental gerontology gave the following picture (A. KMENT and G. HOFECKER, 1977):

The *perichromatin granules* (storage and transport form of the m-RNA) diminish in old age (BERTONI-FREDDARI et al., 1977) same as the protein-synthesis apparatus of the rough endoplasmatic reticulum (GIULI et al., 1977). Using a UTP-H3-tagging on isolated nuclei of rat-brain, SZESZAK et al. investigated the activity of transcription and found a nucleolar and extranucleolar *RNA-polymerase activity* diminished according to the age.

The *adaptive mechanisms* of the RNA-synthesis (H. MARTIN) and the *repairs effected by DNA-polymerase* (SAND-HOFER et al.) are diminished. For the enzyme proteins, SCHOCH and PLATT showed in three 97-year-old persons a declining activity of $Mg^{++}-Na^+$-ATPase and $Mg^{++}-Na^+-K^+$-ATPase in the erythrocyte membranes of old persons. The protein kinase turned out to be independent of age in the cerebral cortex (man, ox), the *cyclic amino-mono-phosphate (c-AMP)* was reduced in old age. (REICHELMEIER et al.).

284

Tissue level

The tissular and organic systems have their own laws of ripening and regression (fig. 265). The central nervous system occupies a special position: it is the only tissular system that has not yet completed the fetal stage at birth but attains it in in the fourth year when the medullary sheath has matured. The numbers of neurons do not increase after birth: in question is an irreversibly post-mitotic condition of the nerve cells. This indivi-sibility is a prerequisite for the stability of the information stored in the brain. The *senile atrophy of the brain* is morphologically characterized by a diminution of volume, by dystrophy of the glia and by accumulations of lipofuscin. According to TREFF, every species of cells in the brain has its « own life history». As far as mobility is concerned, the *supporting tissue* plays a special part. While the connective tissue grows old, the divisibility of the connective-tissue cells is restricted, the heterochromatisation and polyploidisation increase, the synthesis of *collagen and elastin changes* and the spectrum of the glycosaminoglycanes shows aberrations. The proliferation of connective tissue and the *generation of fibroblasts* are prolonged (KRANZ).

The collagen, as the reduction of the cutaneous collagen in old age shows, undergoes changes due to senescence, which NIEDERMÜLLER et al. SKALICKY et al. have summarized as follows:

1. the cutaneous and the tendinous collagen have different metabolic dynamics;

2. the formation of the polymere collagens slows in old age;

3. stabile and labile polymere collagens originate from various tropocollagens; the relation between the syntheses of these two forms changes during senescence;

4. both cellular and extracellular senescent processes account for the changes of the tendinous and cutaneous collagens in old age.

These senescent changes shown for the brain and connective tissue could be discussed at length also for the skin, vessels, heart, liver, kidneys, lungs and bones. The lung shall be picked out as an example. According to P. BRUNNER(1980), the *physiological aging processes* in the lung are accounted for chiefly by the structures of the connective tissue in the respiratory organs, not by their epithelial constituents. The important factor is the changed structure of the elastic fibre system, which reduces the retractability and augments the collagen. Atrophy of alveolar septa, dilation of alveolar ducts, reduction of the alveolar net-capillaries as well as calcareous and osseous stiffness of the skeleton of the bronchial respiratory tracts have led to the morphological term «senile lung», and to the restriction of nearly all parameters of pulmonary functions in old age. The senile lung, therefore, is a sound lung with restricted functions.

The collective term «senile involution» comprises the processes of morphological regression and reduction of functional efficiency in the tissues.

Personality level

The logical evolution, the multicellular organism, which consists of organic systems, does not quite correspond to the concept of human individuality. The forms and functions of the organs, with all their manifestations, measuring and functionary results cannot conceive the properties of the individual. Abilities and shortcomings in the motor, coordinative, social and intellectual fields are more distinctive of the position of an individual than this formal properties (ap-

285

pearance) unless they differ too much from the standard (fig. 266). «Individuality» is more than «organism». Vitality and loss of vitality must therefore be judged from the individuality, the subject, objective findings of organs do not necessarily conform thereto. An «organically» ill person can by discipline and strength of will be a professionally, culturally or socially great personage whereas an «organically» healthy individual may be just the reverse.

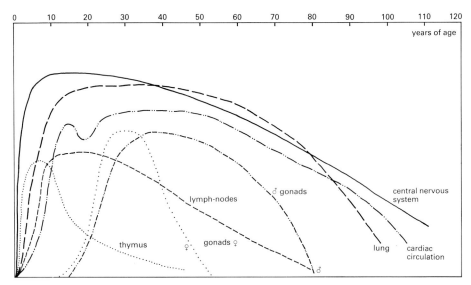

Fig. 265:
Ripening and aging of various tissues in the life-profile, projected on the «genetic» expectation of life.

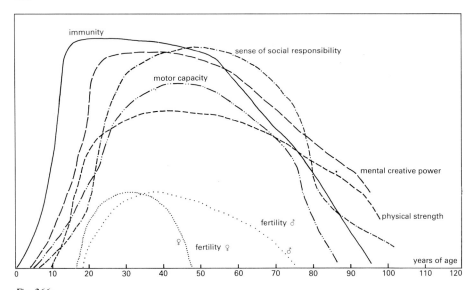

Fig. 266:
Maturation and aging of various individual characteristics.

286

Tab. 39: **Devitalization symptoms**

«Personality»	Loss of interest in
Loss of initiative «debility»	sports
affective «emptiness»	politics
lack of inspiration and experience	acquaintances
general uncertainty	environment
egocentric	hobbies
incapability of acting	
loss of accountability	**Intellectual performances**
	Perceptive faculty impaired
Rough movements	perceptive power permeable
Stiff posture	«senseless» failures
uncertain gait	disturbance of memory
tripping gait	reduced concentration span
reduction of walking distance	memory reduced
trouble when walking up stairs	hard of remembering
walking with expedients	taciturnity
	stereotype monotony (complaints, praise)
	loss of short-term memory
Fine motoric and coordination	reduction of vocabulary
Subsiding mimics	lacking orientation
reduced gestures	
fine tremor	**Old-age regression of organs**
trembling	Senile atrophy of the skin
unsteady hand	vascular sclerosis
restlessness	cerebral sclerosis
	cardiac insufficiency (senile)
	pneumoemphysema
Socio-psych. behaviour	digestive insufficiency
Ill-humour	decline in potency
self-reproach	senile diabetes
loss of social relations	loss of hepatic functions
anxiety for life	insufficient immunity in old age
eremitism	

To perceive the change of individuality is, summarily, an observation, it may be findings for certain characteristics (e.g. arthrosis, emphysema, reduced walking distance). Summing up the regressive senile changes would probably require an analysis of reciprocal development with several hundreds of criteria (see fig. 263). In practice, the judgment of vitality must be confined to important steps of regression, which have been outlined for the various functional spheres in Tab. 39:

From this detailed symptomatological analysis of senescence, conclusions can be drawn especially as to which organs should be selected for the cell therapy (Tab. 42).

STEIN and GIANOLI have drawn up for the practical use a concise list of symptoms, which gives a good idea of the loss of general vitality but does not lead direct to therapeutic consequences (Tab. 37).

Therapy

The treatment and care of aging persons is medically and sociologically in the teething stage. The futile postulate to integrate old people into society, is mostly completed by the doctor's advice «to take longer walks» and by the prescription of combinations of polyvitamin-trace-elements. However, the therapy must same as in cases of retardation in infancy, aim at the entire individuality, and the training of the somatic, social and mental capacities should be given priority.

The function of cell therapy in this field, for which it has earned legendary fame, consists in the regeneration of performances of the organs and organ systems affected by senescence. Experimental data and considerable practical experience are available. The following

typical «combinations for revitalization» are recommended:

for women:

hypothalamus	placenta
adrenal gland female	connective
ovary	tissue

for men:

hypothalamus	liver
frontal brain	placenta
adrenal gland male	testicles

The doses of these preparations are 100–150 mg of lyophilisate. These combinations provide good results in the revitalization but do not meet the differentiation of individual cases. The following survey is intended to show possibilities of rendering the revitalization more individual with regard to the symptoms (Tab. 40). There is a direct relation between the symptoms and the tissues to be selected. Care must be taken that for an

Tab. 40: **Selection of tissues according to symptoms in revitalising therapy**

Symptoms	Selection of tissues
Disturbances of rough movements	cerebrum, cerebral cortex, spinal medulla
Disturbances of refined movements	thalamus, diencephalon, basal ganglia, cerebellum
disturbed coordination	thalamus, diencephalon, basal ganglia, cerebellum
Disturbed impulse, initiative	frontal brain, thalamus, hypothalamus
Disturbed memory	temporal brain, frontal brain
reduced intellect	cerebral cortex, cerebral hemisphere
cerebral sclerosis	placenta, fet. artery, cerebrum
vascular sclerosis	placenta, fet. artery, connective tissue
senile heart-complaints	heart, placenta, artery, liver
hyperuricaemia	kidney, placenta, liver
impaired hepatic functions	liver, gastric mucosa, placenta
senile pulmonary complaints	lung, connective tissue, placenta
disturbed potency	testicles, adrenal gland male, hypothalamus (diencephalon), (liver)
menopause	ovary, adrenal gland female, hypothalamus, diencephalon, placenta of female foet.
degenerative changes of skeleton and joints	cartilage, bone-marrow, connective tissue, placenta, parathyreoidea
insufficient immunity	thymus, adrenal gland, spleen

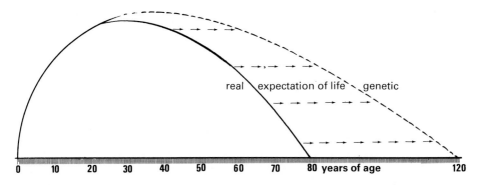

Fig. 267:
Difference between biological «debit and credit». The earlier revitalising measures are taken up, the more vitality persist.

individual treatment usually not more than 5–6 tissue preparations (500–800 mg of the lyophilisates in all) are used as otherwise the stress after the implantation would be too great. These tissues combined can be distributed on 2 simultaneous injections. The more weakened, run-down and emaciated a patient is, the more he needs a good preliminary examination and a methodical aftertreatment (fig. 267). Fatiguing physical work and brain work should be avoided within the phase of stress of 7–14 days. Combinations of medicaments stimulating the metabolism (combinations of polyvitamin trace elements, membrane activators, neurodynamics on a biological basis and enzyme preparations) ought to be included into the aftertreatment. The remarks specially on the enzyme preparations in the chapter «Mental and multi-

ple physical disability» apply analogously.

Repeated treatments as part of revitalization use to be necessary and indicated at intervals of 1–3 years. For the question from what age a revitalization can be looked upon as reasonable, the individuality of the senescence must be taken into consideration. Generally, revitalization will be the more effective the earlier it begins (fig. 267) and the more regularly in the course of senescence it is effected. The 5th decade of life is regarded as the optimal age for the beginning of a revitalizing therapy. Measurable results are obtained also if a treatment is started in the 8th and 9th decades, but it should be realized that already existing degenerative tissular processes may restrict the expected degree of the therapeutic improvement.

Dysfunctions of organ-systems and organs

Maldevelopments and senescence affect certain organic systems more or less but the «individuality» is the central point of the medical measures. The following chapters deal with certain illnesses for which cell-therapeutic measures have proved effective in a considerable number of cases or were applied with encouraging results.

This «special clinic» follows the basic idea that the implantation therapy using fetal tissues must be a constructive-biological method within a wholistic medical concept. The point is not to suggest, as a cookery book, certain tissues for certain diseases or symptoms but to give cell therapy the place it deserves in the groups of diseases. It will then occupy partly a secondary, partly a central position in the scope of therapeutic alternatives.

Central nervous system

The congenital disorders of the central nervous system were a prominent subject on the pages of the preceding chapters. There is no sharp line of demarcation between the symptoms of the innate lesions of the central nervous system and those acquired in early infancy. Extensive experience from 30 years of work in clinic and practice is available under the collective term «brain damage of early infancy» on the innate diseases and those acquired in babyhood and early infancy.

In this connection, the studies of many years by G. DESTUNIS (1957–1960), G. DESTUNIS and E. SCHMIDT (1956), on encephalopathy and debilities of various genesis deserve to be mentioned. The authors worked chiefly on implantations of diencephalon. More reports in this field are available by R. JAKOBS (1960); H. GOLDSTEIN (1961); J. M. DAVID and DAVID, E. A. de AURELIA (1960); P. E. DELONS and J. COUGOULE (1959); W. ZELLER (1957); H. FELDMAN (1961, 1979, 1982). The voluminous literature of DOWN's syndrome is mentioned in a special chapter.

The following diseases have been picked out from neurology and psychiatry; decisive for this selection were the viewpoints of clinical importance and experience in the field of cell therapy.

Infantile cerebral paresis

The forms of infantile cerebral paresis have been outlined in the chapters of «Mental and multiple physical disability». The following survey is just another

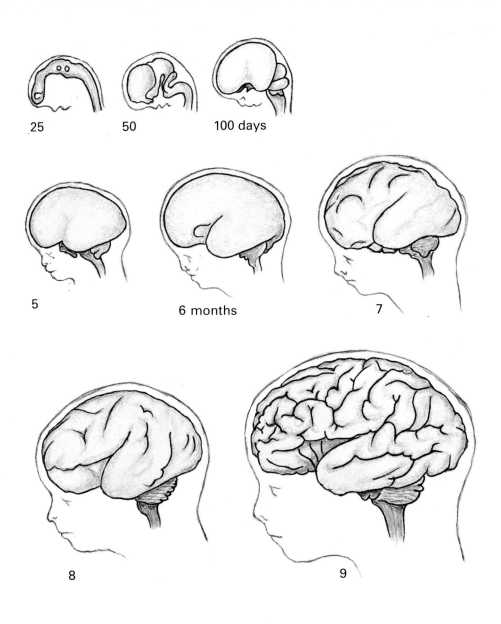

25   50   100 days

5   6 months   7

8   9

Fig. 268:
Embryonal and fetal development of human brain in days (100) and months (till 9).

291

statement of the special aspects of cell therapy with regard to the symptoms:

To the infantile cerebral paresis

belonges disorders of the motor system, which may be combined with sensorial, sensitive, intellectual and psychic pathological deficiencies and cerebral seizures. The causal cerebral lesion constitutes usually a final condition without progression.

The second type is formed by heredodegenerative and metabolic ailments of the central nervous system, which use to proceed in a progressive way:

Whereas in former decades the extent of the intellectual deficit was the centre of considerations and the infantile affections of the central nervous system were divided into debility, imbecility and idiocy according to the degree of the mental retardation, specially the last years have provided other orientation. The influences on the neuromuscular system became the center of considerations as the therapy may be initiated here.

The infantile cerebral paresis can be divided under various aspects; customary is the division according to the form of the motor effects (Tab. 35) and to a symptomatological classification (Tab. 32).

The biological condition of the affected children cannot be perceived unless, besides looking for a label for the diagnosis, the concomitant symptoms in other fields – in addition to the motor effects – are taken into account. This helps to understand the pathobiological influences of the basic process on the child's individuality. Apart from the central neuromuscular symptoms manifesting themselves by spasm, hypotonea, chorea, dyskinesia and ataxia, a wide variety of concomitant symptoms is found in the sensorial, sensitive, psychic, intellectual and somatic spheres; they may influence the fate of the children stronger than the central motor symptoms.

These symptoms include:

a) in the psychic sphere:
   erethism, motor unrest, increased distraction, affective incontinence, tendency to perseveration, apathy, erroneous behaviour and false reactions towards the environment;

b) in the sensitive sphere:
   hypersensitivity, hyposensitivity, trophic disturbances;

c) in the sensorial sphere:
   speech-disorders, hyperkinesia, disturbed coordination, acoustic symptoms, audiogenic dyslalia, deafness of the internal ear with loss of high sounds, motor hearing dumbness, acoustic acnosia; eye symptoms, strabism, visual paresis, nystagmus, defects in the visual field;

d) the intellectual defects are not obligatory but occur very frequently in the course of untreated cerebral paresis. Moreover, a debility with a restricted capacity to develop or serious oligophrenia permitting only a practical formation or constituting a «mere nursing case» may come on.

This incomplete outline of the multiple effects of a lesion in the central nervous system shows that virtually every child has an individual symptom mosaic of his own, which necessarily requires an individual therapeutic scheme.

Residual therapy

In cases of serious multiple disability and if cerebral paresis is taken up in late periods (beyond the second year of age), the causal and symptomatic measures mentioned above are frequently insufficient to provide decisive progress because the lesion in the central nervous system is too deep. Both the callisthenics and the paedagogical measures require a

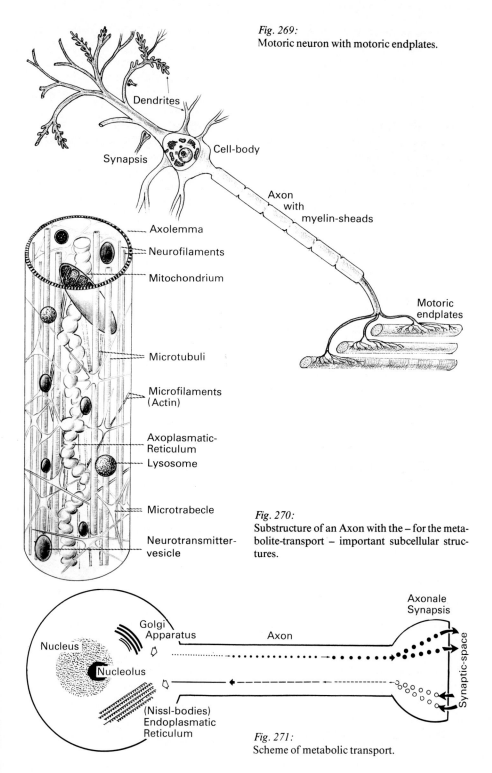

Fig. 269:
Motoric neuron with motoric endplates.

Dendrites

Synapsis

Cell-body

Axon
with
myelin-sheads

Motoric
endplates

Axolemma

Neurofilaments

Mitochondrium

Microtubuli

Microfilaments
(Actin)

Axoplasmatic-
Reticulum

Lysosome

Microtrabecle

Neurotransmitter-
vesicle

Fig. 270:
Substructure of an Axon with the – for the meta-
bolite-transport – important subcellular structures.

Axonale
Synapsis

Golgi
Apparatus

Axon

Synaptic-space

Nucleus

Nucleolus

(Nissl-bodies)
Endoplasmatic
Reticulum

Fig. 271:
Scheme of metabolic transport.

293

minimum cooperation on the side of the child. In the absence of such a cooperation or co-reaction, all measures are wearisome, tedious and unsatisfactory.

Whereas, until a few years ago, doctors were relatively helpless when confronted with such situations, the injection implantations of fetal cerebral tissues provide nowadays a remedy likely to mitigate considerably even these human fates. It may be regarded as a significantly established fact that morphological defects on a cellular or tissular level and dysfunctions can be improved by a specific subcutaneous implantation of cerebral tissues, more so if this method ist combined with the above therapies. Considerable increases of the brain volume index were registered even in general disorders of the brain such as microcephaly or mongoloid brachymicrocephaly.

For practical application (fig. 261, 262) the following remarks must be taken into consideration: *spastic forms* are as a rule, exclusively or prevailingly, lesions of the cortex. Implantation tissues are available as cerebral cortex, cerebral hemisphere or, in localized cortical atrophy, as frontal, temporal, parietal, occipital brain. The effects on the movements are modest beyond the 3rd year of age.

In the *types of choreo-athetosis*, the lesion by nuclear icterus or early infantile encephalitis is in the zones of the diencephalon, hypothalamus or basal-ganglia. The tissues indicates here are the diencephalon, hypothalamus, fetal basal-ganglia. The symptoms indicate whether the disorders encroach upon the neurohypophysis or mesencephalon, and whether parts of the cerebral cortex are involved.

The lesion in the *hypotonic* or *adynamic form* of infantile cerebral paresis is located chiefly in the zone of the mes-encephalon but often exceeds it. The strongest implantations are those of mesencephalon and medulla oblongata; combinations with diencephalon, occipital brain and cerebellum are advisable in certain cases.

Ataxia as a guiding system may be due to an inadequate coordination and thus be localized in the zone of the diencephalon/mesencephalon; very frequently, the cause is a defective development or lesion of the cerebellum (cerebellar ataxia). The most important implantation is that of fetal cerebellum; combinations with medulla oblongata, mesencephalon, diencephalon and, possibly, parts of the cerebrum are necessary in certain cases.

Respecting cell therapy in disturbed hearing and vision, substantial experience has not become known so far. Still, distinct improvements of the general condition of affected children have been obtained with diencephalon, mesencephalon, temporal and occipital brain in reduced hearing capacity, and with occipital brain and diencephalon in *disturbances of vision* caused by the cortex lesions. *Speech disorders* are a complex phenomenon due to disturbances of hearing or to defective coordination in the majority of cases. Tests with diencephalon, basal ganglia and frontal brain are indicated if other remedies cannot take effect.

The therapeutic scheme outlined above for multiple disabilities by cerebral lesions in early infancy constitutes a program that needs completion and refinement in many respects; but evidently it is suited to overcome the reluctant and resigning approach to this syndrome so that many afflicted children can be brought back into their social community.

during the middle and mature age belong to the most satisfying indications of implantation therapy. Above all, N. WOLF has been working at these problems for 20 years (1966, 1969, 1976, 1977, 1978, 1980) and substantiated his clinical findings with psychological tests (W. HENNIG, 1969). N. WOLF's patients included at that time 133 persons who got 2500 individual applications of cell therapy. Each individual treatment of the brain-atrophic processes was an intramuscular injection of 100 mg of frontal brain and 150 mg of placenta of the same sex. A number of patients suffering from obstinate disorders of sleep got additional doses of 100 mg hypothalamus lyophilisate. Unlike the usual cell-therapeutic practice of putting repeat treatments off to a term beyond a time interval of 6 months, 66 patients got several repeat treatments at intervals of 4 weeks in order to intensify the therapeutic effect. Thanks to favourable experience with this intense method and as complications are rare, it is believed that cell therapy of the brain-atrophic processes of the middle and mature age should be started with a intensive treatment i.e. 3–4 treatments as described above are aplied at intervals of 4 weeks. As these initial concentrated therapies have usually improved the state of health considerably, the further applications can be effected at longer intervals.

The complications seen in those 2500 applications were, in two cases, an abscess near the site of injection, which required a surgical intervention; three more cases showed near the site of injection some indurations, which regenerated after conservative treatments. Taking into account these observations, the rate of complications was given to be 2%.

Results of psychological tests

To substantiate the therapeutic outcome, W. HENNIG conducted on 40 patients before and after cell therapy psychological studies, which provided the following summarizing results: the individualities of 50% of the patients were revitalized to normal. In 37% also a revitalization, though less intense, was observed so that positive effects resulted in 87%. The intellectual efficiency improved by about 10 points of the intelligence quotient in 60% of the cases.

HENNIG has completed these figures with the following comment: «One will therefore have to get accustomed to the idea that the heterologous implantations injected to treat brain-atrophic processes take effect on various types of individuality and efficiency, according to the degree and localization of the preceding lesions. Moreover, one cannot ignore the problems resulting from the cognition that, possibly, the brain-atrophic processes do not stop in certain cases, that the disintegration continues, that the intellectual efficiency goes on weakening and that, nevertheless, the patient's vitality, physical efficiency, humour, confidence, sociability and interest appear normal after the treatments. The aspect of vitality makes these patients look healthy and efficient but their intellectual achievements decrease.

As regards sociability, the treated patients can perform tasks and functions learned earlier and achieve again adequate activities when they come back into their old environment. The new vital impulse enables them to achieve the learned behaviour and activities; the limit is usually reached where new tasks requiring independent solution are set.»

Heredodegenerative diseases

In view of the many causes and forms of heredodegenerative diseases of the central nervous system, the question as to whether or not cell therapy shall be applied deserves critical considerations; one is often confronted with the alternative whether an enzyme defect or an autoaggressive destruction of tissue is the cause of the pathological process.

Empirism justifies the ambivalent recommendation to try a therapy with placenta, liver (possibly adrenal gland) because individual observations delay not only the regressive symptoms but also the progress of development. The ambivalence of this trial appears from the fact that cerebral tissue, especially cerebral marrow, is not effective, often entails febrile reactions. Tissue of the white substance, therefore, should not be administered even if just a trace of an autoaggressive tissular process is detected.

Generally, the existing products are not qualified enough to meet the requirements for a treatment of degenerative processes in the central nervous system (Tab. 22). Concentrates of lysosomes and mitochondria are more promising as a more specific use of the cell organelles in question is necessary.

A considerable progress is to expect in this field in the next future.

Degenerative Disorders of the cerebral white matter

It is generally accepted that the course of the majority of degenerative disorders of the central and peripheral nervous system cannot be manipulated by therapy. This view is further supported by the frequently used adjective «heredodegenerative». However, specific observations of a number of different degenerative manifestations in the white cerebral matter (myelin degeneration of the brain and spine) do not confirm the validity of a specific treatment strategy, unless long-termd results gained from a sufficiently large group of observed patients is available.

Nevertheless these individual observations revealed some very striking regeneration features even during the first week and months following the onset of the treatment and they impel us to offer all victims afflicted with this desease not only a diagnostical label, but actual medical help. The discrepancy between the diagnostic display accompanied by various unpleasant annoyances and the therapeutic nihilism produces a red thread which runs through the anamneses of many patients.

Myelin, the predominant component of the cerebral white matter, consists of proteolipid layers surrounding the axons of the nerve cells. While the myelination – as a postponed fetal process – occurs in the first years of postnatal life, the deficiencies of the «marrow-sheat-formation» also starts in the first years of life. This white substance is in an immature state at birth. Even though all cerebral cells are present at birth and no fresh ones appear at a later stage, the brain is the only organ which is not in a position to ensure the sustaining of life independently at this stage. Life sustenance can only be assured by the age of 4 years when the secondary structures (dentrides, synapses, axones, glia) are fully matured and insulation of the nerve fibre conductors with the aid of Myelin (medullary sheath) is complete.

Since the maturing of the medullary sheath (myelinisation), which is in fact a delated fetal process, takes place during the first years of life and is only completed by age 4, initial defects in the maturing of the medullary sheath initially begins during the early years of life. Depending on the actual time at which they appear, we differentiate between the more serious generalised «de-medullisation disorders» which occur at a young age as a result of an insufficient «myelinisation», and the more localised manifestations occurring in older age groups which indicate a «myelin-degeneration».

Somewhere in between we have extensive, but not generalised degenerations which occur in the middle decades of life, such as in Friedreich's ataxia (this disease occurs most frequently between the ages of 10 and 30), or else multiple sclerosis (disseminated sclerosis = scattered focal substitution of nerve tissue by connective tissue), most frequently occurring between the ages of 20 and 40.

Depending on age and localisation we are faced with a broad spectrum of syndromes (= diagnoses) and in specific cases it can be quite difficult to match an individual collection of symptoms with any specific diagnosis. The most important diseases categories are listed below:

Leukodystrophies
Metachromatic leukodystrophy
(sulfatide lipidosis)
Globoid leukodystrophy
*(*KRABBE *disease, cerebrosid lipidosis)*
Spongy degeneration of cerebral white matter
*(*CANAVAN *disease)*
Sudanophilic leukodystrophies
*(*PELIZEUS-MERZBACHER *disease)*

Demyelinating diseases
*Diffuse sclerosis (*SCHILDER *disease)*
Disseminated sclerosis (Multiple sclerosis)
*Neuromyelitis optica (*DEVIC *disease)*

Cerebro-occular degenerations
Amaurotic idiocy – infantile variety
*(*TAY – SACHS*);*
*Late infantile variety (*BIELSCHOWSKY*);*
*Juvenile variety (*SPIELMEYER – VOGT*);*
Tapeto-retinal degeneration.

Spinocerebellar degenerations
Syndrome cataracte-oligophrénie et
ataxie spinocerebelleuse
*(*MARINESCO-SJÖGREN*-syndrome)*
Congenital ataxia, aniridia, mental retardation
*(*GILLESPIE*-syndrome)*
CHARLEVOIX-SAGUENAY*-syndrome*
TROYER*-syndrome*
*Ataxia teleangiectatica (*LOUIS BAR *syndrome)*
FRIEDREICHs *ataxia*
Refsum' disease
Abetalipoproteinemia (Acanthosis;
BASSEN-KORNZWEIG*-syndrome)*
Recessive ROUSSY-LEVY *syndrome*

Recessive type II OPCA *(*FICKLER-WINKLER *type).*
Myoklonus-encephalopathy in children
*(*KINSBOURNE*-syndrome)*

Cerebro-cutaneous degenerations
*Tuberous cerebral sclerosis (*BOURNEVILLE*);*
*Neuro-fibromatosis (*von RECKLINGHAUSEN*);*
*Angiomatosis retinae et cerebelli (*V. HIPPEL – LINDAU*).*

Spino neuromuscular degenerations
Neural muscular atrophies
    (WOLFARTH – KUGELBERG – WELANDER;
    WERDIG – HOFFMANN; CHARCOT – MARIE – TOOTH – HOFFMANN; DEJERINE – SOTTAS);

Progressive muscular atrophies
*(*DUCHENNE; Erb*);*
*Myatonia congenita (*OPPENHEIM*);*
*Myatonia (*THOMSEN*);*
Karnithin myopathia
*Myasthenia gravis (*ERB – GOLDFLAM*);*
*Amyotrophous lateral sclerosis (*CHARCOT *syndrome);*
Syringomyelia.

Degenerations of the basal ganglia
*Hepatolenticular degeneration (*WILSON *disease)*
Dystonia musculorum deformans
(Torsions-dystonia)
HUNTINGTON*-chorea*
PARKINSONs *disease*

Friedreichs Ataxia

Beside the multiple sclerosis the Friedreich ataxia is the most important disease in the heredodegenerative disorders of the central nervous system. The common onset is the late childhood or adolescence. The clinical symptoms are correlated to a progressive cerebellar and spinal cord degeneration and dysfunction. Their base ist a degeneration of the posterior column of spinocerebellar and corticospinal tracs. The main symptoms are:

gait disturbance,
incoordination of upper limbs and speech-motoric,
highly arched foot (caved foot),
hammer toes,
scoliosis,
cardiomegaly (following necrosis of cardiac muscle fibers).

A treatment of this recessive-autosomal disease seemed to be impossible till now and is therefore denied.

By treating a number of cases with degenerative diseases of the central nervous system for the last years, the *Friedreich'sche Ataxia* has only been included recently. So far we have only experience with a few cases, and at this time it is not possible to give a definite judgment on the longterm effect of the treatment. It is remarkable that in these single cases not only a stagnation of the illness could be obtained, but also a restoration of the impaired functions could be registered.

Multiple sclerosis

is caused by a myeline degeneration which presents clinical symptoms most often between the ages of 20 and 40. The most predominant features are impairment of walking, speech and eye-sight as well as numerous neurological outfall symptoms. Periods of progression, remission and even improvements create a mercurial pattern, at the end of which there is usually complete invalidity.

The method of treatment applied now, has not yet been published. The first publications can only be expected when we can look back on an experience of at least two years. Earlier experiences with implantations of fetal muscle of the spinal medulla and tissues of the central nervous system did not bring about a convincing progress, so that the treatment was changed. The basis for this were individual observances. The total concept of the method of treatment, as summarized thereafter, has probably still not reached its optimum result.

Disposition – exposition

Many of the degenerative diseases are hereditary in an autosomal-recessive manner, whereby the pervasiveness of Friedreich's ataxia is particularly great. This hereditary factor very often results in therapeutic resignation. However, in order for a disease to occur on the basis of a hereditary disposition, several *realisation factors,* i. e. additional influences, must be present, which turn the existing faulty disposition into a functional disturbance which ultimately results in disease symptoms. In the context of heredodegeneration of the central nervous system with reference to the interaction between hereditary disposition and the environmental influences which acts as a trigger, the following guidelines can be provided:

1. *Disability caused by predisposition (constitutional)*
   a) of the intestinal resorption and digestive organs;
   b) lysosomalic defects (insufficient production of secretions of lysosomalic enzymes).

2. *Strains produced by environmental factors (expositional)*

which trigger the outbreak of the illness on account of the constitutional weakness. These include:

c) strains caused by de-naturalized foods which cannot be properly broken down, because the inadequate organism lacks the appropriate enzymes;

d) viral illnesses (measles, viral encephalitis, herpes infections and others);

e) immunisations;

f) gastro-entero-colitis with necroses of the intestinal resorption areas.

From the statistical point of view it is practically impossible to evaluate the significance of hereditary predisposition versus triggering factors. On the one hand a family, in which several siblings are afflicted would appear to indicate a dominant influence of hereditary factors, but on the other hand, these members of the same family will have been exposed to the same environmental and nutritive conditions. Even studies on the frequency of distribution in specific geographical areas do not provide an unequivocal answer. Upon discovering that multiple sclerosis occurs 5 × more frequently in the north of England (Orkney Islands) compared with Holland, and 20 × more frequent than in the South of Europe (South of France), then one would be inclined to attribute this to a racial predisposition. In the mixed population of Eastern Canada (Ontario, Quebec) which consists of people of English, Irish, Frenchs, Italian and German descent, the incidence of degenerative diseases of the central nervous system in relation to the population size is probably the highest in the entire world. Thus the significance of the racial factors (predisposition) is put into perspective.

The most convincing arguments regarding the amount of influence exercised by environmental factors are provided by cases occurring in early childhood, in which children of normal development suddenly display symptoms indicating a degeneration of the white cerebral matter following measles, whooping cough, immunisations, herpes infections, entero-colitis and undefined infections.

Cerebral metabolism and nutrition

Studies on the relationship between nutrition and brain development have revealed that the rate of maturity and of intellectual development is adversely affected in the presence of nutrition which is either overall deficient or deficient in protein in the course of the first 3 years. (Summary F. SCHMID, 1981). Much less attention has been paid to the correlation between disorders of the brain and diseases of the digestive tract. Chronic constipation which is not helped by laxatives, which accompanies severe cerebral pareses and degenerative afflictions, and the flatulent spasms following food intake as well as severe anatomical and functional changes in the upper digestive tract (ulcers, scars, mucosal atrophies) which are often quite severe, are frequently regarded as unavoidable consequences of brain diseases (FEHL). The presence of dystrophy with sufficient food intake is also considered to be momentous.

Only upon the discovery of neurohormones (peptides) which are formed in the intestines and in the brain and which include neurotensin, cholecystokinetic-like peptide, somatostatin, VIP (vaso-active intestinal polypeptide and others) SCHMID, F. (1981), it becomes possible to recognize and evaluate the relationship as no longer being a one-way street from brain to intestine, but to view it in the context of its mutual dependency.

The worldwide efforts directed at finding a cure for multiple sclerosis and Friedreich's ataxia have resulted in a number of informative details:

A. BARBEAU's working team (1979, 1980) in Montreal discovered a faulty fatty acid composition (lack of linoleic acid 18:2) of the cholesterol esters in the HDL (high density lipoproteins); they indicated a deficient incorporation of the linoleic acid into the surface phosphaditylic choline of the chylomicrones. Due to an overloading with defective cholesterol esters, there occurs a difficiency of usable lipo protein components which are required for the synthesis of myelin. Secondary consequences are: insufficient activation of the enzyme lipoamid-dehydrogenase (LAD), of the pyruvate-dehydrogenase complex, slow pyruvate oxydation, glucose intolerance, insufficient production of acetyl choline, as well as a drop in the glutamine and asparaginic acid level in the blood.

These intermediary metabolic changes were emphasized by the P. KARK (1976, 1982) working team in Los Angeles.

Parallel to this metabolic lapse which is caused by the mucous membrane of the small intestine, phosphatidyl choline molecules with an abnormal structures can be incorporated into the cell membranes, resulting in disturbances in the calcium-magnesium-taurin interchange and thus leading to a faulty myelinisation. Other reasons include a delay in the absorption of the glucose into the cell, a reduction in the pyruvate oxydation and the presence of diabetic metabolic problems. The linoleic acid deficiency (phospholipids, cardiolipin), particularly when it is located at the interior membrane of the mitochondria, can produce a «mitochondrial energy deprivation», resulting in symptoms such as muscle weakness, scoliosis and cardiomyopathy.

These findings observed in connection with Friedreich's ataxia can also be indications of other CNS-degenerations. Numerous tests on multiple sclerosis cases have revealed an abnormal myelin composition not only in the demyelinised areas, but also in the less obvious tissue parts. (GERSTL, R. B. et al. 1965; BAKER, R. W. R. 1963; CUMINGS, J. M. 1953). SUZUKI, K. et al. 1973; RIEKKINEN, P. J. and CLAUSEN, J. 1969 discovered myelin reductions of healthy parts in about 25–30% of cases.

In spongy degeneration of the central nervous system (CANAVAN-syndrome, V. BOGAERT) gigantic, abnormal mitochondrias with dense, filamentous matrices are present, and also distorted deformed cristae (BANKER, B. Q., et al. 1964), which are entirely in keeping with the hypothesis of Friedreich's ataxia.

These findings, which are somewhat contradictory, are very strong indicators of enzyme defects, whereby many arguments point in favour of a central position of the intestinal food intake and digestion. L. GILKA (1973, 1975) pointed out this correlation. The successes achieved by H. T. R. MOUNT (1973) in treating patients suffering from multiple sclerosis with vitamin B_1 liver extracts and special diets further substantiate this theory.

Treatment strategy

The abundant availability of statistical, biochemical and clinical data can be joined in a network with a firm knot – but with many gaps. Nevertheless, the present stage of acquired knowledge justifies the concept of commencing active therapy in all cases, where
a) deviations in the metabolism are recognized and
b) therapeutic aids are available for treatment.

Based on the expounded strategy, the treatment is based on three columns:

1. Nutrition (diet);
2. Enzyme substitution;
3. Regeneration of the cell functions.

Nutrition and diet

Over the last 3 generations the basis for nutrition under the categories foodstuffs – nutrients – luxury foods has increasingly veered towards the nutrients and luxury foods in most of the industrial nations. Preparation, preservation, colouring and packaging all serve purposes quite removed from nutrition. The preoccupation with calories and protein percentages, carbohydrates and fats in conjunction with the processes required to maintain the foods in a «sterile» condition, have resulted in converting most of the foods (containing «live» ingredients) into pure nutrients (energy suppliers). The essential components required for the synthesis and decomposition of a nutrient product, the so-called ferments (enzymes), are lost at temperatures as low as 45–60° C. These enzymes, which are contained in the «foodstuffs» are effective aids in the nutritional decomposition of the foods in the digestive tract. The de-naturalization of the foods and the destruction of its ferments have resulted in the fact that fresh foods are almost unavailable in certain geographical regions and in areas of industrial concentration, and that all nutrition leans heavily towards canned nutrient ingredients and luxury foods. Thus the organism is expected to cope with a double burden: By eliminating the ferments and natural ingredients (such as minerals, trace elements), the natural assistance required for the decomposition of food is removed, but at the same time the de-naturalization of the nutrients as present in canned foods, puts a burden on the organism by expecting it to digest and decompose nutrients, without being equipped with the enzyme apparatus to cope

with this on its own.

Thus the increased incidence of degenerative diseases in the congested areas of North America, England, Ireland and the Orkney Islands, but also the extreme frequency of intestinal cancer observed in Iceland, is more likely to be due to environmental influences (dry meat, canned foods, insufficient supply of fresh food) than to ethnic factors.

Translated into the field of practical nutrition, the following guidelines are recommended:

The distribution of food intake should be geared towards *«foodstuffs, whilst reducing de-naturalized nutrients and especially luxury foods.»* To achieve this, the following are considered most suitable:

First course consisting of unpreserved, well-ripened fruit or fruit juices: Papaya, mango fruit, pineapple, melons, figs, pears, apples, peaches, apricots, berry varieties in season.

The ferments contained in these fruits will assist in the decomposition of the subsequent main course.

The *main courses* should be low in animal protein and refined carbohydrates (white sugar, white flours, pastries made from white flours). Animal protein should be derived from fresh white meat (veal, fish, chicken, turkey), whereas red and preserved meat should be avoided as far as possible. An exception can be made in serving small quantities of raw liver, spleen or high-quality raw beef mince on salad-diet days. The anamneses of most of the patients revealed that they instinctively removed all fat meat from their nutrition and for this reason pickled, grilled and smoked meats should be left out altogether.

Milk and egg dishes are suitable sources of protein, whereby the milk should be taken in its natural state and the eggs preferably uncooked (beaten or mixed with fruit juices).

The fat intake should be limited to vegetable fats, and fats of animal origin are to be eliminated. The best sources highly unsaturated fatty acids are the following:

Sunflower oil, soya oil, nuts and nut oil. The only known sources of the prestage of linoleic acid (gamma-linoleic-acid) is breast milk and Primerose oil. A linoleic acid preparation which is available in Canada is EFAMOL. Lard and denaturized protein fat complexes should be avoided.

It is most important to avoid canned, de-naturized, coloured, bleached foods and foods to which volume expanders have been added, as much as possible. On or two salad-days with small helpings of milk, cheeses and egg dishes will play an essential role in activating the digestive organs.

Enzyme substitution

As long as the causal enzyme defects in specific degenerative diseases are not known, a broad-spectrum regime of enzyme substitution is recommended during main meals. The enzyme preparations enhance the natural nutrition value of the food and replace it whenever it is not possible to maintain a consistent diet of undenaturized foods. The preparations should contain ferments which decompose fats, proteins and celluloses. The following are recommended:
Wobenzym tablets,
  2 × 2 to 3 × 3 daily as a source of vegetable and bacterial enzymes;
Vitafestal,
  3 × 1 coated tablets, daily as a combination of digestive ferments, vitamins and trace elements;
Bilicombin,
  2 × 1 coated tablets daily as a fat-decomposing enzyme preparation;

Panpur, Panzynorm
  at a dosage of 2–3 coated tablets daily, are also suitable ferment combinations.
Wobenzym may be combined with any one of the above-named preparations. A suitable preparation which is available in Canada is Enzyme Digest. It contains Betaine HCL, Papain, Bromelein and Mycozyme.

The efficacy of the dietetic measures can be increased by the administration of intravenous injections of vitamin B_1 (100 mg/ml), B_{12} (1000 mcg/ml) and raw liver extract such as Reticulogen/ Lilly, as well as Efamol as a source of linoleic acid. At present we do not have any experience with European liver extract preparations as applicable to this field.

Regeneration of the cell functions

In most cases of regenerative disease, cellular metabolic disorders are present in varying degrees, starting from the intestinal mucous cells up to the final segment forming part of the process, the nerve cells. Experiments carried out in the past, when fetal brain tissue was used in an effort to influence the disease, have brought no convincing results. Only the inclusion of the initial elements of the metabolism have lead to a significant breakthrough in this field.

The regeneration of the digestive organs can be approached from two angles:

a) By injection implantations of
  fetal small intestine   100 mg;
  fetal duodenum   100 mg;
  fetal liver   150 mg;
  pancreas   100 mg;
  placenta, according to sex   150 mg;
  suprarenal gland, according
  to sex   100 mg.

These implantations of lyophilisates

should be administered subcutaneously at 6-monthly intervals and usually result in a specific improvement whithin several days. Quite often the peripheral blood circulation is improved after only a few hours. In cases of marked ataxia the combination of fetal cerebellum (100 mg) is recommended and for persistent constipation a combination of lyophilisied colon (100 mg) should be considered.

The use of an ultra-filtrate made from liver-pancreas-placenta-small intestine-mucosa (LPPM) seems to be most beneficial. This preparation is presently not yet available for general use due to the complicating manufacturing requirements and because it has not yet been registered.

Nutrition, enzyme substitution and *cell regeneration* by injection implantations together form the basis for a therapy strategy, which opens new horizons in the treatment of degenerative diseases for which no therapy has been available until now. Although we do not as yet have air-tight evidence at our disposal, the experiences gathered so far nevertheless prove that this concept is far more than just a hope.

The management of the treatment can be summarisized as follows:

1. Injection-Implantations

In order to initiate a amelioration or restauration of the instinal resorption and the cellular utilization functions injection-implantations with fetal or juvenile lyophilisated cells are applied. The following organ-preparations should be injected subcutaneously: →

Fetal small intestine (Mucosa) 100 mg
Pancreas 100 mg
Liver (fet) 150 mg
Hypothalamus 100 mg
Adrenal gland (acc. to sex) 100 mg
Placenta (acc. to sex) 150 mg

At the moment it cannot be determined if and what time-intervals further implantations will be required. The recommended interval is 5–6 month.

2. Regulation of the digestive functions

As substitutions for decreased activities are to be taken enzymes of plant- and animal-origin orally. →

A decisive factor in the restoration of the intestinal-mucosa-function is a cell-free lyophilisate consisting of liver, placenta pancreas and small-intestine mucosa. This preparation is to be taken before the breakfast on the tongue, primarly daily, later on intervals of 2 to 3 days. →

Wobenzym®
   4–8 tablets daily as a source of
   vegetable enzymes
Bilibombin®
   1–3 tablets daily as a fatsplitting
   enzyme
Vitafestal®
   1–3 tablets daily as a combination of
   digestive enzymes, vitamins and
   trace-elements
LPPM - cell-free ultrafiltrate of fetal
   Liver, Pancreas, Placenta and
   Mucosa.

3. Diet

The treatment has to be supported by corresponding nutritional measures. The following rules are recommended:

The nutrition should be low in ✳ animal proteins. If animal proteins are used, they should be taken in small quantities and come from fresh sources. Undenaturated milk and egg dishes are especially suitable protein sources. Three times weekly or daily a raw beaten egg or an egg mixed with juice should be taken. Further not preserved (canned) calv, beef, chicken and fish is recommended.

The ✳ *fat*-composition of the food should contain more plant-fats than fats of animal-origin. The best sources for the hightly-unsaturated fatic-acids are: sunflower-oil, soja-oil. The only known sources of the precusor gamma-linolic acid are breast-milk and prime-rose-oil. To avoid are pork-fat and all preserved and denaturated fats.

To ✳ stimulate the digestive processes fresh, naturally maturated fruits or fruit juices should be taken before the meals. To favour are enzyme-enriched fruits like papayas, mangos, melons, pineapples, grapefruits a. o. If possible, a raw-food-diet (raw salades and vegetables) should be used once or twice a week.

It is very important to avoid all ✳ preserved, canned and denaturated foods including their additives and colors. These agents can probably play a role as releasing noxa.

Morbus Parkinson

Besides the therapeutic principles «stereotactic operations» and «Dopamin-L-Dopa», cell therapy comprises a treatment insufficiently used so far, although already F. ROEDER (1967) and A. C. GIANOLI (1969, 1982) mentioned the effect of lyophilisates of Substantia nigra.

An important condition of cell-therapy for Parkinson's disease is the principle of maintaining morphological structures. Of the 33 patients with evident bilateral Parkinson's syndrome treated by ROEDER, 25 responded with established statistical significance. The first achievement was an improved state of health, a stronger impulse, a retrogression of amimia and of the vegetative symptoms. The gait improved, rigor and tremor subsided. These effects reached their peak 2–3 weeks after the implantation of Substantia nigra and lasted about 2–3 months. The patients responding positively to the therapy got another two injections at intervals of 6 months. Generally, the effect of the second injection was still perceptible though not as distinct as after the first. Remarkably, no noticeable effect was obtained with the third injection. Of 33 cases treated, 8 showed no improvement.

These results are virtually confirmed by GIANOLI, who emphasizes the possibility of combining cell therapy with the dopamin treatment.

From the corresponding infantile dyskinetic diseases it may be concluded that cell therapy using Substantia nigra is not wide enough. Additionally advisable is a combination of basal ganglia (50 mg), cerebellum (100 mg), frontal brain (100 mg) and placenta (150 mg); Adrenal tissue also wins on interest in Parkinsons disease. The partial reconstruction of basal ganglia function meantime could be confirmed in animal trials. This biological therapy can well be combined with the pharmacological treatment (L-Dopa, Nacom® or Akineton) but should be used before a stereotactical operation because after the interruption of structures the effect necessarily remains restricted.

Depressions

According to J. Babillotte (1978), a depression is characterized by disturbances in four fields:

change of the psyche;
disturbances of the vegetative system;
changes of the hormone balance;
so-called somatic sensations in the organs.

The changes of the psyche are defined by a depressed, anxious mood, accompanied by listlessness, insomnia, joylessness, uninterestedness, lack of resoluteness, feeling of absurdity, discouragement; associated with these symptoms are anxiety, internal tensions and worries about the future.

The vegetative symptoms are much differentiated, with insomnia at the beginning and in the centre. Vegetative false regulations affect also the cardiocirculatory system and the digestive tract.

No doubt, cell therapy for depression is more biological and causal than drugs, let alone electric shock. The tissue of choice is hypothalamus, but the spectrum ought to be completed by tissues from germ glands, placenta and liver, according to the symptoms.

As regards the hormones, depressive women suffer from a loss of libido with anorgasmy, uninterestedness in sexual life, often amenorrhoea, dysmenorrhoea. The endocrinic effects in men make themselves felt by loss of libido, disturbed potency, which may increase to complete impotence.

The somatic sensations often so difficult to interpret clinically, which Barth found in 247 patients of 298, are registered in nearly every region of the body. Complaints in the zone of the head are reported for about half of the cases, for 40 % in the extremities and for $\frac{1}{3}$ of the cases in the chest and abdomen.

Migraine

The many causes and pathological reactions of migraine make the subject of a comprehensive study by F. Sulman (1979). After exhausting the medicamentous measures, Sulman recommends cell therapy where other methods have failed. According to him, cell therapy is still promising in such cases. J. Babillotte extends the indication of cell therapy for migraine by placing cell therapy over medicamentous measures in cases of migraine. The tissues of choice are: placenta, thalamus, frontal-temporal-lobe, adrenals, gonadal tissue.

The apallic syndrome

Apallic syndrome (term created by Kretschmer) means central nervous lesions with loss of the pallic functions (pallium = cerebral cortex). Whilst the vital reflex mechanisms in the brain stem (circulation, breathing) still work, no sensory or sensitive stimuli enter consciousness so that no reactions controlled by consciousness can take place; the function of the «cerebral cortex» has been lost, the functions of the brain stem are, partly, maintained. The full aspect corresponds to a «decerebration» with the clinical consequences of the decerebration rigidity. If certain reactions of the cerebral cortex – though abortive – are still traceable, the term «Coma vigile» is more adequate.

In the clinical aspect, the apallic syndrome is characterized by general listlessness and immobility due first to muscular atony, later muscular hypertonia. In serious cases, there are no corneal reflex and light reflex of the pupils, no deglutition-reflex and no buccal reflex. The functions of the central nervous system are reduced below the reactivities existing at birth. The eyes are open, vacuous, staring, mostly directed to one side above (fig. 260, 262). Optical and acoustic stimuli are neither registered nor answered, tactile stimuli may be perceived but cannot be answered either.

The course

is characterized by the rigor of decerebration. Part of those affected by acute insulti die within hours or days. In question are usually lesions reaching beyond the pallium i.e. involves the brain stem. The artificial control of breathing, cardio-circulatory function, heat-balance and nutrition, has in the majority of cases temporal limits, which cannot be mastered by methodical techniques.

If the vegetative functions continue and the pallium functions subside, the chronic condition corresponding to the full aspect of the apallic syndrome develops: no reaction to optical, acoustic and tactile stimuli, tetraparesis or tetraspasm (fig. 272), growing marasm, trophic disorders (incl. cutaneous ulcers), lowered resistance to infections. The condition may be complicated by focal or generalized spasms, vomiting attacks, constipation difficult to influence.

The shorter the apallic condition the greater the chance of a rapid and complete return of the central-nervous functions. But only few are likely to have such a favourable course i.e. the short apallic conditions are seldom referred to as «apallic syndrome». The latter term ought to be reserved to apallic lasting conditions, namely the cases that stay apallic for weeks and months remain stationary or grow worse. Unconscious motor-automatisms (bending and extensor synergies, motions of the look and head, wiping and lacing-up movements, F. BROSER) and primitive answers to stimuli may occur, without any fundamental change of the condition of decerebration. The apallic syndrome fixed for weeks and months passes for a therapeutically uninfluenceable final stage.

As to the genesis

of the apallic syndrome, 2 mechanisms have to be distinguished as a matter of principle:

1. *Acute lesions of the central nervous system* cause serious destructions of the cerebral architecture and extinguish the functions of the cerebral cloak (decerebration); in the case of survival, a neurological final stage likely to be individualized by secondary symptoms is reached.
This form is caused mainly by traffic accidents, incidents due to anaesthesia, acute encephalitis, strangulation, anoxia (especially in stenosing laryngotracheobronchitis). Remarkable is the fact that among 22 observations anamnestically in 5 cases the onset of the apallic condition coincides with a cerebral angiography. The possibility of an additional cerebral lesion by extravasating high-percentual opaque matter from the (injured, ruptured) vessels should be included more ex-

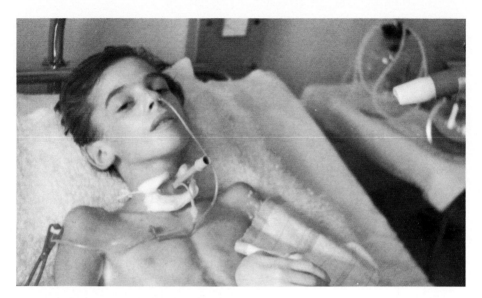

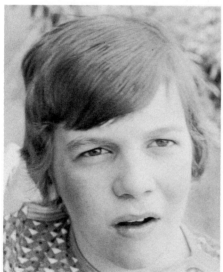

Fig. 272:
Courses of an apallic syndrome: physiognomy.

a) R. M. after a five-month apallic condition with nasal tube for nutrition, trachea-canula and bladder-catheter.
b) Condition of the boy 8 months after the therapy described in the test.

Haben einige Kinder, oder auch Erwachsene das Apallische Syndrom, wie ich? Wenn recht, dann ist es auch nicht schlimm. Ein ¼ Jaar war ich dort im Stadinischen Krankhaus von Asch affenburg, geplegen. Und ich danke Ihnen dafür, daß sie mich gesund gemacht haben.

Fig. 273:
Specimen of hand-writing by a 12-year-old boy, who was in a complete apallic condition for 5 months; finished the teaching matter of the 5th elementary school after 3 years of treatment.

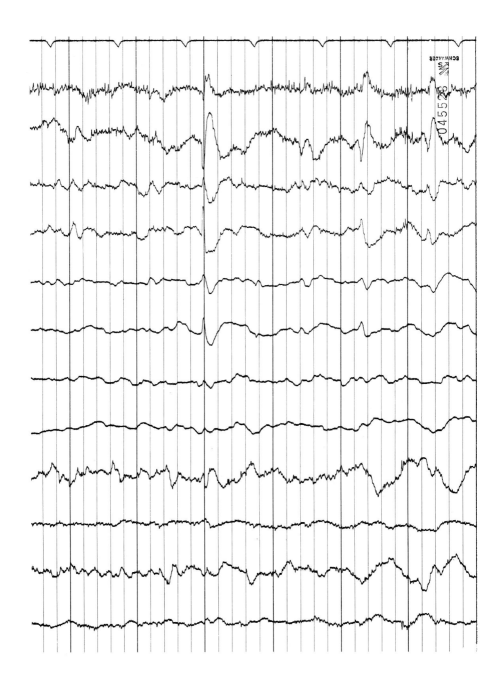

Fig. 274 a, b:
Differences of EEG in amplitude and ground rhythm after 11-month apallic condition (a) and after 17 months of treatment (b); case as per fig. 283.

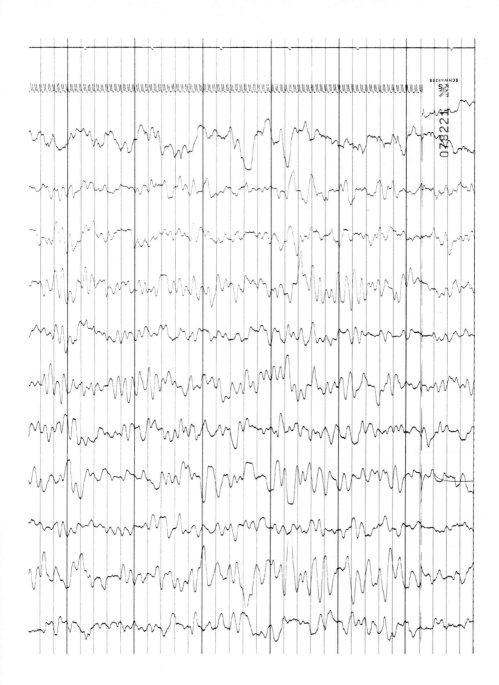

actly into the indication of angiography.

2. *Owing to chronic diseases of the central nervous system,* the apallic syndrome develops slowly and often constitutes the final stage after the lapse of years.

This form originates mostly from heredodegenerative metabolic or chronic inflammatory systemic diseases of the central nervous system. Tuberous cerebral sclerosis, leukodystrophy, cerebroretinal degenerations, leukoencephalitis, hyperammonemia, final stages of Louis-Bar's syndrome constitute the most frequent initial diseases.

Whereas in the acute form no stimuli are perceived or answered, the perception of stimuli lasts long in the chronic form, with respect to the earlier extinguished possibilities of answering stimuli.

Apart from the characteristic clinical findings, the EEG gives valuable diagnostic data (fig. 274 a, b) as the activity of the cerebral cortex is reduced or extinguished (zero-lines EEG).

Therapy

As described above, the apallic syndrome is looked upon as an irreversible final stage, which cannot be influenced by therapies. Observations and findings on 22 children and adolescents aged 2–19 years, however, have shown that chances of regeneration are there even after months of apallic condition if the treatment is based on a wide fundament. This applies only to the acute apallic conditions, not to the heredogenerative final stages: The therapeutic outcome varies and seems to depend on the patient's age. Unfavourable is the age up to the ripening of the medullary sheath i. e. the second and third years. In 2 children

of this age (1 × strangulation; 1 × anoxia by stenosing laryngotracheobronchitis) spasms were considerably alleviated, the deglutition reflex and buccal reflex as well as answers to tactile and acoustic stimuli were restored, but a fundamental improvement of the general condition was not achieved. In other cases, remarkable improvements up to the re-establishment of the learning and school capacities were reached after 5 to 9 months of apallic condition. One of the main problems is the re-learning of speech. Four of 21 cases died, after various intervals in the stationary state, of acute dysregulations of respiration, temperature and circulation.

The therapeutic conception

took shape after reluctant attempts within 8 years and comprises the following measures:

1. Elimination of all dispensable residues of intensive therapy, among them the removal of esophageal tubes for feeding (nasal, oral, operative gastric tubes), tracheal canules, permanent catheters for the bladder.

2. Regulation and re-establishment of the deficient functions of the digestive tract: preparing the pathways of the buccal and deglutition reflexes, medicamentous treatments of (frequently unmotivated) vomiting and of inveterate constipation.

3. Injected implantations of lyophilised fetal cerebral tissues (200–300 mg of the lyophilisate) with 150 mg of lyophilised placenta as initial measure for the regeneration of the central nervous system.

4. Injections of cerebral hydrolysates (cerebrolysin 1–3 ml daily for 3–4 weeks) combined with amino-acid and lipid infusions at intervals of 2 days. Lipid infusions are sometimes

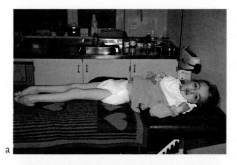

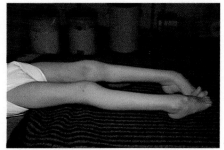

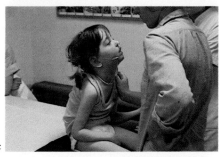

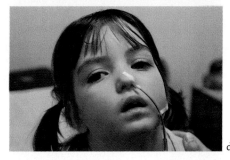

Fig. 275 a–d:
Metachromatic leukodystrophy in a 5-year-old girl. After a regression period of two years loosing the most centralnerveous functions no reaction to the environment, severe tetraspasticity (a, b). 6 month after starting a multidimensional treatment (physiotherapy; diet; digestive enzymes; liver-pancreas-placenta-intestine extracts; implantations of fetal liver, intestine-mucosa, placenta) partial recovery: head control, sitting with support, reduced spasticity, some directed sounds (c, d).

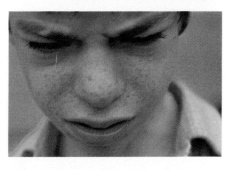

Fig. 276: Tuberous sclerosis with adenoma sebaceum; 13-years-old boy.

poorly tolerated and must then be stopped.

5. Consistent preparing the way for stimuli from the periphery by gymnastics (2–4 × daily for 15–20 min), initiating speech, optical and acoustic stimuli (music, television, conversation).

6. Posture measures adequate to the stage of regeneration and supply of auxiliary apparatuses.

For the break-through of the apallic state, the biological measures mentioned under 3 and 4 are not only starting conditions but of decisive importance; they can create the prerequisite for the achievement and results of the other measures (1, 2, 5, 6). Cerebral lyophilisates and cerebral hydrolysates should not be used if apallic states as part of heredodegenerative diseases of the central nervous system are in question.

The therapeutic outcome
depends on the consequency of the measures described, on the kind and extent of the lesions and on the age. The

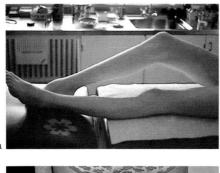
a

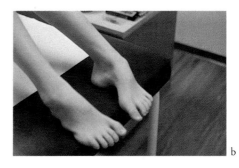
b

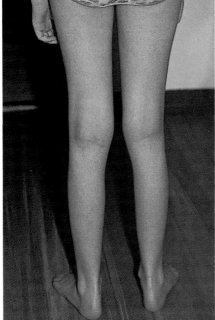
a

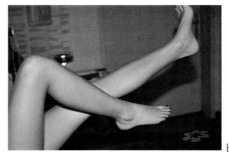
b

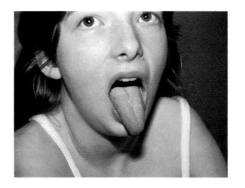
b

Fig. 277:
Caved foot and periphereal muscle atrophy in a 15-years-old girl with *Friedreichs Ataxia*.

Fig. 279:
Carnithin-deficiency-disease with muscle atrophy, reduced walking and lost stair-going capacity in the age of 14 years (a); During 2 years of a multidimensional treatment a satisfactory recovery of the muscle functions (b).

Fig. 278:
«Snow tongue» as a symptome of intestinal disorders in many degenerative diseases of nervous system and muscles. 14-years-old girl with progressive muscle dystrophy, scapulo-facial type.

duration of the apallic syndrome seems to be of minor importance as in certain cases (fig. 272, 275, 277) apallic «final stages» of 3–11 months can still bring about astonishing restitutions. Exactly, every individual case ought to be represented separately; but the observations made in the stage of regeneration provide very valuable conclusions on the topographical points of apallic lesions.

312

In contrast to the opinion that chiefly nerve cells perish and the condition is irreversible, the long-term observations specially of the traumatic forms suggest that mainly the secondary structures of the neuropils (dentrites, neurites, medullary sheaths, synapses) are affected. The following arguments may substantiate this:

a) The re-establishment of the functions follows much the sequence of the acquirements of these functions in infancy and babyhood; the speech provides more difficulties than the rough statomovements whereas words are well understood.

b) The memory, which must be supposed to be seated in the cytoplasm of the neuron, persists largely and in many details even if interrupted for several months by the apallic state.

c) Even abstract areas remain (a boy e.g. learns to speak only indistinctly after 5 months of apallic condition with zero lines EEG after acute dysmyelinisating encephalitis, but reckons quickly and with reliable correctness using dominoes).

d) The memory returns up to the time of the loss of consciousness and sets in three weeks after the beginning of the treatment (examples fig. 272, 275, 277).

The therapeutic results are influenced by the final failure of important perceptive organs e.g. by atrophy of the optic nerve. Focal onsets, which may call for anticonvulsive treatment, occur frequently in the stage of regeneration. Ground activity and re-ripening of the graphic elements in the EEG do not correspond to the clinical findings.

Neurocrine-endocrine synopsis

Neurosecretion means the production and output of hormones and their prophases by nerve cells of the diencephalon. As these synthesis products of the nerve cells are secreted direct into the portal circulation of the hypophyseal stalk, this function of certain areas of the central nervous system is also called «neurocrinia», its products are referred to as «neurincretes». The regular and very narrow connections between the central nervous and endocrine systems have so far been chiefly the subject of studies by anatomists, histochemists and endocrinologists, but their importance for the clinic has not yet been sufficiently appreciated. The following synopsis of the organismic connections is based upon data by SCHALLY and KASTIN; BARGMANN; HAGER; NOETZEL as well as E. L. SCHÄFER.

The diencephalon regulates a number of vital functions such as body-temperature, blood-pressure, rhythm of sleep and awakeness, balances of water and electrolytes. In particular, the hypothalamus is the central switch-board for the coordination of the endogenic regulatory mechanisms and for the processing of environmental influences. Whereas the latter are led to the central nervous system through afferent nerves (fig. 280), the endocrine and metabolic processes are regulated by reactive mechanisms. The system seems to be secure enough in many respects to reduce clinically relevant real «dyscrinia» to a minimum, provided that the central nervous system is intact.

The many symptoms of innate dysplasia and metabolic disturbances of the development of the central nervous system, however, indicate considerable relations between the disturbed development of the brain, the endocrine regulation with its somatic influences on the growing organism. They become perceivable in the area of the glandotropic hormones (fig. 282); the growth hormone (GH = growth hormone; STH = somatropic hormone), the thyroid hormones and sex hormones are of primary interest.

The tubular survey is to show by simple data the interrelations between the central nervous system and the endocrinium (fig. 280–282) and gives an outline of the clinical main effects (fig. 282). Under these aspects, somatic influences and functional disorders as part of disturbed cerebral development cannot be understood unless the connections are clear. They include all symptoms that can occur only through the endocrine system i.e. not direct but indirect are consequences of the disturbed cerebral function:

> *nanism; high growth; aberrations of growth proportions* (e.g. acromegaly,

acromicria).

«Diencephalic symptoms»: erethism, disturbed rhythm of sleep and awakeness; lability of the water-electrolyte balance; circulatory lability with reduced compensation; tendency to salivation, alopecia, cushingoid cheek-erythema (cheeks of a clown), abnormal ossification: disturbed sequence, asymetry, accelerated differentiation, and the like.

«Thyroid symptoms»: clumsy lineaments, thick skin; hoarse voice; large tongue; tendency to constipation; dry, strawy hair; retarded ossification.

«Sex-gland symptoms»: general infantilism; hypogenitalism (penis, scrotum, labia); absence of sexual characterization and of puberty.

Neurincretions

The 7 incretory glands (epiphysis, hypophysis, thyroid gland, parathyroid gland, adrenal glands, male and female sex-glands, pancreas) produce increts, which are divided into 4 biochemical groups:

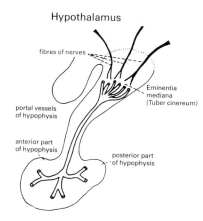

Fig. 280:
Functional connection between nerve fibres of hypothalamus and portal vessels of hypophysis into which the secretory products of the nerve-cells (neurosecretions are ingested direct, thus becoming neurincretes.

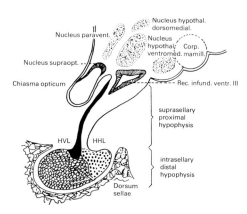

Fig. 281:
Diencephalic and hypothalamic centres. Hypophyseal stalk and hypophysis.

Neurotransmitters

Monoamines
  Dopamin
  Noradrenalin
  Serotonin
  Acetylcholin
  Histamin
Aminoacids
  Gamma-aminobutylacid
  Glycin
  Taurin ?
Neuropeptides
  Carnosin
  TRH
  (Thyreotropin-releasing-hormone)
  Methionin-Enkephalin
  Leucin-Enkephalin
  Angiotensin II
  cholecystokinin-like Peptid
  Oxytocin
  LHRH
  (Lutein.-hormon-releasing-hormone)
  P-substance
  Neurotensin
  Bombesin
  Somatostatin
  Vasoactive intestinal polypeptide (VIP)
  β-Endorphine
  ACTH (adreno-corticotrope hormone)

Derivatives of amino-acids (adrenalin, noradrenalin; thyroxin, triiodothyronin – as thyreoglobulin bound secondarily to protein).

Polypeptide hormones (oxytocin; ACTH; most of the hypothalamic neurohormones, so-called releasing factors).

Proteohormones (prolactin; choriongonadotropin; somatotropic hormone; insulin, glucagon; parat-hormone).

Steroid hormones (hormones of adrenal cortex: hydrocortisone, corticosterone, aldosterone, hydroxyandrostendione, sex hormones: testosteron, oestron, oestriol, oestradiol, progesteron).

The neurincretions originating from the hypothalamus are, as shown by recent analyses (SCHALLY and KASTIN), not only releasing factors but real hormones or their prophases. They belong to the group of polypeptide hormones and have very low molecular weights.

These hormones regulate the function of hypophysis, which therefore can no longer be regarded as the endocrine «control room» but as a «relay station» between impulses of the central nervous system and metabolism.

Endocrine disorders

Implantation of *calf's hypophysis* for nanism belong undoubtedly to the oldest methods of cell-therapy using xenogenous tissues. Looked upon as the hour of birth of cell therapy is that dramatic occasion when P. NIEHANS (1931) implanted dissected tissue of parathyroid gland under the abdominal skin of a woman writhing in tetanic spasm immediately after strumectomy whereupon spasms subsided before long. Meanwhile, comprehensive experience and documentation in many fields of endocrine disorders and diseases involving endocrine organs are available (STEIN, J. 1982).

Nanism

Nanism (more than 10% below average) and dwarfishness (more than 20% below average) are clinical collective names for stature deficits of various causes. The most important forms have been compiled in Tab. 41 (after O. MAR-GRAF, 1979). The forms of endocrine nanism are disorders of the axis: hypothalamus – hypophysis – thyroid gland – adrenal gland – gonads. Forms of endocrine nanism use to be less proportionate than constitutional or metabolic forms, but better proportionate than most of the skeletal forms of nanism. Enchondral

dysplasia and dysostosis call for other therapies and are treated separately (Tab. 49–50).

The *hypophyseal nanism* is caused by lack of STH (somatotropic hormone = growth hormone). The standard therapy consists in a permanent parenteral application of this hormone. It is doubtful whether the results of this expensive con-

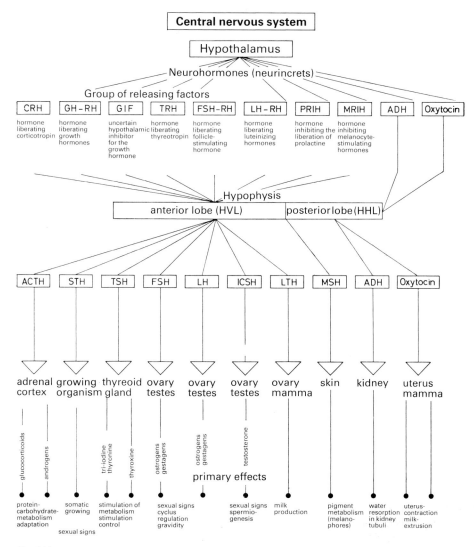

Fig. 282:
Synopsis of neurocrinia and of the endocrine system and glandotropic glands; relay stations, substrates, target organs and primary effects.

316

Tab. 41: **Survey of nanism** (after O. MARGRAF, 1979) (= etiologically different clinical forms of the symptom «nanism»)

hereditary factors	neuro-endocrine nanism	metabolic nanism	Ossary nanism (defective bone growth)	N. with chromosomal aberrations and genopathies
Familial nanism	**dycerebral nanism** innate or acquired brain defects mongolism microcephaly cerebral, malformation Laurence.-Moon-Biedel-S.	**Renal nanism** deformities congenital tubular nephropathies Phosphat-Diabetes (Vit.-D-Def. Rachitis) Vit.-D-resist. Rachitis Debré-de-Toni-Fanconi-S. serious chron. nephritis	= congen. skeletal dysplasia with short limbs Chondrodystrophy = Achondroplasia hereditary dysostosis diastr. nanism chondroectoderm. dysplasia metaphys. dysostosis Osteogenesis imperfecta dyschond. nanism	the most monosomies trisomies and chromosomal deletions
Constitutional retardation of development				
Primordial nanism				
Hereditary, brachy-meta-carpal nanism (Pseudo-Hypo-Parathyreoi-dism)	**hypophyseal nanism** isolated lack of growth hormon			
	nanism in partial growth hormon deficiency	**Intestinal nanism** Coeliakia, Megacolon Pancreasfibroses Kwaschiorkor-S. Andersen-S.	**Nanism with prevailing shortening of trunk** Spondyloepiphys. Dysplasia Morquio-disease	
Progeria	Somatomedin-deficiency lack of ACTH combined hormon deficiencies			
(= hered. const. **nanism** defective growth potency of bones)		**Hepatic nanism** Starage disease Glykogenosis Lipoidosis Mucopolysacchari-dosis Cystinosis	**Further dysprop. dysost. nanism** Pfaundler-Hurler-disease Hunter's disease Sanfilippo disease (all mucopolysacch.)	
	Hypothyreotic nanism precipitation of TSH			
	nanism in Hypopara-thyreoidismus **Adrenal nanism** M. Cushing	**An-or hypaxemic nanism** cardial nanism pulmonal nanism. anaemic nanism rachitic nanism	**Proport. dysostot. nanism** marble bones Dysostosis cleidocranial.	
	Dysgenital nanism Pubertas praecox Pseudo-P. p. Ulrich-Turner-S. Hanhart-S. (hereditary nan. with lack of STH and retarded ripening) **Pancreas** ill controlled diabetes with lack of insulin	**Alimentary** Hypocaloric hanism (prot. vit. trace elements)	**Nan. with multiple varieties** Laurence-Moon-Biedel-S. Männl.-Turner-S. Pseudo-Hypoparathyreoi-dism. **Pseudoforms** (= false nanism) phocomelia rachitic curvetures	

tinuous therapy are better than the former implantations of calf's hypophysis and oral substitution because immunological reduced effects bring about less convincing growth rates in later years.

The evaluation of 14 own cases treated with subcutaneous implantations of calf's hypophysis under the skin of the abdomen revealed rather different results. Apart from non-reactions with growth rates of 2–3 cm per year, some cases showed enormous growth impulses of 11–18 cm per year. As regards the concomitant oral substitution-therapy or cell-therapeutic concomitant therapy, it must be taken into consideration that hypothalamus and hypophysis have leading conductor's functions in the finely coordinated symphony of endocrine glands. From this it appears that the effects on the secondary glands must be tested and disorders be included in the therapeutic conception. The use of thyroid gland, adrenal glands, gonadal tissue justifies these considerations by the demonstrable effect where implantations of hypophysis alone failed to bring about the growth impulse desired.

Hypophyseal – hypothalamic disorders

The axis of hypophysis – adrenal glands – gonads plays in adults a part that often escapes the doctor's notice. RÜMELIN (1970) demonstrated the effect of implantation therapy in 2 filigree-like analysed cases of post-partal *Sheehan syndrome*. The part of the hypophysis-hypothalamic system in the loss of weight during puberty – socalled *anorexia nervosa* – and various forms of *obesity* is surely less circumscribed. It is advisable to consider the use of hypothalamus, diencephalon, hypophysis, adrenal gland and gonadal tissue when the «classical» i. e. customary methods fail. A. C. GIANOLI (1968) reported on the combined treatment of obesity with diet-choriongonadotropin-cell therapy. According to recommendations by SIMEONS, the best results were obtained after 21–30 days of treatment with a 500 cal.diet, 125 int.units of human choriongonadotropin i. m. and implantations of hypothalamus or diencephalon. This study relies on 165 observations. The implantations are said to have a long-term effect regulating the metabolism.

Furthermore, articles on cell therapy in diseases of hypothalamus/hypophysis were written by: G. DÖDERLEIN, (1953); MAISCHEIN (1955); JANSON 1955); F. E. BIRCHER (1953); BLUME (1957); EHNI and DUDE (1957).

A. KMENT (1968) and J. BABILLOTTE (1979) dealt specially with the central position of hypothalamus in the endocrine system, F. G. SULMAN (1975) with the neurohormones.

In *Diabetes insipidus*, the balance of water and electrolytes is disturbed owing to dysregulations of the posterior part of the hypophysis and hypothalamic centres. No verified reports on cell-therapeutic treatments of human patients are available so far because the nasal substitution makes usually adequate permanent treatments possible. K. ULRICH (1960) reported on the successful implantations of diencephalon in 7 dogs; the substitution of hormones of the posterior part of the hypophysis alone was not sufficient.

Irrespective of the classical diseases with constellations of distinctive symptoms, the diencephalon-hypothalamus system is involved in many disturbances of growth, cerebral affections, forms of obesity and loss of weight, and can characterize the secondary and concomitant symptoms. The inclusion of these tissues into the therapeutic conception should be taken into consideration wherever the symptoms seem to suggest so (e. g. Down's syndrome).

Thyroid insufficiencies

constitute, primarily as athyreosis or hypothyreosis with a frequency of 1 : 4000 new-born, a numerically minor problem, which however is significant from the sociological point of view. Still more important is a mostly unrecognized secondary dysfunction of the thyroid gland among the cerebral diseases, namely the *secondary hypothyreosis*.

Hypothyreosis manifests itself according to the functionary deficit of the thyroid gland during the first weeks of age – in athyreosis – or are detected in infancy. The early diagnosis for the newborn adopted in many countries is likely to reduce henceforth the number of cases recognized later. Of course, the diagnostic safety of the TSH-determinations leaves doubts, which often are covered with the mantle of «transient hypothyreosis», probably however imply wrongly positive diagnoses. The determination of the bone-age should be included in the diagnosis, in new-born the degree of the ossification of the talus, calcaneus, distal femur – and proximal tibiaepiphysis. These are found in a mature new-born.

Hypothyreosis is a classical indication for the substitution-therapy with thyroid-hormone preparations. The fractions T3 and T4 are used more frequently nowadays as integral preparations on a base of thyreoidea sicca; the correctness of this method ist doubtful. If the thyreoid substitution is applied too late or by inadequate doses, the whole organism is affected, especially the development of the brain. The forebrain is the part to suffer most, which can often be noticed alone by the narrow, flat forehead, a low-descending growth of hair and a narrowed bitemporal diameter of the skull. The individuality lacks chiefly initiative and the capacity of abstracting and combining. Increases of the thyroid substitution cannot neutralize these effects on the brain; frontal brain, temporal brain, thalamus, hypothalamus, possibly combined with thyroid implantations, in total doses of 200–300 mg of lyophilisate per series of implantations bring about effects that cannot be obtained with any other therapy. The substitution therapy and the implantations should be completed by long-term medications with vitamin-B complexes and trace elements, especially as long as macroglossia and thickenings of the skin as clinical symptoms indicate this deficiency.

Research workers dealing specially with the cell-therapeutic problems of thyroid disorders are H. KURTZAHN and H. HÜBENER (1927) as well as A. STURM (1955).

Parathyroid insufficiency

Although the implantation of parathyroid tissue by P. NIEHANS in 1931 for a dysfunction of this organ is a spectacular individual case at the beginning of modern « cell therapy», only little substantiated reports such as by A. STURM (1955) and A.C. GIANOLI (1971) were added. The small number of cases may be accounted for by the fact that the substitution-therapy is easier to apply in practice. A.C. GIANOLI describes the case of a 53-year-old woman, who suffered from postoperative hypoparathyroidism with tetanic syndrome, trophic disorders and vegetative symptoms. In spite of many years of intense and careful treatments with AT10, vitamin D and calcium, the condition grew worse into incapability for work. Already the first cell treatment with parathyroid gland, thyroid gland, hypothalamus and placenta provoked soon a marked improvement; the tetanic attacks did not occur any more. After another two treatments at intervals of 13 and 12 months, no complaints were seen during an observation of 3 years.

Diabetes mellitus

Diabetes mellitus (= diabetes, from Greek «sweet honey passing through») constitutes a first-class sociologico-medical problem, with respect to its frequency and therapeutic problems. Although the therapeutic conception with the two columns « diet» and «insulin substitution» appears well-founded theoretically, every clinician knows the practical difficulties of the long-term treatments, the shortcomings of which are readily imputed to a defective diet discipline of the patients. Diabetes is generally looked upon as «a factor of risk» for many other diseases because the vascular and circulatory lesions predispose the organism to other serious affections:

circulatory dysregulations; hypertonia, vascular occlusions;
infarctions; apoplexia; ophthalmological lesions to the retina, lens and iris;
degenerative lesions of liver and kidneys; disturbed gastric, intestinal, vesical and sexual functions;
degenerative lesions of the skeleton and joints, and trophic discorders.

Diabetes is believed to be caused by a genetical disposition. Accumulations of the tissular antigens HLA-B8 and HLA-DM3 were found in diabetics with organo-specific autoantibodies (GROMET et al., 1974). Diabetics needing insulin have antibodies against parietal cells of the gastric mucosa and against thyreocytes more frequently than diabetics independent of insulin. When diabetes manifests itself, autoantibodies against islet-cells will appear, but persist only in 20 % of the cases, especially in patients depending primarily on insulin (R. LENDRUM et al., 1976). This has caused suggestions that the diabetes type I, which depends on insulin, should be classified among autoimmune diseases and be di-

vided into the types I a and I b. To the type I a belongs the diabetes developing in infancy and which needs insulin at once; perhaps viruses (mumps?) react with HLA-specific areas of the B-cell cytomembrane and lead to immuno-cytotoxic cellular lesions. Whereas the autoantibodies against islet-cells disappear here, they persist in type I b; accumulations in families, predisposition in women and occurrence of other organospecific autoantibodies indicate a «primary» autoantibody disease.

Even if the main function of the insulin is to infiltrate glucose through the cytoplasma membranes into the interior of cells, it must be realized that the transporting and intermediary metabolism is also affected in the area of the electrolytes (potassium, sodium, magnesium, phosphorus, zinc), the proteins and lipids.

The inadequately solved problems called for methods constituting a causal principle against the symptomatic substitution (insulin) and the restriction therapy (diet). Though this way has been taken experimentally and clinically, it is not yet generally practicable.

Casuistical reports on cell-therapeutic treatments of Diabetes mellitus are available already from the period of 1950–1960 (NIEHANS; RIETSCHEL; SPRADO; FELDWEG; UHLENBRUCK; SCHENCK). They were insufficiently substantiated and recorded. NIEHANS himself was nearly possessed by the cell therapy of Diabetes mellitus and sacrificed large sums for the experimental research in order to reach the therapeutic use of «isolated B-cells». Recently overviews were given by STEIN, J. (1982) and NEUBERT, H. (1982).

The first experimental studies by DUBOIS and GONET (1961) proved that injected pancreatic cells can produce in subtotally pancreatectomised rats sufficient insulin to normalize the blood-sugar. Remarkable in this case and for alloxane diabetes was the intensive proliferation of the remaining B-cell areas. These first results have been confirmed widely as an effective principle in many variations these last few years (FEDERLIN et al. 1978; RUMPF et al., 1977, 1978; W. MEYER, 1979; W. KÖSTERS, 1979).

The following results must be emphasized:

1. Intraperitoneal and intraportal injections of islet-cells work better than subcutaneous or intramuscular transplants.
2. Fetal, juvenile and adult tissues develop heterotopically in the organism of the receiver into areas of fully functioning islet-cells.
3. Isogenous implants (of inbreeding strains) function for months, allogenous (homologous) implants are disintegrated.
4. An immunosuppressive therapy can keep allogenous implants functioning for months. How far diabetic secondary changes can be remedied by transplantations of islet-cells, appears from the detailed studies by KÖSTERS on changes of glomeruli.

Genetically isologous male Lewis-albino-inbreeding rats were used to produce diabetes through want of insulin by intraperitoneal injections of acqueous solution of streptozotocin (65 mg/kg of body-weight). Part of the animals got intraportal transplantations of isologous pancreatic islet-cells 7 months after the onset of diabetes. The islet-cells were isolated manually with a stereomicroscope following the methods described by LACY and KOSTIANOVSKY (P. E. LACY and M. KOSTIANOVSKY: Method for the isolation of intact islets of Langerhans from rat pancreas, Diabetes 16, 35 (1967) and SHIBATA et al. ; (A. SHIBATA, C. W. LUDVIGSEN, St. P. NEBER, M. L. MCDANIEL: Standardization of a digestion-filtration method for isolation of pancreatic islets, Diabetes 25, 667, 1976). The parameters for the clinical assessment were: weekly determinations of the blood-sugar, tests for the tolerance to glucose, body-weight, quantities of beverages, volumes of urine, secretion of glucose in the urine. Ten months after the beginning of the tests, renal tissue was taken from healthy and diabetic animals and such treated with transplantations for the light- and fluorescence-microscopic studies. Seven months after producing the diabetes, 34 of the 35 diabetic animals tested had a diabetic glomerular sclerosis, and incorporations of pathognomonic nodular mesangium were traced in 13 animals. Immuno-histologically, IgG, complement beta 1 c fibrinogen and albumin were detected in the mesangium and along the basal membrane in nearly all diabetic animals.

Already 2 days after successful transplantations of islet-cells, the level of the blood-sugar was normalized. The increase in weight corresponded for the animals treated with transplantations to the physiological course in healthy animals. Ten weeks after the implantation of islet-cells, a distinct regression of the histological glomerular changes was observed. Impressive was the regression of the immuno-histological changes: only a third of the animals treated showed minor, mostly fine-grained deposits of protein of the categories described above. The mean width of mesangium in the animals treated with transplantations came to 9.18%, in the diabetic animals to 13.38%.

Compared with these broadly founded experiments, the clinic lags behind. The most comprehensive studies in this field were submitted by H. NEUBERT (1978, 1982), J. STEIN (1982). Of 179 diabetics that got cell theryps in 1977, 94 (61 women, 33 men) were evaluated catamnestically. Their ages varied from 14 to over 80 years, most of the patients i. e 75 were 60–79 years old. In 38 cases (= 40% of the patients) an improvement of the carbohydrate metabolism was observed. It ranged from the stabilization of the blood-sugar with equal medication, through the reduction of the tablets to the reduction of the dose of insulin (in 3 cases).

The favourable influence on diabetes as part of the so-called revitalizing treatments has been confirmed repeatedly.

More difficult are the problems with the insulin-depending diabetes in children and adolescents.

The author's own experience in this respect is restricted to individual cases of instable diabetes difficult to treat in the first five years. The metabolism is stabilized (blood-sugar, acetone, exretion of sugar). The requirements of insulin may increase in the first days after the implantation, to drop in the 2nd to 3rd week below the initial requirements before the implantation. This calls for an exact – preferably clinical – observation in order to conform to these changes pending the stabilization.

For the old-age diabetes, the following viewpoint is noteworthy: if trophic disorders and serious changes of vessels are in question, the conditions of absorption for the implantation are often unfavourable so that a broad, deeply subcutaneous injection is advisable.

Treatments of Diabetes mellitus with xenogenous tissues cannot be recommended generally for the following still not yet sufficiently cleared up reasons:

1. The instability of metabolism in the insulin-dependent diabetes of children in the stress-phases after the implantation must be analyzed thoroughly and regularly.
2. The therapy with pancreas or pancreas-hypothalamic tissue is not extensive enough as the gastric mucosa, liver and adrenal gland must be included into the clinical aspect.
3. Careful attention should be paid to the reduced absorption in advanced diabetes of old age.

However, a cell-therapy prepared by an experienced expert according to individual symptoms of a diabetic cannot only stabilisize the metabolism but also influence heterotopic symptoms (fig. 291).

Adrenal insufficiency

The adrenal cortex with its cortical hormones constitutes an important switch point in the endocrine system. The isolation and therapeutic use of corticosteroids belong to the greatest medical progress of the last decades – with many draw-backs. The adrenocortical hormones stimulate the gonads so that the third (= puberal) phase of growth is initiated and controlled by the adrenal and sexual hormones. The retarded appearance of the secondary sex characteristics (beyond the 16th year in boys, beyond the 15th year in girls) is due to an insufficiency of this part of the endocrine chain in the majority of cases.

Primary and secondary hypogonadism justify the use of endocrine glandular tissue; the organs must be selected in accordance with the diagnostic results incl. the analyses of hormones and the clinical outfall symptoms. The earlier in the hypophyseal phase of growth (between the 3rd and 10th years) the outfall symptoms manifest themselves, the more hypothalamus-diencephalon-hypophysis must be involved. If the development of stature and genitals is not retarded before the prepuberty and puberty, the adrenal glands (of the same sex), ovaries, testicles should preferably be used, along with homosexual placenta.

General medical treatments are recommended especially for complex aspects. For the *Prader-Willi-syndrome* (fig. 283), the absence of the secondary sex characteristics is the main criterion, though obesity and retarded mental development are not less important. The observation shown in fig. 283 demonstrates, how astonishing effects a complex long-time treatment may have (and cell therapy as central point cannot be replaced by anything); this case is one of 7 treated so far, which had different initial situations and different therapeutic results.

The *secondary lesions* of the adrenal glands are more frequent nowadays than the innate hypofunctions. The broad therapeutic spectrum of the corticosteroids in inflammation, allergies, as cytostatics and externals has augmented the atrophies of the adrenal cortex due to therapeutic measures; they are referred to as *hypercorticism, secondary Cushing's syndrome, cushingoids*, etc. The basic process is the functional immobilization of the adrenal glands by hormones supplied from outside for some time, with higher doses and unfavourable intervals between the (daily) applications. The functional non-use is followed by the morphological atrophy of structures so that, from a certain time, the adrenal glands can no longer produce sufficient quantities of their own hormones. This

situation is also of major importance for many prolonged allergies so that the application of adrenal tissue should be taken into consideration, in spite of contraindications.

Prolonged therapies with corticoids in allergies, asthma and generalized neoplasms (leukemia) cause this secondary adrenal insufficiency; its treatment involves serious practical problems, more so if it is accompanied by leukopenia or even panmyelopathies. Implantations of adrenal, hepatic, splenic and bone-marrow tissues may bring about remarkable changes (fig. 306), though the risk of the stress phase after the implantation must be taken into consideration.

A relative indication for a combination of thymus and adrenal gland is the *deficient resistance to infection* and *severe allergic conditions* including *autoimmun diseases*, which can be mastered neither with biological nor with antibiotic remedies.

Puberty

is the third phase of growth after the genetic and hypophyseal phases; it is controlled by the adrenal-sex hormones. Accordingly, the sex characteristics are the main point of the puberty, besides the dimensions and proportions of the body.

The medical problems of the puberty have been characterized largely by the secular process of acceleration these last decades. The beginning and end of puberty have considerably moved to younger ages in the course of the last hundred years. According to the exact criterium «Menarche», the mean values have been shifted from a mean age of $16\frac{1}{2}$ years to $12\frac{1}{2}$ years. The earlier onset of puberty proceeded with an acceleration. This means it is now more difficult to

overcome the changes of the pubertising body as puberty manifests itself earlier and proceeds faster than in former generations.

Somatic-physiological problems of puberty

The commencing function of the sexual glands promotes the growth unharmoniously, often impetuously. This process is identical with the so-called «change of stature» after W. ZELLER. During the second half of puberty, the arms and legs, especially the hands and and feet grow faster than the body. Legs and arms are relatively longest at the beginning of menstruation in girls, at the first production of semen in boys (H. R. STOLZ and L. M. STOLZ). Adolescents of

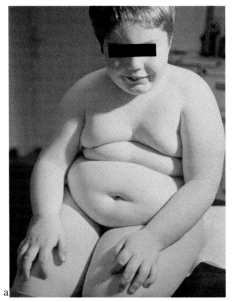

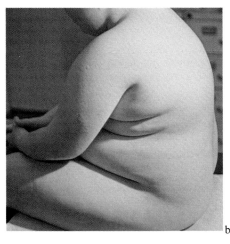

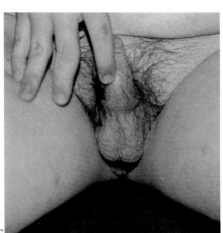

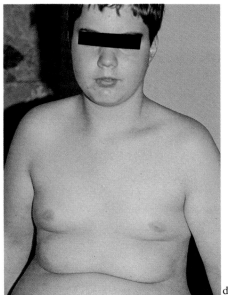

Fig. 283:
Prader-Willi's syndrome

The boy is presented for the first time at $6\frac{1}{2}$ years.
127 cm (+ 7 cm), 53.1 kg (+ 27.5 kg = about
110% overweight), apron obesity (a, b), genital
hypoplasia, flat scrotum, testes only palpable as
a fluffy texture.

The parents are chiefly worried about the lack of
impulse, absence of striving for performance
and abnormally deep sleep; he cannot be sent to
school.

From $6\frac{1}{2}$ to 12 10/12 years, at half-year intervals,

implantations of hypophysis, hypothalamus
diencephalon temporal brain, frontal brain,
male adrenal gland and testes, by double combinations of 200 mg of lyophilisate.

At this time 170 cm, 82.8 kg (the weight had been
up to 100 kg), attends the 6th class of elementary
school, mean performance, testes palpable and
adequate to age, the genital hypoplasia has been
remedied, pubes (c, d).

324

that age do not know what to do with their extremities. The harmonious-natural movements become more clumsy, more abrupt, reluctant to anxious, before in the second half of puberty the harmonious coordination of movements is restored.

According to the sex, the body gives the adolescents different problems:

Girls are more often afraid of growing too big rather than of remaining too small. The form of the body, needed with new movements, is paid more attention. Girls do not like to be too fat, are afraid that their breasts might remain too small. The frequently assymmetric budding of the breasts makes mothers and daughters suspect that some disorder might be the cause. The hairs on the body are the subject of apprehensive observation. Girls do not like to wear glasses.

Boys would like to be taller, to have more muscles and broader shoulders, use more consciously their newly acquired physical capacities (sport). At the beginning of puberty, the question of small genital organs arises frequently, later the impurity of the skin (acne) will prevail. The stronger and more specific effluvium proceeding with the hormonal change may provoke uncertainty in both sexes when getting into touch with the environment.

With the speed of growth and the hormonal change, circulatory problems and inconstancy of temper caused by hormones proceed. Among them are:

lability,
easy fatigability,
lack of concentration,
unsettlement,
wayward reactions,
nervousness.

Phases of dislike alternating with phases of showing off. Physiologically, in part, a «change of shift» results in the secondary schools. Whereas boys have difficulties mostly between 11 and 15 years of age, and the girls are usually better, well-behaved and less problematic, the girls slow down in their work during the second phase of puberty or find it hard to maintain their reputation of being «good pupils». For boys, however, their achievements at school stabilizes between the 15th and 19th years of life unless the physiological break as secondary schools stops them.

Pathology of puberty

With sexual-specific clinical aspects, the following principles of pathological variants of puberty result:

1. premature puberty;
2. retarded puberty;
3. missing puberty.

The premature appearance of the characteristics of puberty makes up

1 a) a *constitutional-geographical variant.* In warm countries and regions nearer to the equator, puberty occurs usually earlier than under northern latitudes and in humans with light pigments.

1 b) The *premature appearance of single secondary sex characteristics* as alpha-premature, mostly transitory budding of the breasts, beta-premature puberty (before the 7th year of age).

1 c) *Pubertas praecox vera* with appearance of the secondary sex characteristics before the 8th year, and of the menarche before the 10th year of age. The causes are usually not traceable, sometimes a hamartome of Tuber cinereum or a Weil-McCune-Albright syndrome (Pubertas praecox + fibrous, polystotic or monostotic skeleton dysplasia + Café au Lait spots on the skin) is found.

1 d) *Pseudopubertas praecox* with appearance of secondary sex characteristics in cases of adrenal or ovarian tumours.

Retarded puberty is seen:

2 a) in constitutional maldevelopment,
2 b) in malnutrition and unfavourable environmental conditions,
2 c) in hypoganadism (most serious primary form: Ulrich-Turner's syndrome, 45XO-chromosome aberration),
2 d) missing hypophyseal gonadotropins with secondary hypoganadism

(in panhypopitutarism, hypophyseal nanism, serious hypothyreosis).

Missing puberty is a rare event in

3 a) Dystrophia adiposo-genitalis;
3 b) Prader-Willi syndrome (fig. 284);
3 c) other forms of intersex.

Special somatic problems result as hypertrichosis in girls and in hirsutism. Hypertrichosis is usually familial, occurs often in cerebral dysplasia, sometimes owing to medicaments (cortison, antiepileptics).

Infertility

Disorders of fertility in males are due to various causes (Tab. 42); their effects are listed in the spermiogram. Accordingly, the forms as per Tab. 43 are distinguished. The diagnostic measures must take into consideration the roughly anatomic analyses and hormone analyses. Attention must be paid to cryptorchisms, undescended testicles, varioceles or hydroceles, size of the testicles and (diminished) consistency of the testicles. Testicle biopsy, analyses of hormones (gonadotropins, androgenes), analysis of chromosomes and possible test

for the patency of the spermatic ducts; vesiculography and epididymography complete the number of diagnostic possibilities. The assessment of the spermiograms is not based on the number alone; motility of the sperms, pathological forms and the content of fructose are further criteria.

The practical experience in this field exceeds by far the literary records, which are restricted to few authors: W. CAMER-

Tab. 42: **Causes of male infertility** (to be ascertained anamnestically)

---

mumps-orchitis
orchidopexy
testicular trauma
herniotomy
gonorrhoea
urogenital Tbc
chronic prostatitis
urethritis
varicocele or hydrocele operation
strong smoker
alcoholism

Tab. 43: **Cell therapy indicated:**

---

if spermiogram normal
  – or oligospermia I
  – or oligospermia II
    in case for azoospermia
if testicular biopsy normal
  – or diffuse tubular testicle atrophy
  – or focal tubular testicle atrophy
  but reproductive epithelium still
  exists.

If the spermiogram shows aspermia or the histological findings reveal total fibrosis, cell therapy is not indicated.

ER (1958, 1978, 1982); NIKOLOWS-KI (1956), JANSON (1952, 1953, 1957); A. C. GIANOLI (1971). At the congress of therapeutists held in Karlsruhe (1957), W. HEUBNER dealt with the subject («Cell therapy and endocrinology»). H. RONNEBERGER (1961) and TUCHLINSKI confirmed the therapeutic effects seen in man with the results of cell therapy obtained in infertile bulls and results established in stallions by AEHNELT (1960).

W. CAMERER conducted a subtile double-blind study on 10 men suffering from fertility disorders (with 2 simultaneously infertile women) and an infertile woman. The case histories (W. CAMERER, 1978) are worth reading for the multi-dimensional diagnostic and therapeutic measures, moreover for the long times of subsequent observation. Conception occurred in 8 cases of 11, including 2 patients with serious, bioptically proved changes of the testicles. Used for each series of injections were lyophilisates of testes (ovary in hypofunction of the ovaries), placenta of male and female feti, hypothalamus.

The cells of the testicular tubuli are very regenerative and favour the metabolism. According to A. C. GIANOLI, striking improvements of spermiogenesis may be anticipated in oligospermia, tests should be conducted in asthenospermia. No results are likely to appear on the spermiogram in aspermia nor can be expected in total fibrosis.

Ovarian insufficiency

G. LEWANDER (1941, 1957) and J. BERNHARD (1958, 1963) demonstrated the induction of implanted endometrial tissue on the uterus of castrated rabbits. The specificity of the effect was inferred per exclusionem because implantations of fetal liver, spleen, lung, heart and placenta caused no endometrial new formations. In 4 test series, castrated rabbits got injections of lyophilisates of endometrium from a pregnant rabbit; in all series, a regeneration of mucosa with a distinct formation of glands in the recipient was observed. Fresh tissue and lyophilisates had the same effect; oestrogens were not traced in the tissues.

Papers by W. CAMERER (1957, 1978, 1982), GOOS and MAISCHEIN (1957), VORSTER (1958), HOLMER (1958), J. BERNHARD and W. KRAMPITZ(1963, 1967), RÜMELIN (1970) deal with partly experimental, partly clinical problems of the female menopause and amenorrhea.

Therapeutically, it is expedient to distringuish *amenorrhea* and *oligomenor-rhea*, as expressions of functional insufficiencies in the mature age of the woman, from the physiological concomitant symptoms of the subsiding ovarian function in the menopause.

For the chromosomal *ovardysgenesis* as part of *Turner's syndrome* (fig. 246), questions of the growing stature and of the properties of the body are more important than the fertility. During the maturation of the woman, however, the problem of fertility prevails. Non-biological habits (contraceptive pill) and ideals of beauty (Twiggy-types) have augmented this field of gonadal dysfunctions during recent years. The cell therapy does surely more for the *menopausal involutionary symptoms* and has better physiological and more lasting effects than a hormone-substitution therapy.

Central tissues for cell therapy to treat *gonadal-ovarian insufficiency* are the ovaries and adrenal glands. Considering the general medical aspects of the outfall symptoms, the selection of organs should have an adequate scope. Hypothalamus, placenta, liver, connective tissue ought to be use in certain cases, too, according to the clinical symptoms.

Cardiac and vascular disorders

The foremost indication in practice for injected implantations of placenta, fetal arteries, myocardium are the degenerative changes of the vessels. Although approximately more than 2 million people with peripherous circulatory disorders, cerebral coronary sclerosis were treated by cell therapy during the last 30 years, the clinical records are scarce as against the practical empirism.

Experimental studies on these pathological complexes were conducted by DORNBUSCH(1956, 1963, 1967); KUHN and KNÜCHEL (1954); KLEINSORGE (1954, 1956); STEPANTSCHITZ and SCHREINER (1956, 1966). The effects on the peripheral blood circulation proved unanimously by the research workers were not found by KANZOW (1957) alone.

The tests on animals are supported for the peripheral circulatory disorders by extensive clinical experience: KUHN and KNÜCHEL (1954, 1955); E.A. MÜLLER (1953); H. KLEINSORGE (1956); C. VIDAL SAPRIZA and M. GAYOSO (1956); J. OETZMANN (1956); R. BRANDNER (1957); A. PICOURET (1958); G. SPRADO (1957); VALLS CONFORTO (1961); F.E. BIRCHER (1959); R.B. HENRY (1961); J. STEIN (1974); A.C. GIANOLI (1980).

Peripheral circulatory disorders, arteriosclerosis

Whoever has seen repeatedly the action visible after 3–10 minutes of 150 mg of placenta on the livid-cool acres of peripheral circulatory disorders, has remarked with astonishment this rapid though temporary immediate effect of a cell injection. This may be accounted for by the hormones contained in the placenta, perhaps also other vasoactive substances; the factual action on the vessels after cell therapy sets in later.

KUHN and KNÜCHEL (1954), KNÜCHEL and KUHN (1955) saw in fundamental clinical studies the lipoprotein and cholesterol level subside in 64 patients with arteriosclerosis within 4–6 weeks after injections of placenta; on the other hand, these readings changed little in 100 patients of a control group. The 17-ketosteroids in the urine augmented – as analyses with various injections showed in more than 700 patients – after injection of placenta more than after hypothalamus or hypophysis, although significant results were obtained here, too. The mean daily secretion of the total-17-ketosteroids came from 8.45 ± 5.5 mg before the treatment, to 19.61 ± 8.0 mg after the treatment, the significance of the secretion was established at P = greater than 0.001. These results were not confirmed by H. HAENEL, W. SCHNEIDER and H.J. STAUDINGER (1962); they were not able to demonstrate any specific effect by changes of the 17-ketosteroid and corticoid secretion in the urine when applying dry cells (siccacell) of endocrine and non-endocrine tissues (adrenal cortex, testes, liver). The small number of «ulcus sufferers confined to bed but healthy in endocrine respect» were not suited for this parameter as the effect of cell therapy depends essentially on a disorder (hypofunction) of the tested organs.

STEPANTSCHITZ and SCHREINER found objective and subjective improvements in 8 patients of 15 with vascular sclerosis treated with placenta. The ergometrically, oscillometrically and rheographically registered improvements persisted for at least 8 months. Of 3 patients suffering from Morbus Reynaud, 2 improved. The cholesterol level did not respond in 11 patients, in 5 it declined. KLEINSORGE used the walking distance, the registering of skin temperature and oscillography to substantiate the therapeutic results. General conditions and nocturnal calf-pains were assessed subjectively. The walking distance was doubled within 4–12 weeks after injection of placenta among 21 patients (45–76 years) in 8 cases, and tripled in 3 cases; 3 persons were virtually free from complaints. These improvements persisted for 13–16 weeks in the majority of cases

(14 of 21 patients), and up to $\frac{1}{2}$ year in 4 cases.

Of 72 cases treated by OETZMANN in part with placenta, placenta + liver + testes, 58 showed improvements. Reactive hyperemia, changes of the skin temperature, lowering of the cholesterol level, increased walking distances were registered. BRANDNER divides his observations into 19 cases of general sclerosis. For average ages of 66 (57) years and in cases of preceding complaints of 3–4 years, the results in coronary sclerosis were better (15 cases free from complaints, 1 temporary improvement, 1 failure) than in general sclerosis (9 free from complaints, 6 improved, 4 failures). As «rates of success», OETZMANN gives 73.2 % of 150 patients, KUHN 67 % of 700 patients and RIETSCHEL 72.1 % of 93 patients.

For coronary sclerosis, BRANDNER examined 9 of 17 patients 1 year after the cell implantations: 5 showed improved ECG, 4 no changes of ECG, though they were free from complaints.

Cardiac insufficiency

Whereas certain authors regard cardiac insufficiency as a contraindication against cell therapy because the stress by the injection alone constitutes an additional strain for the organism (GIANOLI, 1977); H. J. OETZMANN 1956) relying on his many clinical patients drew more differentiated conclusion. In the classical postulate for limitation of cardiac activity (rest), strengthening of the myocardium (glycosides), diet and diuretics he does not see any contrast to cell therapy.

Doses of fetal myocardium (100 mg), fetal liver (150 mg) and placenta (150 mg) reduced in degenerative disorders of the myocardium the time of recompensation in the stage of decomposi-

tion. After a short phase of lassitude, the patients revived. As massive diuresis was observed during the active phase even in so far glycoside-refractary cardiac insufficiency, cell implantation seems to be the very cause of the glycoside effect on the decompensated heart in many cases; OETZMANN presented 5 casuistic reports.

Normalizations of the blood-protein pictures, the calcium, sodium, potassium metabolism and, probably, influences on the metabolism of the adenylic acid proceeded with the clinical effects.

Papers on this subject are published by B. SCHWEERS (1956), RAWER (1959) and UHLENBRUCK (1960).

Cardiac infarction

Fresh cardiac infarctions are improper to cell therapy (J. STEIN, 1974; A. C. GIANOLI, 1977). After an interval of 3–6 months and a clearly proved identification of scars, cell therapy does good for the blood circulation and promotes the contraction-regulating mechanism of the heart. The regenerability of the myocardium by new buddings of vessels has been substantiated by impressive studies.

Contraindications against cell therapy are, according to unanimous judgments, all inflammatory heart diseases as the inflammatory processes might be stimulated. Also advanced cases of coronary sclerosis need critical consideration, especially if the following changes of ECG are there (J. STEIN, 1974): graduated ST-lowering, convex descendent or inverted T-wave tempering into isoceles negativity, trouble in the conductive nerves of the heart and absolute arrythmia.

Pulmonary diseases

A connection between chronic-obstructive pneumo-emphysema and an enzymopathy, the lack of *alpha-1-antitrypsin*, is said to exist in that persons affected by this anomaly suffer 15 times more frequently from chronic destructive pulmonary diseases than the average population; however, the alpha-1-antitrypsin is not supposed to influence the so-called senile emphysema.

Alpha-1-antitrypsin, a glycoprotein having a molecular weight of about 60000, inhibits trypsin, chymotrypsin, plasmin as well as elastolytic and collagenolytic enzymes, including those of leukocytary origin. It is supposed that in cases of lacking alpha-1-antitrypsin the proteinases are not inhibited and that the latter can freely exert a destructive effect on structures of pulmonary tissues.

W. v. LANGENDORFF's (1974) tests on female Sprague-Dawley rats weighing 200–250 g were based on these ideas. A pulmonary emphysema was produced by injecting intravenously 1–2 mg of thermolysin in 0.2 ml of physiological saline solution. *Thermolysin*, a proteolytic enzyme from thermobacteria produces a high elastolytic activity at a neutral pH. The injuries are irreversible.

Fetal pulmonary tissue (30 mg/kg of bodyweight) injected into these rats 2 days before the destructing injection of enzymes brought about a protective effect persisting for 2–3 weeks even if several doses of thermolysin were applied. More injections of pulmonary tissue repeated at intervals of 14 days extended this elastin-protective effect for prolonged spaces of time. Tests for the pressure volume and histochemical qualities (hematoxilin-eosin; elastin staining after VERHOEFF) provided identical results. Injured pulmonary tissue was not regenerated by the injection, developed emphysemata resisted every influence. This protective effect was not seen with cells of fetal connective tissue.

Developmental biology

The lung develops like a gland from a tube of cylindrical epithelium separated from the mesenchyme by a basal membrane (P. BRUNNER, 1982). In the first 4 years of age the structures present at birth develop only few bronchial ramifications and alveoli are formed anew. The organism must for the whole life have enough of what is present at birth (HIERONYMI, 1960). The total of alveoli is estimated at 60 million to 1 milliard, their surface at $5\,m^2$–$200\,m^2$.

Senile processes in the lung affect chiefly the fibre system so that the loss of elasticity is the crucial point. According to P. BRUNNER (1982), the changed structures of the elastic fibres with the dwindling retraction power and the growing constituent of collagen are of primary importance. The decrease of the alveolar septa, dilation of the alveolar ducts, reduction of the alveolar net capillaries, calcareous and bony stiffening of the bronchial breathing skeleton form the «senile lung» morphologically. The decreasing spectrum of functions causes the clinical symptoms.

Clinical data

on the possibilities and indications of cell-therapeutic methods for pulmonary diseases are scarce and vary. The authors agree as to that acute, inflammatory diseases of the lungs and respiratory passages constitute contraindications.

Bronchial asthma

is regarded by many as contraindication for its chiefly allergic genesis; others, above all experienced practicians, think bronchial asthma one of the fields in which cell therapy brings about results that cannot be obtained with the classical methods. A final judgment cannot yet be given as cell therapy has so far been used for a merely negative selection i. e. when all other methods had failed. If one decides on cell therapy, the choice of tissues to be used ought to be sufficiently wide. Apart from the fetal pulmonary tissue, adrenal gland, thymus, fetal connective tissue or placenta should be taken into consideration. J. BUSCHA gave 1981

a catamnestic report on the clinical results following cell-treatment in bronchial asthma.

Contrary to the belief, widely held until now, that asthmatic subjects should not be treated with fetal cells because of the high risk of allergy, such patients have in fact been treated for more than 15 years. The author reviews, from her own point of view, 88 patients with asthma, in some cases severe and often in combination with multiple allergies, treated over the past 3 years. None of the patients of this group showed a higher risk of allergy than other completely non-allergic patients, and in fact they reacted rather less frequently. Asthma attacks occurred on only three occasions after the treatment while the patients were still hospitalized and under observation, and a status asthmaticus was never observed.

Fifty-six of these 88 patients themselves reported on the effect of the treatment.

Thirty-six patients reported an improvement in their asthma, while 11 patients showed improvement in other pathological conditions and in their general wellbeing, but no effect on their asthma. One patient reported definite deterioration of his asthmatic condition. The remaining 8 patients showed no effects of any kind after the treatment.

These experiences encourage the inclusion of asthma in the indications for cytotherapy, since a proportion of these patients can apparently be helped by this treatment, successfully and without any significant risk.

Obstructive pulmonary emphysema

is also the subject of new studies (A. C. GIANOLI). The significance of the few results substantiated by the pulmonary-function test must still be established.

331

The senile emphysema of the lung is part of the involution. As far as the vitality of the aged is impaired essentially by the reduction of pulmonary functions, it is advisable to include pulmonary tissue in a general combined revitalizing therapy.

Renal diseases

In continuing his studies on the induction of the organic growth in chicken embryos (MURPHY and DANCHAKOFF, 1916), NEUMANN (1963, 1967) tested the effect of spleen, liver and kidney for the organic growth of chicken embryos.

According to Tab. 44, 45, spleen and kidney implants in hen's eggs show better and more specific growth-stimuli than e.g. liver.

Increases of diuresis were not obtained in any tests on animals (GORDONOFF, 1960).

Only few experiments have been conducted e.g. those by MOENCH (1955), MOENCH and BURKHARD (1957) on the influence of heterologous tissular lyophilisates on the experimental nephritis in rabbits and on the neosalvarsan nephrosis in white rats.

In proportion to the clinical importance of the renal diseases and dysfunctions, little useful material on cell therapy in renal diseases is available. The reservedness shown so far in this respect may be accounted for by partly occa-

Tab. 44: **Influence of splenic, hepatic and renal tissue on the weight of these three organs**

transplant	embryos	spleen			kidney	liver
		weight	over 16 mg			
		mg	const.	weight	mg	mg
controlls	76	10,4	1%	16	87	347
spleen tissue	90	14,2	22%	22	104	365
liver tissue	19	10,9	2%	21	86	351
kidney tissue	69	12,4	17%	19	129	352

Tab. 45: **Induction of the organic growth**
Weights in % of spleen, liver and kidney after implantation of splenic hepatic and renal tissues.

transplant	Effective organ increases in weight as against control animals		
	spleen	kidney	liver
spleen	36%	20%	2%
kidney	19%	48%	1%
liver	4%	1%	1%

sional reports on «nephritis» or « autoimmune phenomenon» of the kidneys after cell therapy. Verified casuistics on immunological changes of kidneys after cell implantations, however, do not exist.

The author's own experience is restricted to a few individual cases. In two cases of *Lowe' syndrome*, no demonstrable effect was reached. Aminoaciduria and the total development in *cystinosis* were influenced favourably for a short while of just 4 weeks, without any lasting effect. Convincing, however, was the outcome of an intraperitoneal injection of fetal kidney and placenta in a case of decompensated steroid-resistant nephrosis, which had caused a hydropic deformation of the whole body. Diuresis, which effected an extensive restitution, set in already on the second day after the implantation.

Hepatic diseases

Basing upon the results of injected implantations after experimentally produced hepatic lesions by HARBERS (1954), HARDEGG and MAAS (1958) and STÖWER (1956), major clinical studies on hepatitis and consequences of hepatitis were conducted already in the 1950s by RIETSCHEL (1955) and OETZMANN (1958, 1959). Not few physicians engaged in cell therapy were induced by therapeutic results in their own chronic hepatic disease to change to this method. NEUMANN (1963, 1967) has methodically dealt with the experimental fundaments.

H. TEIR (1951, 1957) and his team succeeded in augmenting the rate of mitosis in hepatic cells by injecting hepatic tissue if the recipients were young (2-month-old-rats) whereas old animals showed no effect augmenting mitosis, no matter whether the material came from young or old animals. The effect augmenting mitosis ceases when the suspensions of liver are heated to 60° or 100° C. As back as in 1945, MARSHAK and WALKER demonstrated that chromatin from cellular substance of rat liver augments the rate of mitosis in the liver cells of recipient animals.

HARBERS (1954) provoked the hepatic lesion with carbon tetrachloride twice per week for 10–12 weeks produced in the Wistar rats a hepatic necrosis, which developed into an aspect resembling the cirrhosis of the liver. HARBERS concluded from the course of the function tests and from the time of survival that «the very serious manifest hepatic lesions are favourably influenced both with fresh cells and with dry cells». High doses of implantation material (63 mg per injection) did not provide better results than low ones (17 mg).

HARDEGG and MAAS (1958) studied, under slightly changed conditions, the influence of homologous fetal hepatic tissue on the lesion caused in the liver of rats by carbon tetrachloride (females 0.5 ml/kg of CCl 4 three times per week for 2 months); parameters were the general behaviour, loss of weight, formation of ascites, activity of the serum-choline-esterase; the latter subsided during the injections of CCl 4 to 30%–35% of the initial values, but recovered in the animals treated with cell implantations more obviously than in the controls.

OETZMANN produced with thiocetamide a slighter lesion similar to cirrhosis of the liver. The group treated with hepatic lyophilisate had the highest rate of survivors (36.5%), in contrast to that of the control group (13.3%).

HÖTZL (1956, 1960, 1961), LAUDAHN

and LÜDERS (1960) as well as L.F. MÜLLER (1961) conducted extensive studies using *suspensions of hepatic mitochondria* in cases of chronic hepatitis and cirrhosis of the liver. These experiments referred to as «new biologicotherapeutically highly effective principle» by HÖTZL were unfortunately not continued.

Clinical reports
on cell therapy in hepatic diseases were written by P. NIEHANS, BURCKHARD-(1956), KALK (1957), OETZMANN (1958, 1959) and A.C. GIANOLI. The clinical statistics by OETZMANN (1959) comprise only part of the patients whose number grew later but are useful as regards the numbers and controls. OETZMANN divided his patients into 3 groups.
Group a):
The patient got only the basic therapy: choline, hepsane, vitamins and diet.

Group b):
The treatment was based on choline, hepsane, diet and prednison.
Group c):
Treatment with choline, hepsane, diet and injections of tissues i.e. in all cases: liver, adrenal gland and placenta. This group includes 210 patients.

In question were diseases treated with «classical-conservative» methods (a), a second group (b), which got in addition prednison, and a third one with additional implantations of tissues (c). The results obtained in group c) with examinations 2 years later are shown in Tab. 46. Both for the chronic hepatitis and cirrhosis of the liver, the best results were obtained in the group on implantations, the worst in the prednison group.

Subsequent bioptic examinations were conducted later, though not evaluated.

Tab. 46: **Hepatic diseases**; summary of the clinical results by OETZMANN. Explanation of the therapies denoted as a), b), c) in the text. n = number of patients. The figures in parentheses give the results of subsequent examinations conducted about two years later.

Clin. aspect	therapy	n	improved	unchanged	worsened
Chronic	a	116	57%	39%	4%
hepatitis	b	54	50%	9%	41%
	c	99	67%	33%	0%
	(c)	(62)	(18%)	(47%)	(35%)
Transitional	a	45	39%	39%	22%
stages	b	19	42%	16%	42%
	c	38	65%	29%	6%
	(c)	(22)	(23%)	(41%)	(36%)
Compensated	a	54	33%	45%	22%
cirrhosis	b	27	37%	45%	18%
	c	63	48%	43%	9%
	(c)	(51)	(21%)	(28%)	(51%)
Decompensated	a	–	–	–	–
cirrhosis	b	22	14%	14%	72%
	c	12	0%	50%	50%
	(c)	(5)	(0%)	–	(100%)

Most clinicians and practitioners agree in stating that

a) implantations of cells are not indicated for acute hepatitis;
b) indicated are: *chronic aggressive hepatitis, transition forms of liver-cirrhosis and compensated cirrhosis of the liver.*

Agreeing with OETZMANN, the implantation material should not be restricted to fetal liver but include moreover gastrointestinal mucosa, placenta, adrenal gland, in case also pancreas. Beyond these approved indications, implantations of liver ought to be taken into consideration for

all congenital disorders of protein metabolism,

enzymopathies,
dysbacteria,
ulcera,
degenerative disorders of central nervous system,
liver complaints due to alcohol,
achondroplasia,
osteogenesis imperfecta.

The central position of the liver within the protein and glycogen metabolism, its part of a fetal place of hematopoesis make this organ a neuralgic point in most of the metabolic disturbances, in cases of abnormal hematopoesis and in cardiac decompensation. Fig. 257, 258, 259, 302, 303, 305, 308, 309, 314 show examples of including implantations of liver in a general therapeutic scheme.

Alcoholism

Liver damages are a central problem in chronic alcoholism. A wholistic concept for this important socio-medical question offered H. BRAMMER (1982).

A catamnestic study on 87 alcoholic patients subjected to combined therapy. The physical part of the treatment consists of cell therapy, autohaemotherapy and ozone; the non-physical involves psychotherapy, individual interviews and group therapy. Overall condition, capacity to act productively, and ability to concentrate had improved by 95–100% at the time of post-study, 13 months later, and the relapse frequency was reduced from 85% to 44%.

Skin diseases

The use of cell therapy was proclaimed nearly an euphoriant in early years. But enthusiasm calmed down because the indications were too wide and it was not possible to reproduce individual success in other cases. Publications of that time are by G. ACKERMANN (1956); R. ECKSTEIN (1955); H. HASSELMANN (1959); P. H. JANSON (1953–1957) and a survey by G. W. KORTING (1957). Reference is made to the following indications: *systematised elastorhexis sarkoid* DARIER-ROUSSY; *cosmetic lesions; Kera-* *tosis palmaris et plantaris hereditaria; rosacea, Acne vulgaris, Lichen chronicus simplex, sclerodermia.* The reports contradicted each other especially for the therapy of acne, and varied from prompt success to failure.

As many skin diseases are based on internal and, specially, metabolic disorders, the therapeutic scheme for the indications was probably not broad enough so that failure had necessarily to be anticipated. Since the skin is a superficial organ, it is recommended to apply the skin

Tab. 47: Indications for fetal cutaneous extract in 109 tests

Objective control and recording were possible for the skin diseases (fig. 284–292) whereas only subjective data are available for the «internal» tests.

Symptom	Cases	Effect proved	Without effect
Burns, scalds	34	34	0
keloid scars	21	17	4
epidermolysis-Lyell's syndrome	3	3	0
eczema acute, dermatitis seborrh.	3	0	3
ulcus cruris	3	2	1
«senile skin»	4	3	1
dermatitis by irradiation	1	1	0
anhidrosis syndromes	3	2	1
hyperkeratosis	8	6	2
alopecia	6	6	0
acne	4	2	2
affections of joints and ligaments	7	7	0
mucopolysaccharidosis	1	0	1
colitis	3	3	0
epicondylitis	8	8	0

preparations locally; however, it is difficult to find the proper degradation-size of the skin derivatives.

Many attempts indeed have been made to cover major cutaneous defects with transplants of skin and other organs. Used were *omentum transplants* (A. NISHIMURA, 1973), *skin of dead bodies* (B. KÖRHOF, 1973), *wraps of amnion* (M. C. ROBSON, 1973) and *epidermic suspensions* (W. D. F. MALHERBE, A. MEYER and J. VAAN DER WALT).

Relying on own experience with *large burns* and *scalds* in children, the author developed a fetal cutaneous extract suitable for prolonged local applications in various skin diseases. Two multicentric studies were conducted to determine the spectrum of indications. Later, the fetal cutaneous extract was put on the market under the reg. trade-mark *Cellcutana®*. It constitutes an ultrafiltrate, which is prepared by extraction of fetal skin, fetal connective tissue, placenta and adrenal gland.

This composition was chosen to favour the physiological connections between the epidermis and subcutaneous tissular formations and to promote the regeneration of cutaneous lesions also from beneath. The preparation is available in two pharmaceutical forms, as a lyophilisate and as a suspension, is stable if dissolved at temperatures of 2–8°C for more than a week without losing anything of its efficiency, but should be used immediately after resuspension in Ringer's, Tyrode solution or in the suspension liquid supplied along with the preparation. The local effect can be improved by warming and cleaning the skin. In cases of extensive scalds, burns and irradiation burns it is advisable to disperse the extract or the lyophilisate on thin layers of muslin soaked with Ringer's solution.

The results of the two tests are represented in the Tab. 47, 48, and it must be pointed out that a total of 47 physicians, 15 of Switzerland and 32 of the Federal

Tab. 48: **Fet. skin extract: multicentric study Switzerland – Fed. Rep. of Germany.**
In the Swiss group, 51 tests were positive, 5 doubtful, 7 negative. In the Fed. German group, 41 tests were positive, 2 doubtful, 4 negative. All in all, positive results were seen in 92 cases of 110, 7 were doubtful and 11 negative; the indications had been chosen in part by the treating physicians themselves.

Indications	Switzerland Result			F. R. Germany Result			Sum Result		
	+	?	−	+	?	−	+	?	−
Acne (various stages)	3	1	1	7	1	1	10	2	2
Acrodermatitis		1							1
Alopecia areata	4		1				4		1
Alopecia totalis		1						1	
Diabetic gangrene	1						1		
Epicondylitis			1	2			2		1
Epidermolysis bull. hered.	1						1		
Eczema				1			1		
Hair dystrophy	1						1		
Cutaneous metastasis in mammal carcinoma					1			1	
Hyperkeratosis	1			2		1	3		1
Keloids	10	1		7		1	17	1	1
Mult. cutaneous ulceras in Pyoderma gangraenosum	1						1		
Ulcer on the tip of the nose				1			1		
Neurodermitis	1						1		
Pigment-variations	3						3		
Pruritus senilis			1						1
Psoriasis		1	1					1	1
X-ray skin	2						2		
Ulcus cruris	13			8			21		
Sequels of burns and scalds	10			8			18		
Vitiligo		1	1					1	1
Secondarily healing skin transplantation				1			1		
Ichthyosis				2			2		
Erythema solare				1			1		
Herpes zoster				1			1		
Reticulo-sarcoma						1			1
	51	5	7	41	2	4	92	7	11
	63			47			110		

Republic of Germany, participated in the 2nd test, which took place between January 1st, 1978, and June 30th, 1979. The following indications crystallized for the fetal cutaneous extract: *scalds, burns* (fig. 286, 287), *irradiation burns on the skin physical injuries* (fig. 290), *explosion injuries* (fig. 289), *keloids, hyperkera-*

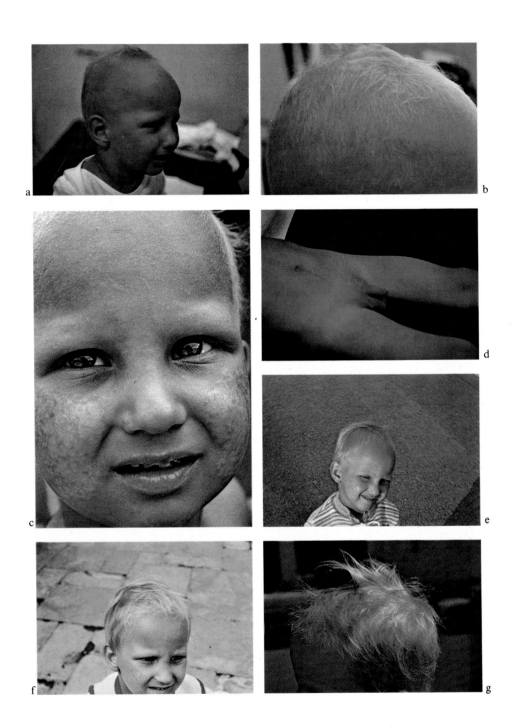

Fig. 284:
Rothmund's syndrome with downy hair at the beginning of treatment at 3 years. Development of the hair of the head within a year (e) and after 3 years (f, g).

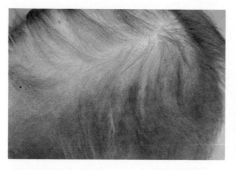 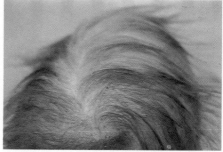

Fig. 285:
Christ-Siemens-Tourraine's (anhidrosis) syndrome. First nearly invisible, thin downy hair. Condition after 3 years of treatment.

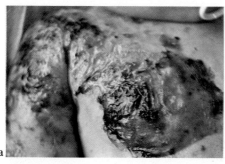 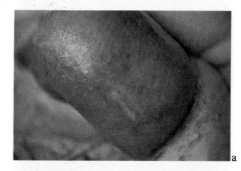

Fig. 286:
Scald with hot water, 2nd–3rd degree a) after 3 days; b) after 2 weeks. Nearly scarless regeneration of the skin.

Fig. 287:
Scald with hot water, 3rd degree. Course of a week (a–c).

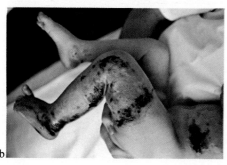 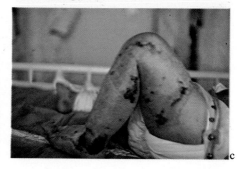

339

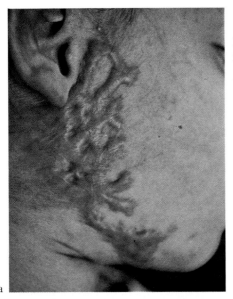

a

Fig. 288:
Keloid scars of a 9-year-old girl after burn by exploding spirit. Course:
a) treatment initiated with fetal skin extract;
b) after three months;
c) after nine months.

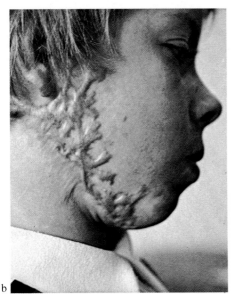

b

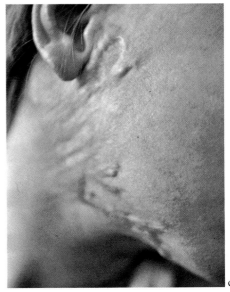

c

tosis (fig. 291, 292), *anhidrosis syndromes* (fig. 284, 285), *ulcus cruris* (fig. 293, 295, 296), *senile atrophy of the skin; trophic disturbances in circulatory trouble; Lyell syndrome; cosmetic lesions; keloids* (fig. 288); *sclerodermia.* Different were the results of the treatment of *acne* in various stages, of *Alopecia areata* and of *psoriasis* (W. SCHUCK, 1982).

Contraindications for the local application of fetal cutaneous extract are acute inflammatory affections of the skin, above all the acute wet eczema, which may grow worse by applications

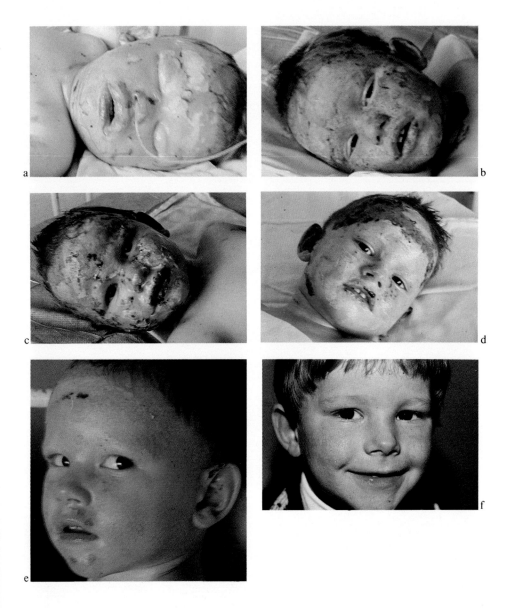

Fig. 289:
Burns of 2.–3. degree in face and neck by gas-explosion.
a) condition on admission in the hospital
b),c) cleaning and rejection of the necroses on 7th and 10th day
d) 16th day
e) 19th day; nearly complete healing
f) 18 month later skin without scars

of Cellcutana, and acute viral skin-diseases, especially herpes.

The optimal treatment of innate and chronic skin-diseases, however, may be some combination of cell-therapeutic remedies supplied parenterally, and their application to the surface.

For parenteral doses of lyophilisates, especially fetal liver, placenta, connec-

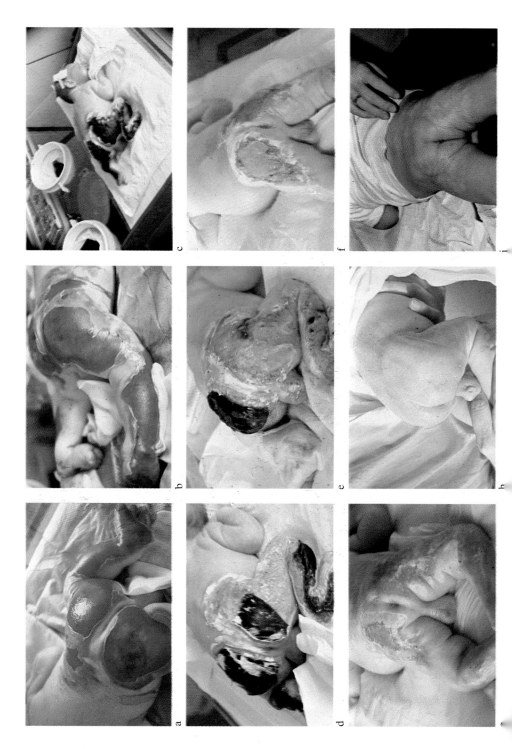

Fig. 290: Text see page 343.

Fig. 291:
Fig. 291:
Ichthyosis congenita, pictures of the lower leg (a, b) and central abdomen (c). After application of fetal cutaneous extract, the hyperkeratotic scales disappeare sometimes within days (d, e).

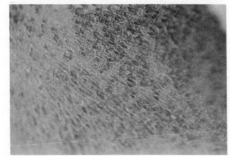

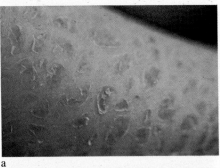

a

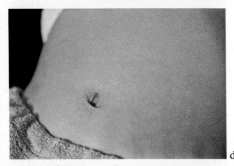

d

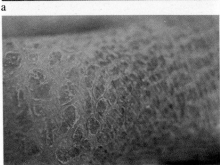

b

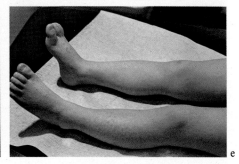

e

c

◀ *Fig. 290:*
Third-degree burns through defective
a) gummibattle in a newborn baby; about
b) 30% of body surface are involved
c) and d) Demarkation of the «coaled» tissue-necrosis on the 10th and 13th day
e, f, g) progressing cleaning and healing after 3, 5 and 7 weeks
h) and i) relativly minor scars and recovered functions after months

tive tissue and, as far as hirsutism on the body is concerned, sex-specific adrenal preparations, besides fetal skin, should be taken into consideration. HAGMEIER (1978) presented impressive results with fetal mesenchyme – Resistocell® – even in long-lasting skin defects resistant to other remedies (fig. 293–296).

343

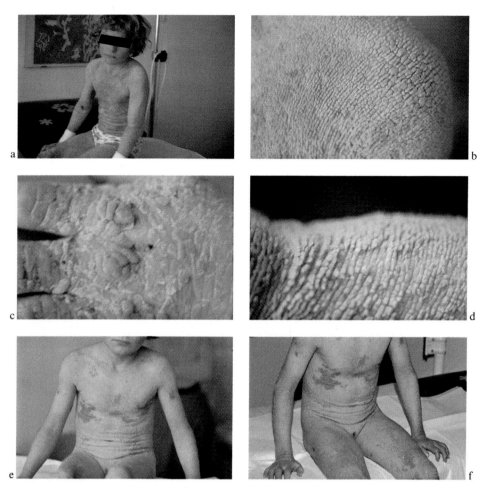

Fig. 292 a–f:
Serious Ichthyosis cong. (Hysterix) in 8-year-old girl. Practically all therapies were exhausted, fetal cutaneous extract brought improvement but no essential change. Initial situation with injection implantations of 150 mg of liver, 150 mg of placenta (781 220); after 5 weeks (790 129) extensive scaling, an effect that persisted only 6–8 weeks even after repeated implantations.

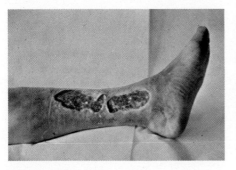
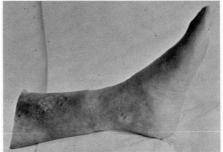
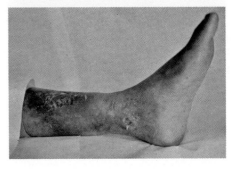

Fig. 293:
Ulcus cruris with phlegmon in diabetes
Ulcus on left leg open for more than 20 years, with phlegmon on lower leg in Diabetes mellitus.
On admittance, a smeary palm-sized ulcer, moreover ulcerations about the size of a piece of money (∅ 25 mm) on the inner ankle.
Cell therapy with fetal mesenchyme.
After a few days already, astonishing cleaning of the wound, the improvement of which can be followed nearly with the naked eye (HAGMEIER, 1978).

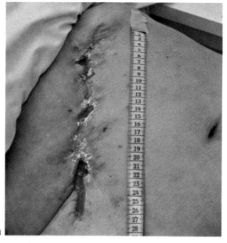

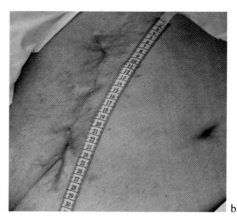

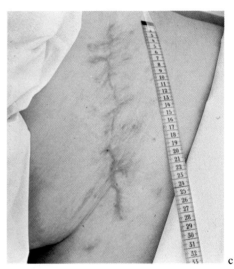

Fig. 294 a–c:
Secretion of wounds (HAGMEIER, 1978)
A patient with highly intense adipositas (125 kg, 162 cm), serious gall-bladder emphyema, stenosis of cysticus and cholithiasis.

After extensive operation still after 6 months highly intense wound secretion in spite of all conventional therapeutic measures. In this condition – i.e. after 6 months – implantation of 1 ampoule (= 100 mg) of Resistocell.

After 10 days already essential improvement of general condition, visibly increasing healing of the large surgical wound, proceeding with completely stopping secretion and rapid, entire epithelisation.

Fig. 295 a–c:
Burn with remaining ulcus cruris
Extensive burn on right lower leg with remaining leg ulcer above the edge of tibia, no healing for 5 months.

Then 100 mg of Resistocell®: after 8 days already complete cleaning of wound so that skin could be transplanted. Complete epithelisation. Consequently, recovery after 5 months of vain treatment with one injection of Resistocell®. Observed for more than 2 years (fig. c: 2 years after injection).

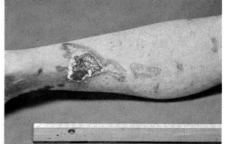

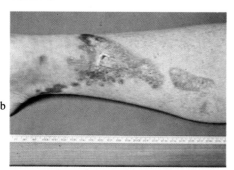

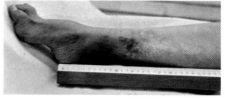

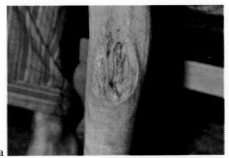

a

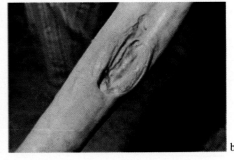

b

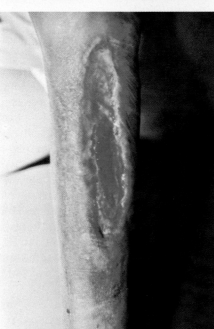

c

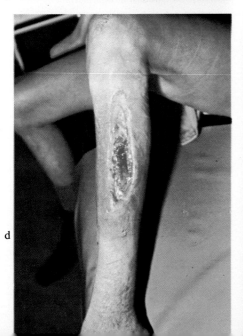

d

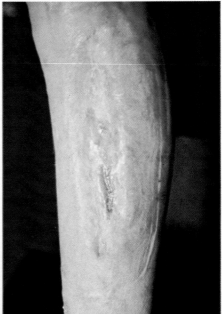

e

Fig. 296 a–e:
Ulcus cruris through wound inflicted in war
Most serious ulcer on the lower leg persisting for more than 30 years as a sequel of a wound afflicted in the war, in a patient now 63 years old.

The patient's general condition had worsened to an extent bad enough to justify the idea of amputation for vital reasons. To this, however, the patient resists, because he heard about cell-therapeutic alternatives.

Injection of 1 ampoule of Resistocell® (= 100 mg of fetal mesenchyme) (fig. 296 c).

Two months later, the extensive ulceration appeared virtually clean, without any additional surgical measure applied (fig. d). Three months after initiation of cell therapy (fig. e) and after a total lapse of 4 months, the leg, which had persisted in a damaged condition continually for more than 30 years owing to a wound inflicted in the war, was completely healed so that the patient was discharged from the clinic and can now take his daily walks without any complaints (HAGMEIER, 1978).

Diseases of supporting tissues

The value and limits of cell-therapy cannot yet be defined for the many skeletal abnormalities and diseases. With the exception of some orthopedic reports, the pertinent literature is very sporadic so that the following data are based on the author's own recorded observations.

A concise outline of the skeletal development must be given first to arouse the understanding of the possibilities and initial points for cell-therapeutic measures and necessary additional treatments.

Development of the skeleton

The supporting tissue develops from the embryonic mesoderm and includes the following tissues (W. BARGMANN):

Unformed supporting tissues:

1. mesenchyme
2. gelatinous connective tissue
3. reticular connective tissue
4. adipose tissue
5. loose connective tissue
6. tight connective tissue

Formed supporting tissue:

1. tendinous tissue, elastic tissue
2. cartilaginous tissue
3. chorda tissue
4. bone-tissue, dentin
5. vascular system.

Whereas the unformed supporting tissues retain partly the pluripotency of the embryonic structures and represent much of the active mesenchyme (reticulo histiocytary system), the formed supporting tissues have already taken special functions.

Up to the final differentiation, the skeleton passes a mesenchymal, a cartilaginous and a bony stage. In the mesenchymal stage, the mesenchyme develops, generally via the pre-cartilage, the model of the prospective supporting tissue. Disturbances affecting the growth of the skeleton in this stage are usually aberrations from the ground-plan. Tab. 49 is a list of the most important of these aberrations. In the cartilaginous stage, the mesenchymal pre-cartilaginous rudiments are rebuilt first into cartilage. The transformation begins in the second month of embryonic life between the stages of 10 mm and 26 mm of the embryo via the chondrification centres. On the 60th day of pregnancy, the rudiments of the cartilaginous skeleton are completed up to the terminal phalanxes of the toes, and the cartilaginous skeleton is then successively replaced by bones (= substitution bones). This process sets in as from the 7th embryonic week and is accomplished at the end of the somatic growth between the 15th and 20th year of age.

Cartilage is a special form of connective tissue; its consists of cells (chondrocytes) embedded in a matrix. The matrix is composed of a fibrillary meshwork of collagenous fibrils and an amorphous ground-substance; the latter is rich in sulphates containing mucopolysaccharides (chondroitinsulphate). The gelatinous ground-substance is polyanionic, highly polymerised. Cells and ground-substance are carriers of the highly *metabolic activity* distinctive of the growth, and of the *plasticity* of the cartilage. The collagenous fibres effect the *rigidity* and *elasticity*. Cartilage has no vessels, contains only canals resembling vessels. The metabolic processes pass through the diffusion, which is rendered the more

1. Craniosynostosis (= premature suture synostosis) by maldevelopment of the cranial sutures in the mesenchymal stage: Dolichocephaly, Turricephaly, Oxycephaly, Plagiocephaly, Microcephaly
2. Dysostosis craniofacialis (CROUZON)
3. Dysostosis mandibulofacialis (FRANZESCHETTI; TEACHER-COLLINS)
4. Oculo-mandibulo-facialis syndrome (FRANCOIS, HALLERMANN-STREIFF)
5. Acrocephalo-syndactily (APERT)
6. Acrocephalo-Poly-syndactily (CARPENTER)
7. mandibular hypoplasia (PIERRE-ROBIN)
8. Rubinstein-Syndrome
9. Aglossy-adactyly syndrome
10. Dysostosis cleidocranialis (cleido-pelvico-cranialis)
11. Sprengel's deformity; innate scapular elevation
12. Klippel-Feil syndrome and other vertebral segmentation disorders
13. Cranio-Rachischisis centaurica (iniencephaly)
14. Cervico-oculo-acusticus syndrome (WILDERVANCK)
15. Oculo-vertebral syndrome (WEYERS)
16. Oro-digito-facialis syndrome
17. Dysostosis spondylocostalis
18. Pectoralisaplasia-Dysdactyly syndrome
19. Osteo-Onycho-Dysostosis (Nagel-Patella syndrome, TURNER-KIESER)
20. Radiusaplasia-Thrombocytopenia syndrome
21. radioulnar synostosis
22. carpal and tarsal synostosis
23. Syndactyly-Polysyndactyly-Spoonhand
24. Ectromely
25. Polydactyly
26. Oligodactyly
27. Brachycarpie-Brachyphalangie-Brachytele-, meso-, -basophalangy
28. Dolicho-steno-carpia
29. Sirenomelia
30. Arthrogryposis multiplex (Arthromyodysplasia congenita)
31. Dystrophia mesodermalis congenita (MARFAN u. a.)

difficult the more the maturity continues (= gel condensation). With these properties, cartilage is a tissue that has lost the pluripotency of the mesenchyme but still retained many functions of the origin tissue e. g. the metabolism, the dividing activity, plasticity and elasticity. Cartilage is formed through prechondroblasts, highly synthetic chondroblasts and chondrocytes. Hydroxylapatite is embedded in the growing zones.

Disturbances in the cartilaginous stage provoke modelling abnormalities of the skeleton. The essential abnormalities are listed in Tab. 50 and 22.

Bone is a specific calcified derivative of connective tissue; its architecture depends on its function. Bone consists of cells (osteocytes) and of a lacunar meshwork. The organic ground-substance (30%–40%) consists chiefly of collagen (90–95%) and sulphate-mucopolysaccharides. The mineral salts (60–70%) constitute a homoiostatic reservoir for calcium, phosphorous and citrate ions, and are formed into hydroxyl apatite by the ossification. The ossification (osteogenesis), too, is an active cell performance of specialized cells of connective tissue, the osteoblasts, which are derivatives of the pluripotent cells of connective tissue. The initial process of ossification, the formation of crystal nuclei along the collagen fibres requires certain biochemical and inorganic substances; some of them are the cells and cell derivatives, organic and inorganic substances listed in Tab. 51.

The *collagen fibres* formed by the osteoblasts are an aggregate of subunits, the so-called tropocollagen. Every molecule of tropocollagen consists of 3 peptide chains. The hydroxylation of the prolin depending on the ascorbic acid takes place when prolin unites with a nucleotide or with soluble RNA. The fibrillation is caused by a crystallization process.

Osteogenesis is either desmal or chondral, according to whether the bones are formed from the connective tissue direct or through the cartilage.

The fig. 297 a, b, outline by means of examples the relations between the derivatives of the connective tissue under physiological and pathological conditions.

Therapeutic conceptions should take into consideration these connections.

The development of the skeleton is a process regulated by cells; it undergoes

Tab. 50: **Modelling anomalies of the skeleton**

1. Achondrogenesis
2. thonatophorous nanism
3. Achondroplasia (= Chondrodystrophy)
4. Hypochondroplasia
5. Dyschondrosteosis
6. metatrophic nanism
7. diastrophic nanism
8. asphyxiating thoraxdysplasia
9. Chondrodysplasia punctata (Chondroangiopathia calcarea)
10. chondroektodermal Dysplasia (ELLIS-VAN CREVELD)
11. mesomel nanism
12. Spondylo-epiphyseal dysplasia
    a) congenita (SPRANGER)
    b) tarda
13. Spondylo-metaphysary dysplasia
14. metaphysary dysplasia
    a) Type Murk-Jansen
    b) Type Schmid
    c) Type McKusick (cartilage-hair-hypoplasia)
    d) with neutropenia and malabsorption
    e) with thymic lymphopenia
15. multiple epiphysary dysplasia (FAIRBANK)
16. Acrodysplasia epi-metaphysaria (BRAILSFORD)
17. Dysplasia epiphysealis hemimelica (FAIRBANK)
18. Enchondromatosis (OLLIER)
19. multiple cartilaginous exostosis
20. Enchondromatosis with haemangiomatosis (Maffucci syndrome)
21. fibrous dysplasia
    a) without abnormal pigment anomalies (JAFFÉ-LICHTENSTEIN)
    b) with abnormal pigment anomalies and pubertas praecox (ALBRIGHT syndrome)

Tab. 51: **Essential factors of osteogenesis**

Tissues, cells, cellular derivates	Organic substances	Inorganic substances
Mesenchyme embryonic connective tissue	Amino-acids (prolin) nucleotides	calcium phosphorus
procartilage	soluble RNA	sodium sodium citrate
cartilage	ATP	potassium
vessels	Mucopolysaccharides	magnesium
chondroblasts	Vitamin D	iron
chondrocytes	Vitamin C	fluor
	Vitamin A	
osteoblasts	carbonic acid	sulphur
osteocytes		
osteoclasts		
tropocollages	Phosphatase	
collagen fibrils		

350

many stages and is therefore exposed to a richly differentiated scale of maldevelopments. The effects of such failure depend chiefly on the time, then on the character of the malregulation. The following points must be distinguished:

1. *Aberrations of the architecture* originating up to the end of the somitic stage (28th–30th day of embryonic life); they are somitic i. e. axillary, constitute more or less gross aberrations from the architecture and form of the body. Aplasia, hypoplasia, synostosis and slots belong here (Tab. 49).
2. *Modelling abnormalities* originates after the somitic stage till the end of the somatic growth i. e. from the 5th week of embryonic life till puberty. As they include the mesenchyme and cartilaginous stages, they ought to be called dysplasia, not dysostosis (Tab. 50, 22). During this long time, the bones grow much more rapidly at the metaphysical ends than by periosteal apposition. Disturbances manifest themselves chiefly in the metaphyseal-epiphyseal zones of growth, transverse to the bone axis. Whilst the number of bone-elements is regular, the form is affected, which means that the moulding is abnormal. In question are *osteogenesis imperfecta, meta- and epiphyseal dysplasia, achondrogenesis, achondroplasia, mucopolysaccaridosis and many syndromes with skeletal dysplasia.*
3. *Structure disorders.* Changes of the bone-structure in the preformed skeleton should be summarized under the collective term «dysostosis». In question are local or generalized dis-

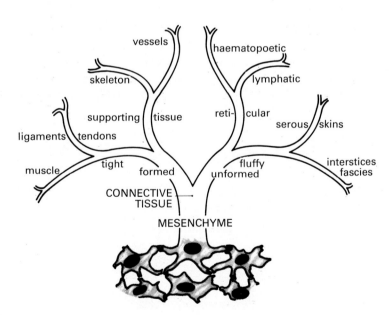

Fig. 297 a:
«*Mesenchyme tree*». The embryonic mesenchyme brings forth the formed and unformed connective tissues, which specialize in the nearest branching (muscles, ligaments, tendons, skeleton, vessels; haematopoetic, lymphatic system, serous skins, interstitia, fasciae). The following differentiation has been omitted for better survey (from F. Schmid: Pädiatr. Radiologie, volume I).

351

turbances of the distribution between organic bone-matrix and inorganic deposits; simultaneously, the relation of elasticity: stability is changed. The spectrum ranges from the *osteomalacia* over *osteoporosis* to *osteosclerosis* and *osteopetrosis*. Disturbed metabolism, lack of vitamins, immobilization, hormonal influences are the main causes for aberrations of bone-structure. Senile osteoporosis belongs here. Of the rare cases of innate dysostosis, osteopetrosis is best known.

Therapeutic remedies

The following tissues are suited to treat skeletal dysplasia and dysostosis with cell-therapeutic measures:

Tissues of first choice: cartilage, fetal mesenchyme, connective tissue, osteo-blasts, bone marrow.

Tissues of second choice: placenta, liver.

As to third quality, the use of endocrine organs ought to be considered in each particular case e.g. hypothalamus, hypophysis, adrenal gland, gonads for forms of nanism, and parathyreoidea and kidney for abnormal structures.

The *implantation therapy* can be completed by *hydrolysates* and *enzyme preparations*. Of the hydrolysates, arumalon® is the best-known. Enzyme preparations in the form of Wobe-mugos, Wobenzym® are available for oral and rectal applications. More effective parenteral or mucosal preparations are Oculucidon®, Rheumajecta® and Vaselastica®.

The biological substitution therapy should be completed by quantitative trace elements and vitamins to be deter-

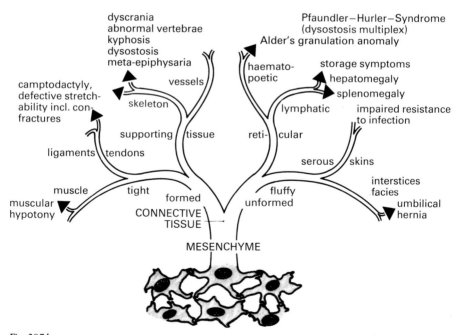

Fig. 297 b:
Development, specialization and differentiation of the mesenchyme («mesenchyme tree»); participation of the mesenchyme derivatives in Pfaundler-Hurler's disease. Besides the formed connective tissues, essential parts of the unformed connective tissues are also affected; consequently, a «mesenchymosis» in the strict sense is in question (from F. SCHMID: Pädiatr. Radiologie, volume I).

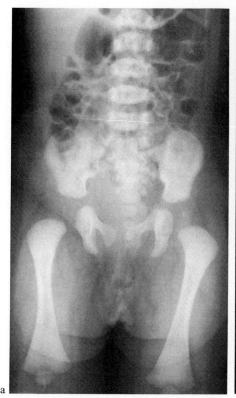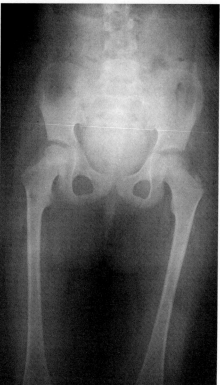

a   b

Fig. 298 a, b:
Arthro-Myo-Dysplasia
a) Shoulders, hips and knees cannot be stretched in new-born on account of articular dysplasia. Besides physiotherapy, implantations of cartilage, bone-marrow, placenta, liver and cerebral tissues are injected combined by 200–250 mg of each at intervals of 5–6 months.
b) Shoulders and hips are moved freely at the age of $9\frac{1}{2}$ years, the hips are well moulded; the static development and speech are still retarded, same as the stature.

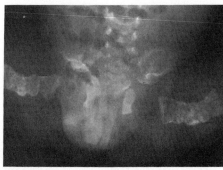

Fig. 299:
Osteogenesis imperfecta, Type Vrolik.

mined in each particular case. Vitamin C is of importance for the tropocollagen synthesis, vitamin D for the incorporation of hydroxylapatite (= calcification).

To find a proper preparation of quantitative trace elements, hair analyses may be more useful than tests on sera. In achondroplasia and osteogenesis imperfecta the calcium-content in the hair is markedly elevated, selenium lowered.

Physiotherapy, massage, gymnastics

353

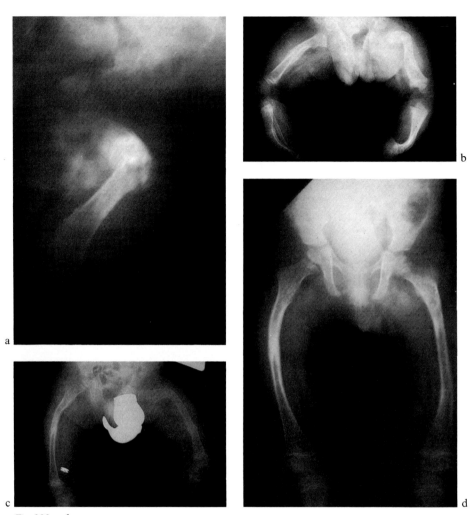

Fig. 300 a–d:
Osteogenesis imperfecta, severe Vrolik-type.
Till 5 and 6 month of age multiple bone fractures (a) and skeletal deformities. After starting the treatment less and faster healing fractures, but still deformed left femur (c) in the age of 16 month. Good reconstruction of the bones in the age of 25 month. Treated with various mesenchymal tissue-implantations.

or special physical exercises constitute an important factor to support structural processes by functional activities.

Further, a *dietetic promotion* should not be underrated. Raw vegetables and sufficient supplies of calcium by milk, salt-water fish, crabs are well suited to balance the calcium-phosphorus metabolism. Colostrum milk and raw epiphyseal cartilage added to the food have special indications. It must, however, be emphasized that all these measures relate to treatments of disorders considered as untreatable, and that the results in all must still be denoted as unsatisfactory.

As regards the skeletal abnormalities and diseases, just little can be said about the usefulness of these therapies, all the

354

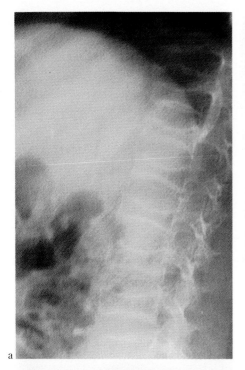

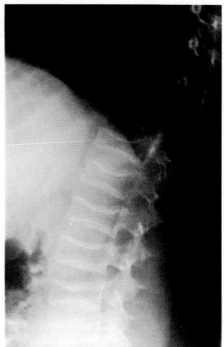

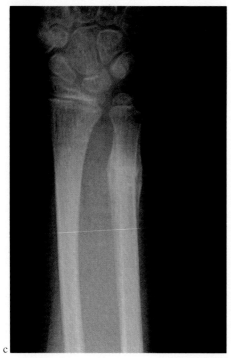

Fig. 301:

Osteogenesis imperfecta

The 8-year-old girl, who had suffered many fractures (so far 13 large, many small ones) was im-
mobilized for over 2 years, unable to walk, increasingly depressed.

a) at 8 7/12 years, with serious dysplasia and
    deficiency in calcium of the entire skeleton
    incl. the vertebrae, she got the first implanta-
    tion of 100 mg of cartilage, 75 mg of bone-
    marrow, 150 mg of placenta; basic treatment
    with 500 mg of vitamin C daily, coliacron.

b) on half-year implantations no fracture for 2
    years, good mineralization, walking up to $\frac{3}{4}$
    hour; only after immobilization due to
    Genua valga operation, new fractures occur.

c) healing ulna-fracture.

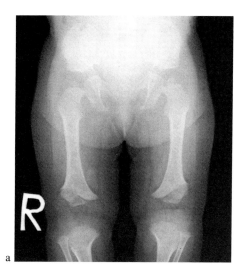

a

Fig. 302 a–d:
Achondroplasia
P. W. comes to be treated at 1 7/12 year with the classical symptoms of achondroplasia.

a) The pelvic shovels are low, roundish, the acetabula horizontal, the necks of the femora are thick, distal meta-epiphyses laterally ground off, medially drawn out like beaks, proximal tibia-metaphyses mushroom-like blown out, concave irregular calcified zones.

Gets cartilage, osteoblasts, bone-marrow, placenta and liver in combinations of 200–250 mg of lyophilisate each, at half-year intervals, at times arumalon (hydrolysate) and oculucidon (combination of enzymes).

b) At $7\frac{1}{2}$ years, short but straight femora, horizontal calcified zones on the distal femur, solidified metaphyseal structures, epiphyseal cores nearly regular.

c) At $9\frac{1}{2}$ years virtually straight hollow bones, fibula slightly curved, smooth calcified zones, regular epiphyseal cores.

d) Curve of growing stature　　　▶

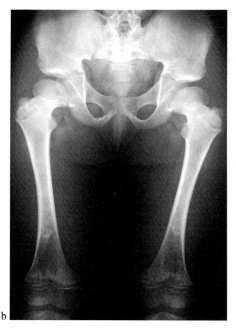

b

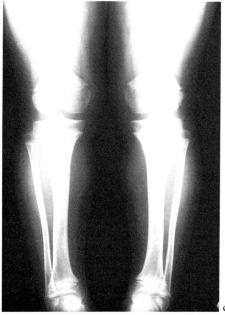

c

more since the number of the aspects under concern is often restricted.

Arthrogryposis multiplex (arthromyodysplasia) constitutes a serious syndrome, with malformed rudiments of the joints, tendons and muscles with considerable functional restrictions as main characteristics. Four long-time observations during 6–12 years have shown that the

356

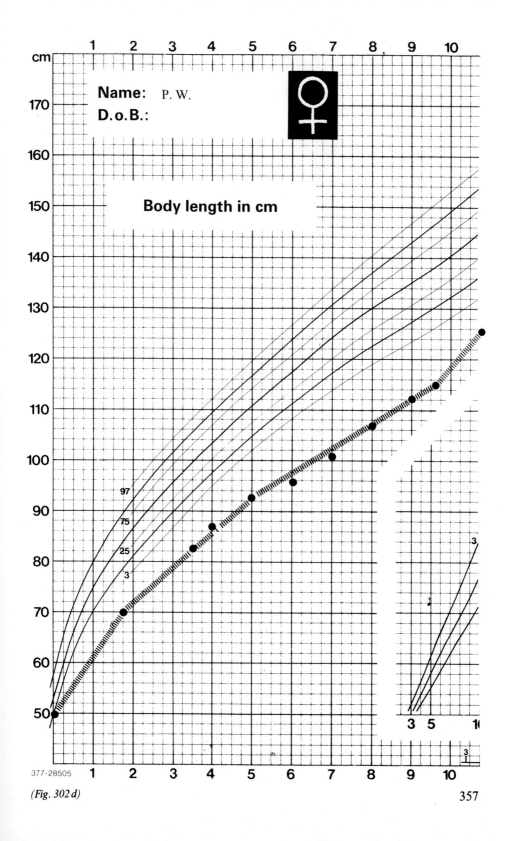

cm

Name: P. W.
D.o.B.:

Body length in cm

97
75
25
3

3
5
10

3

(Fig. 302 d)

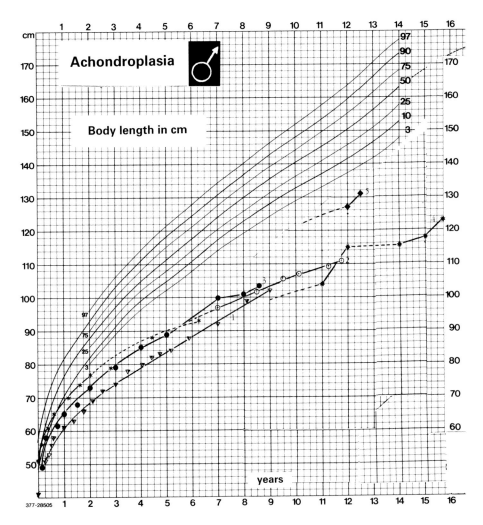

Fig. 303, 304:
Achondroplasia, growth curves of 5 boys and 5 girls. The solid lines symbolize the times of implantation treatments, the interrupted lines the periods exempt from treatments. The influence of implantations is evidenced mainly by the cases treated late (4, 5, 10). In the case 6, which was treated consistently from early infancy and evidenced a serious condition, the X-ray symptoms on later radiographs do not exclude hypochondroplasia.

skeletal and articular functions can essentially be restored even in cases seeming hopeless on account of articular dysplasia (fig. 298).

Osteogenesis imperfecta
is divided into the serious form (Vroliktype) and mild form or retarded manifestation (Lobstein-type); other subtypes are discussed. Irrespective of the severity, the disposition to fractures can be remedied by injection implantations for 3 months in infants, for 4–6 months in older children. Seven observations by the author for in part up to 10 years have shown that multiple fractures heal within 3 weeks after the implantations, with

358

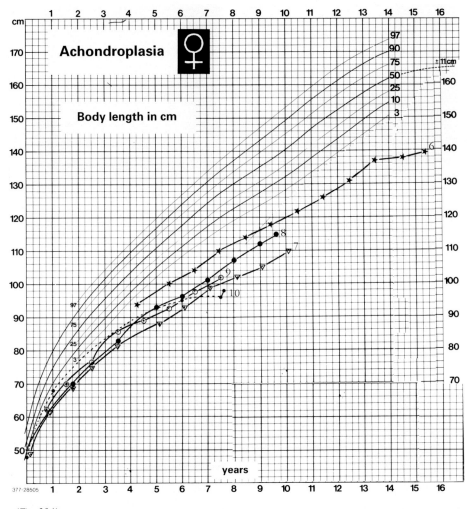

(Fig. 304)

pain (breathing after fractures of ribs, extremities) subsiding rapidly. The quantities of implants used so far (200–250 mg of lyophilisates) are probably too low. The proper combinations are: cartilage + placenta; liver + osteoblasts (fig. 299, 300, 301).

For *achondroplasia (chondrystrophy)*, experience of many years (15 observations) is available. Though a final statement cannot yet be made, certain findings are worth mentioning. The yearly growth rate is 3–5 cm during the treat-

ment, the final result may exceed the expected rates of untreated patients by about 10–15 cm. Untreated girls reach an average tallness of 119 cm, boys 127 cm. The growth curves in fig. 303, 304 give some individual courses in treated children. Interruptions of treatments show more clearly their positive influence on the growth of the body. It must be pointed out that treated children have no problems with the hydrocephalus, that their members are more straight in spite of their shortness, and the calcification zo-

359

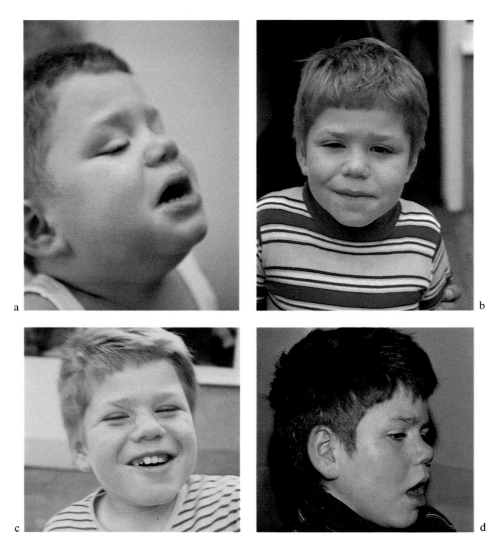

Fig. 305:
Mucopolysaccharidosis, type II
a) The boy was presented first at 3 6/12 years (670,609–701,208); diagnosis had been made else-where, and a short prognosis for life had been given.
b), c) In the course of regular implantations with cerebral lyophilisates, placenta, liver, not only the retrogression of the early years is stopped; the boy learns to walk, cycles on a tricycle, uses a few words, but the results won by the implantations subside again after 3–4 months.
b) 6 years, c) 8 years.
d) Beyond the 10th year, the motor functions of cleanness and the physiognomical control retro-gress.

nes and metaphyses, originally uneven and often bizarrely deformed, are transferred into increasingly regular structures (fig. 302).

Mucopolysaccharidoses (see Tab. 22) proceeds with more or less serious skeletal dysplasia. The therapeutic measures have brought about so far only temporary improvements (fig. 305) and retarded the progredience. The causal principle of lacking lysosomal enzymes can be influenced with the available preparations only for a short while and insufficiently. The same restrictions apply to *spondylo-epiphysary dysplasia*.

Individual observations suggest that the healing processes in *aseptic necrosis* and *fractures* can be accelerated by cell implantations, which constitutes a prerequisite for the healing of *chronic osteomyelitis* (HERBERT; HAGMEIER; EICKSCHEN; fig. 294, 296, 306.

Most of the practical experience is available for *arthrosis* and chronic from of *arthritis* (R. ORTIZ, 1973, 1980; HERBERT, 1982). The tissular combination comprises connective tissue, cartilage, osteoblasts, placenta and liver. The clinical effect, of course, depends on the stage of the regressive changes; that is why the therapy should not be put off till the function of a joint disappears and osteophytes, calcified tendons and secondary deformations create irreversible anatomic conditions.

Skeleton and growth

The growth of the stature is the result of skeletal growth and takes place in 3 phases, namely

a) *a genetic phase*
b) *a «hypophyseal» phase*
c) *a «gonadal» phase.*

The first, genetically regulated phase ranges from birth till about the 3rd and 5th year and characterized by a high speed of growth. The second phase (from about the 4th–5th to the 8th–12th years) is regulated chiefly by the hypophyseal diencephalic system and stimulated by the somatotropic hormone (STH). In this phase, growth is slow-steady, with an annual increase between 4 and 6 cm. The third phase leads to another augmented growth under the influence of the adrenal-gonadal system (the so-called puberal growth outburst).

The *adrenal glands* undergo an involution after birth; after the 6th–8th years of age, the adrenal glands and gonads grow rapidly, reaching simultaneously a culmination between the 14th and 18th years. Whereas the corticosteroids show a nearly linear rise from birth, the production of gonadotropins, 17-ketosteroids and sexual hormones begins also between the 6th–8th years, but in the concentration proceeds virtually parallel to the growth of the adrenal glands and gonads (PRADER).

The growth of the stature and the development of bones are influenced usually in the same way by adrenal and sexual hormones. The physiological function of these hormones is to initiate the third growth outburst in the beginning puberty and to finish the growth by closure of the epiphyses at the end of puberty.

The earlier this group of hormones acts, the earlier the puberal growth outburst sets in, but of course is earlier finished. The final stature, therefore, is lower in girls and among certain races of southern regions than in boys, who reach puberty later, and in most members of northern races.

Suite text page 364

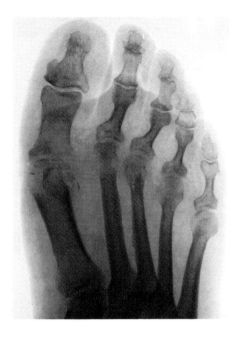

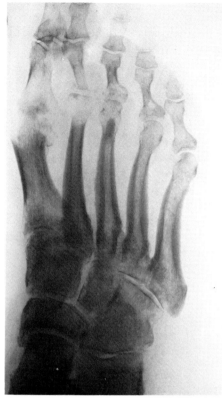

Fig. 306 a:
Focuses of *osteolysis* and destructions of all metatarsal and phalangeal joints, specially on the second ray (23. 7. 1977).

Fig. 306 b:
Advanced osteolysis of the metatarsal-phalangeal regions, spreading of osteomyelitis on the other tarsal bones (24. 10. 1977).

Chronic osteomyelitis (H. EICKSCHEN)
Anamnesis and course: E. W. born 30.3. 1894:
27-XI-76: strong, obese man of 82 years, with Adam-Stokes' syndrome. Complete AV block. R. R. 150/90, pulse 40, disturbances of peripherous blood circulation, acrocyanosis, foot pulse right cannot be confirmed. 5. XII. 76: fractures of 4 ribs owing to downfall, admitted to Bethesda Hospital, Mönchengladbach, from there moved to Düsseldorf clinics, heart pace-maker. 15. I. 77: relative well-being, RR 150/90, pulse 72. Hallus valgus right, hammer-toe, suppurative ulcer on this toe. Blood circulation still disturbed. Operation on hammer-toe. Exostosis chiseled away. 6. V. 77: patient is presented again, suppuration on right big toe, surgical area not healed, elimination of bone-splinters, pain,

walking impossible (fig. 306 a).
Admitted again after ambulatory treatment. Hospital surgeon recommended, after conservative treatment with absolute rest in bed for weeks, to amputate the right leg in the thigh. 1-VIII-77 to 13-IX-77: refusal of this suggestion, discharge from clinic, the patient was cared for in bed by his wife at home. Diagnosis: osteomyelitis in the area of right big toe (fig. 306 a, b).
Increased pain, extension of suppuration, a second fistulous opening with profuse suppuration is seen on sole at proximal phalanx of 3rd toe. Another fistula lateral on heel, with less suppuration. Increased inflammatory swelling of the foot, sharp pain. Placing on splints, daily dressings with diverse ointments, baths, highly dosed antibiotics, ampicillin, eusaprim, tetracyclin, and after tapping

362

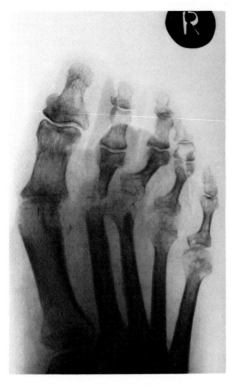

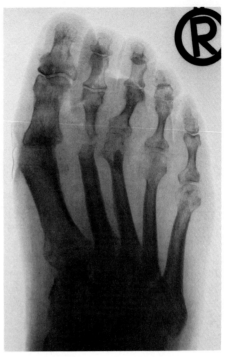

Fig. 306 c:
Beginning restructuring of the osteolysis areas, especially clear in metatarsal I; on the other metatarsals still many focuses of osteomyelitis (14.4.1978).

Fig. 306 d:
Restored bone-structure on the metatarsal I distal defective substance of the proximal phalanx II, extensive healing of the osteomyelitic focuses of osteolysis (4.8.1978).

the pus and test for sensitivity, adequate further treatment. No improvement, on the contrary, slow continued increase of findings. 27-X-77: roentgenographic examination (fig. 306 b). 23-XI-77: no change of findings, further daily changes of dressing, profuse suppuration, sharp pain.
Resistocell® fet. mesenchyme
First dose of 1 ampoule (100 mg of lyophilisate). Simultaneous cessation of all antibiotics, further changes of dressings, placing on splints, rest in bed, injection tolerated without local reaction.
21-XII-77: suppuration subsided considerably. Pain clearly diminished. The foot-relief seems to be restored. Edema and inflammatory secondary reactions subside.
23-I-78: Foot bears weight for the first time after a year. Patient ist out of bed. Suppuration stopped completely! Slight pain. 25-II-78: Resistocell® 2nd dose of 1 ampoule (100 mg of lyophilisate).
22-III-78: lasting improvement. Patient can walk, climb stairs, foot bears full weight. Suppuration dries up.
14-IV-78: roentgenological examination of right foot (fig. 306c): restructuring of osteolysis.
4-VIII-78: roentgenological control (fig. 306 d): extensive healing of osteomyelitic focuses.
Ater injected implantation of 100 mg of fet. mesenchyme (Resistocell®) decisive change of illness – after 1 year chronicity with progression. During the following months steady clinical improvement with reconstruction of skeletal lesions (fig. 306 d).

363

Physiologically, adrenal androgens promote the growth moderately, the skeletal development strongly; ovary oestrogens during adolescence do not promote the growth but favour obviously the skeletal development.

Hyperfunctions have more distinct aberrations: adrenal androgens accelerate much and usually finish earlier the growth and ossification when used for the adreno-genital syndrome; an overproduction of adrenal glucocorticoids inhibits growth, skeletal maturation and mineralization in the combination of Cushing's syndrome. Testicular androgens (e. g. Leydig cell tumour) accelerate growth and skeletal ripening more distinctly than increased ovary-oestrogens (granulosa cell tumour).

Hypofunctions of the adrenal-gonadic system work less intensely than hyperfunctions. Lack of adrenal steroids *(e. g. Morbus Addison)* influences the structure more than the skeletal ripening; slight retardations of skeletal ripening without influence on the growth of the stature may be caused during puberty by deficiencies of testicular androgens and ovarian oestrogens *(hypogonadism)*.

The gonads not only correlate with the adrenal glands but are influenced also by the hypothalamus-hypophysis system, its hormones and releasing factors. Gonadotropins, follicle-stimulating hormones and luteinising hormones are decisive. Before deciding on a therapeutic plan for special aspects, one should consider the interactions within the endocrine system as shown in the synoptic survey of fig. 282.

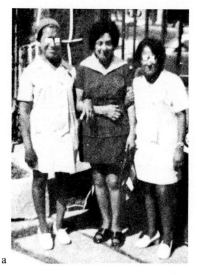
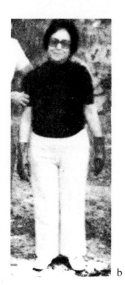
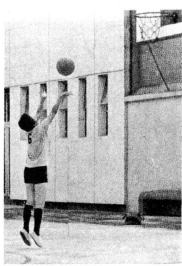
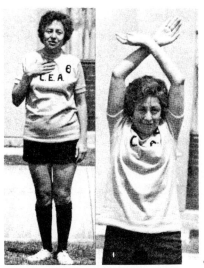

Fig. 307:
Chronic polyarthritis in a case of Lupus erythemadotes visc. (case F. Ramos ORTIZ, 1973).
The woman of 40 years falls ill of generalised articular swellings, fever, loss in weight (24 kg), can move only if supported by two persons (a). Hypercorticism after cortison treatment (b). The first cell-therapy is conducted after $1\frac{1}{2}$ year, causes an exacerbation of pain in the joints and fever, the second implantation follows half a year later and initiates a slow improvement and remobilization (c, d), which persists during a subsequent observation of 6 years.

Hematopoetic diseases

Bone-marrow and blood constitute an organic system, for which «cell therapy» is an excellent therapeutic method: *blood transfusions, transfusions of erythrocyte-concentrates, leukocytes, thrombocytes* belong to the standard treatments. In order to improve the tolerance and to reduce complications, the immunological criteria were refined in the course of the last decades. Another trend aimed at the differentiation i.e. attempts were made to substitute the lacking cellular ingredients of the blood by corresponding concentrates (e.g. erythrocyte-concentrates, thrombocyte-concentrates) without using also the «ballast substances» of the whole blood.

As blood and bone-marrow are not accessible to contact transplantations owing to their distribution over the whole body, implantations by injection (transfusion) have always been applied in these cases.

During the last 3 decades, impulses came chiefly from the radiation biology and from the therapy of systematized tumours.

Irradiation lesions

In thinking over the further perfection of the protective effects of *parabiosis* (BRECKER and CRONKITE, 1951), JACOBSON (1949–1952) protected various parts of the body during irradiation. When the spleen of a mouse was protected while its entire body was exposed to irradiation, the LD 50 increased from about 550 r to 1025 r. This protective effect was reached also by intraperitoneal injections of splenic tissue, and the spleen of new-born animals showed the greatest effect.

LORENZ (1951), relying on tests by REKERS (1948), maintained the idea that the protective effect was caused by a cellular mechanism. Mice treated with their whole bodies exposed to 900 r irradiation, got intraperitoneally or intravenously vital bone-marrow from long bones of untreated mice. The rate of survivors was 75%, the erythrocyte values did not decrease; islets of active hemopoetic tissue were found in the liver of the irradiated animals, and also in the Omentum maius after intraperitoneal injections. The protective effect was about equal with isologous and homologous tissues, and weaker with heterologous tissues.

The statistical significance for the survival of the donor cells in the recipient organism was established by extensive tests (FORD, 1956). Mice of the strain CBA (recipient) showed, three weeks after 950 r complete irradiation and transplantation of bone-marrow from mice of strain T 6, the chromosomal characteristics of T 6. When bone-marrow of rats was transmitted, is got a little touched. From this, the term *«irradiation chimera»* was derived. (The chimera is a fabulous being in Greek mythology, consisting of a goat's body, with a lion's head and a serpent's tail.)

The results certified repeatedly thereafter have proved that after the elimination of immunoresistance foreign cells can survive and function in the organism. The donor cells effect a «colonisation» and repopulation of the bone-marrow. If the recipient's immunity is not quite eliminated, mutual immunological reactions may come on. A variant with the clinical symptoms of autoaggression is the *Runt-disease* (runt = dwarf cattle); this term is to express the stunted growth in connection with changes of the skin and mucosa, diarrhea and disturbed absorption.

Generally, the following alternatives are given:
1. Complete and lasting substitution of the recipient's bone-marrow by the donor's bone-marrow.
2. The implanted bone-marrow disappears gradually and is just as promptly substituted by the recipient's regenerating bone-marrow.
3. Hematopoetic tissue of the donor and recipient coexist so that an irradiation chimera originates. The formation of a chimera can proceed to such an extent that a kind of cells (e. g. granulocytes) originates from the donor, another one (e. g. erythrocytes) from the recipient.

After the practical use of fetal cells by Paul NIEHANS and others between 1931 and 1960, FEREBEE (1957, 1958) tried to avoid the immunological problems by using fetal tissues. UPHOFF (1958) tried to achieve this with undifferentiated lymphatic tissues.

The first case of application to man was the involuntary experiment by the nuclear research centre of VINCA (1958). An accident in the nuclear reactor affected 6 persons, 4 of them with a lethal dose of 700–1000 r, one with a supralethal dose between 1000 and 1200 r, and the 6th with a sublethal dose of 300–500 r. These persons were taken the next day by air to the hospital of the Curie-Foundation, Paris, and treated (JAMMET, MATHE, SALMON, 1959).

The clinical course showed 3 phases:
1. In the *initial shock phase*, which began 1 hour after the accident and persisted for the first day, there was a general alarm symptom with adynamia, vomiting, paraesthesia and profuse perspiration. The experimentator who had got a supralethal dose, suffered moreover from diarrhea.

2. A *latency period* followed and lasted 2–3 weeks. The general conditions were not too bad, but the affected persons showed loss of weight, general debilitation and disposition to profuse perspiration, sleeplessness and splitting headache. The disorders were seen also in the blood-count, skin and intestinal tract. The person who had got a supralethal dose suffered from attacks of fever on the 14th and 15th days.

3. The *crisis* lasted from the 4th to 7th week, with serious general collapses of health and diffuse drowsiness, decreasing diuresis, anorexia, very serious nausea, profuse perspiration. Only the person who had got a sublethal dose of 300–500 r did not show these symptoms. In that period, the patients had moreover marked conjunctivitis, dry and cracked skin as from the 20th day, and lost nearly all of their hair, including the beard as far as they were male. The patient who had got the supralethal dose died on the 32nd day, after invaginations, ileus and anuria.

The blood-count showed the following changes: Immediately after the irradiation, leukocytosis of 9000–11 000 leukocytes/mm^3 with lymphopenia developed. The various kinds of blood-cells decreased gradually during the latency period. Affected first were the lymphocytes. The myelogram showed a bone-marrow atrophy, which changed into a bone-aplasia at the beginning of the 7th week. Connected therewith were gingival bleedings, hemorrhages from the nasal mucosa, stomach and intestine. After

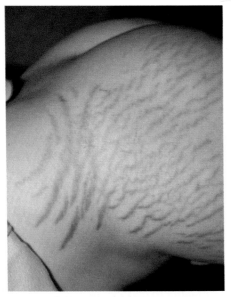

Fig. 308

Panmyelopathy; hypercorticism

The 12 8/12-year-old boy suffering from thrombocytopenia had been treated with 100 mg of urbason for 6 months. He developed more-over anemia, leukopenia, granulocytopenia and serious hypercorticism with Cushing's face and extensive striae.

When 60 mg of adrenal gland (male), 75 mg of spleen and 150 mg of liver-lyophilisate were implanted, the blood-count was as follows:

Hb 8.4 (52%), Ery 2.75, HbE 30.5, leukocytes 1700; segmented 24%, lymphocytes 69%, monocytes 7%.

The following day already, the granulocytes make 45%, on the second day 49%, and 68% on the 5th day. The changed numbers of the thrombocytes, leukocytes and erythrocytes seen in the following months appear from the diagram fig. 298 hereafter. Distinctive of the therapeutic outcome is the rapid response of the myeloic series, followed by the retarded reaction of the thrombocyte apparatus though weeks after the erythropoesis.

The hypercorticism decreases within a few weeks.

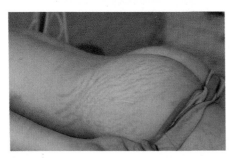

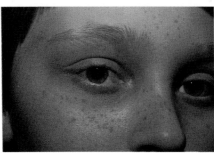

Fig. 309:

Pancytopathy of Fanconi-type with severe anemia and steady nose-bleedings since the 5th year of life. Till the age of 13 40 bloodtransfusions were necessary, when the hemoglobin dropped down to a level between 2.7–3.5 g%. Admission to the hospital with following values: hemoglobin 5.1 g%, erythrocytes 1600,000, white blood cells 2700; 19% granulocytes, 80% lymphocytes, 1% monocytes; sedimentation rate 56/100. The Panmyelocytopathy includes anemia, leukopenia, granulocytopenia and thrombocytopenia. 6 month after implantation of 75 mg fetal spleen-, 75 mg fet. bone marrow- and 150 mg fet. liver-lyophilisate no further blood-
◄ transfusion was necessary.

Schwarz

bridging the critical phase with small blood-transfusions, first hematopoetic fetal tissue from the liver of a human fetus was implanted by injection. The number of cells was about 4,2 × 10⁹ fetal liver cells. The effect was obviously small so that the next therapeutic measure was injections of adult bone-marrow cells from donors of similar blood-groups. The bone-marrow was taken from the sternum and injected intravenously. Transfused were 180–300 cm³ of

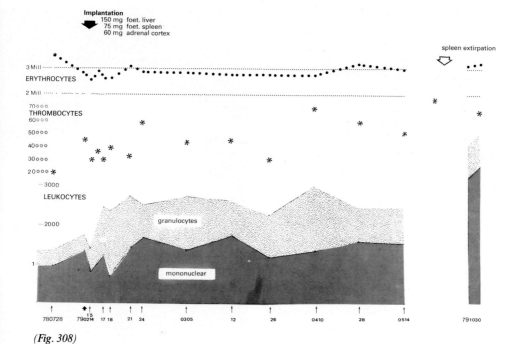

(Fig. 308)

bone-marrow, the number of the cells came to about $8{,}5–14 \times 10^9$. After a short transfusion shock, the general conditions of the moribund patients improved. The sensorium came back, dynamics, appetite and increase in weight showed recoveries.

Under the special conditions of the elimination of immunity, implanted tissues of bone-marrow seem to take the functions in the recipient's organism till the own bone-marrow is active again. As the erythrocytes and the cells of the myeloic series as well as the thrombocytes recovered after the implantation of bone-marrow though they were not transfused direct, a general colonization can be presumed.

Implantation by injecting hematopoetic tissues in leukemia and systematisized blood-deseases

The second column of our knowledge of the effect of implantations by injecting hematopoetic tissues is constituted by the experience in the field of systematisized tumours and disorders of the apparatus of blood formation. The fundamental tests will be described in detail hereafter.

Effects and specific effects of various tissular lyophilisates on aberrations of the leukemic blood-count

Objects of trials for a possible therapeutic effect on cell suspensions on leukemic aberrations were AK-mice, which have been bred at the Dr. FURTH-laboratory, New York, since 1928. In question

369

is an inbreeding strain of animals, which shows a high rate of leukosis in their 6th–9th months of age. Extensive observations corresponded to the classical aspect described by other research workers (LEVEVRE, HOGREFFE, PEDERSEN and others); examinations of blood, marrow and tissues, however, can only demonstrate a marked «myeloic reaction», which has just a faint resemblance to human leukosis (W. SCHUSTER, H. SCHUSTER, 1954–1957).

The progenies of our strain bred from two braces sickened spontaneously with a high frequency (70–90%) in the 6th–8th months of age with this «myeloic reaction» and died within 4–8 weeks of a uniform aspect, which takes a course much like leukosis in children.

This hereditary disease occurring at the same age and in the same form can be outlined as follows:

Whilst these vital white mice thrive well in the beginning, their coat becomes dry and rough and turns yellowish, they shed hair in the course of the 5th or 6th months of age (fig. 311); 2–3 weeks later, the animals have no appetite, they become weary. Finally, the hair falls out entirely in the area of the snout and in the anal-genital region (fig. 312), thick infiltrates grow into the size of hazel-nuts, and colliquate, disintegrate, discharge pus, become incrusted. The tail shows knot-shaped thickenings, which ulcerate seldom.

In the blood count, the numbers of leukocytes increase by 2–5 times, the juvenile and segmentary granulocytes as well as immature myeloic forms augment whereas the lymphocytes (which make 60–80% of all white blood-cells in healthy white mice) decrease relatively or absolutely. These changes in the white blood-count proceed with a progressive anaemia, the blood grows thin, shows a lighter colour; bleedings can often hard-

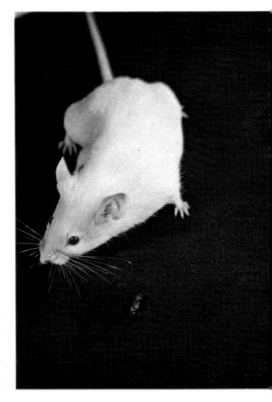

Fig. 310:
AK-mouse without manifestations of illness.

ly be stopped in the advanced stage. The condition of the animals worsens very rapidly, and they die of general cachexia within 4–8 weeks after the onset of the first symptoms. Autopsy reveals enlargements of liver, spleen and lymph-nodes in most cases. Liver and spleen are soft, fragile, show stained patterns and are difficult to separate from their physiological concrescences with neighbouring organs as they are easily injured. Histologically, attention is attracted by cell infiltrations and amyloid incorporations.

This hereditary aspect manifesting itself at a relatively constant age and accompanied by changes of the blood-count was used to examine the following questions:

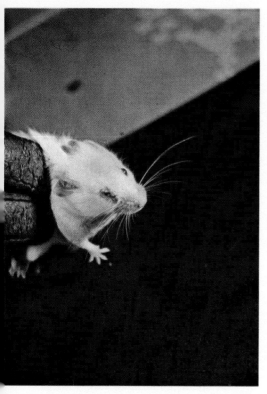

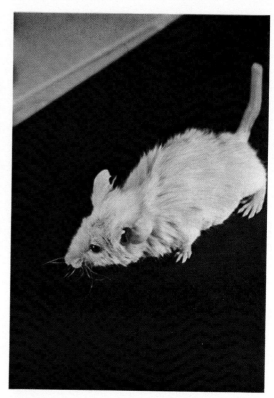

Fig. 311:
AK-mouse with beginning diagnostical symptoms. Shedding of hair and ulceration on snout, eyes and ear.

Fig. 312:
Florid pathological manifestations without leukaemoid changes of blood-count in a 7-month-old AK-mouse.

1. Can the progressive disturbances of the blood-count and general disorders be influenced by cellular suspensions?
2. If so, have the kinds of cells used equivalent effects?
3. Is the effect temporary or lasting?
4. What side-effects do occur after intraperitoneal administration of the cell suspensions?

These questions are examined in four test-groups.

In the *first group* consisting of seven test series on various cubes, heterogeneous dry-cell preparations of various mesenchymal organs (spleen, liver, bone-marrow, thymus) were used.

In the *second group* consisting of four test series, homogeneous, fresh fetal cell-suspensions (whole and organic suspensions) of a strain of healthy albino mices were studied.

The *third group* comprised four control series; in one of them, the effect of dry cells of bone-marrow on healthy mice was investigated, while in two more series some protein substances (sera) were used to find out whether the results observed constitute non-specific protein effects or not.

In a *fourth series* treated with dry brain cells, the question was whether also ectodermal tissues can influence the blood-count.

371

Another *test group* consisting of four test series was to clarify the question concerning the effect of cell suspensions of sick animals of the same strain.

The four test groups therefore comprise 19 test series. A total of 313 animals was tested, 250 of them AK-mice, 63 were healthy white mice. 63 AK-mice were used as controls in the test series, each comprised 4–20 animals according to the litters; mostly one litter was used, sometimes two.

First, however, 30 healthy mice had to be examined to know the numbers of leukocytes and the differential blood-count. It appeared that the results vary considerably according to how the blood is taken. The ends of the tails were cut off by scissors and the blood was taken from the stump. The results differed even if the tails, to promote the bleeding, were put into warm water before they were cut. Moreover, the numbers of cells were influenced by pressing and squeezing the stumps, which was probably accounted for by the tissue fluid. It was also worth mentioning that the readings of blood taken from the heart of a killed animal were by up to 100% lower than in the blood of its tail.

To obtain comparable results, it was necessary to apply always the same method. It appeared favourable to give the animals a slight etherization before their tails were cut. The resulting relaxation permitted to obtain blood without squeezing and pressing the stump. The numbers of leukocytes were counted in the Thomas' chamber, the blood-smears were uniformly stained after PAPPEN-HEIM. Blood-smears had to be prepared in preliminary tests also from considerable numbers of sick animals to coordinate the sometimes not easy classification of pathological cells in the test series. To prepare the suspension of dry cells, the cellular substance was dissolved in Ringer's solution; to prepare the suspensions of fetal cells, pregnant animals were killed immediately before the bearing, their abdominal cavities were opened and the embryos taken sterile from the uterus; then the embryos in toto or only certain organs were reduced to small pieces with scissors and ground into a pulp in a mortar. The pulp was diluted with Ringer's solution and made into a suspension, then filtered through sterile gauze.

All cellular suspensions and test substances (sera) were injected intraperitoneally. The quantity of suspension was $0,4–1,0 \, cm^3$ uniformly within the series.

Blood examinations were performed before every injection in all test series, but were restricted to counting and differentiating the white blood cells. The first control followed three days after the injection. Further controls were performed not before long intervals (3–4 weeks) because too frequent takings even of small amounts of blood alone would have provoked considerable anaemia. The animals experimented upon were observed permanently and the times of survival were exactly recorded.

Results

Relying on the theoretical premises that gave occasion to the tests, namely the transmission of the biological potencies of fetal tissues to an insufficient system of blood-formation, we get the following results:

Mesenchymal tissues exert, at different degrees, a concrete, often deep, influence on the blood-count and on the disease of obviously ill AK-mice.

Within three days after the intraperitoneal injection, the numbers of leukocytes decrease to a maximum of more than 80% of the initial values. The differential blood-count is moved towards a normalization (fig. 317), the granulocytes, juvenile and early forms of the myeloic series, are reduced by about 30–40%, the lymphocytes augment relatively, often also absolutely. While the blood-count changes, the general conditions improve, the animals eat more, become more vital, their coats grow thicker and brighter, the formations of nodes

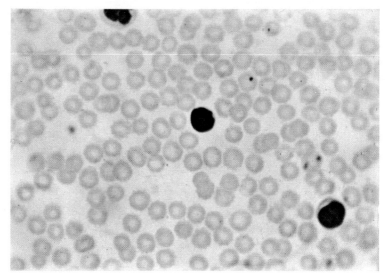

Fig. 313:
Blood smears of AK-mice without diagnostical symptoms. Small quantities of cells, chiefly lymphocytes.

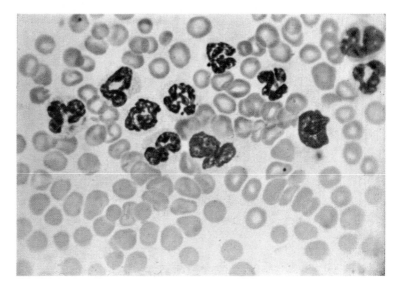

Fig. 314:
Blood-smears of AK-mice at the maximum of the leukaemoid blood-count aberrations. Considerable augmentation of cells. Atypical juvenile forms of the granulocytary series prevail. Scarce numbers of atypical monocytoids.

373

and ulcers are stopped or even decrease.

The average duration of life of animals treated with effective cell suspensions exceeds by about two months that of the untreated young or of the non-injected controls of the same litter. *Anaphylactic reactions were observed only after injections of sera.*

The different effects of the mesenchymal tissues on the numbers of cells appear from fig. 315. Fig. 316 compares the control series (brain substance, serum) with the effect of splenic suspensions. The different numbers of cases in the various series results from the use of litters, in order to guarantee the homogeneity of the material. Of special interest and theoretically hardly explainable is the observation that after injections of effective cell suspensions the numbers of cells were «normalized», irrespective of how high they were before. The considerably different results of injections of fetal «bone marrow» were explained later: the tissue was coarse osteoid splinters without any functioning bone-marrow.

Changes of the blood count and the influence on the general condition are passing phenomena, which persist 4–8 weeks after an injection, 6 weeks on an average. The effect is reproduceable though subsequent doses of cells seem to exert a less lasting influence on the general condition.

The basic idea that the biological potencies of fetal tissues could be transmitted to animals, turned out to be correct, but the result meant a disappointing restriction of the practical therapeutic consequences.

It appears that the affected organism utilizes temporarily the biological potencies of healthy tissues but after consuming them continues the specific course of its disease at least in tumorous processes.

Limited though the results respecting the initial questions were, yet they enlightened considerably the effect of injected cells:

1. The effect of injected cells as ascertained by our tests is caused by an *induction* but does not provide *lasting*

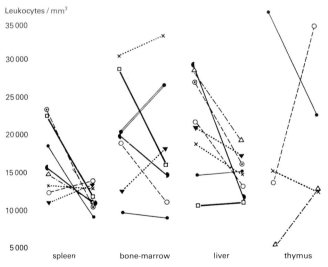

Fig. 315:
Different effects of various mesenchymal tissues on the cells of AK-mice of the same litter 3 days after intraperitoneal tissue-injection.

374

regeneration. Experiments on animals, therefore, have substantiated what clinical experience with the usual therapeutic fresh-cell methods (blood-transfusions, concentrates of leukocytes, transplantations of bone-marrow, implantations of hypophysis) foreshadowed.

2. The effect of injected cells is *specific*, does not rest upon a non-specific effect of protein. No effects are seen on cell-free protein carriers.

3. The effect of injected cells and tissues depends on germ-layer-dependant, and its extent is even *organ-specific*. Whereas the tested mesenchymal tissues provoked without exception the described changes of the blood-count, the latter were not seen after injections of ektodermal tissues. The effect of the mesenchymal tissues, however, is not equivalent. In our tests the changes of the blood-count were most distinct and constant after injections of spleen and liver, less constant after doses of bone-marrow and thymus.

4. The specific effect of the homogeneous and heterogeneous tissues cannot be obtained by homogeneous fetal general suspensions. In certain cases, the injections of particularisized feti of a healthy strain of mice, especially of the AK-strain, worsened the blood-findings.

These long-term tests

a) demonstrated the different specific effect of suspensions of heterologous and homologous tissues,

b) showed the temporary influence of leukaemia-like changes of the blood-count,

c) revealed no criteria for the antigenicity of heterologous fetal cells whereas homogeneous homologous tissues of adult animals provoked repeatedly shock symptoms.

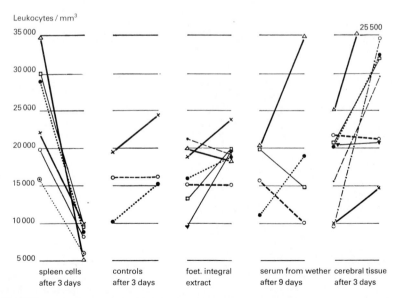

Leukocytes / mm³

Fig. 316:
Controls of specific effects (e. g. splenic cells) with heterogenous sera and fet. integral extracts of healthy strains of mice as well as ectodermal tissues. Numbers of cells 3 days after injection.

Transplantations of bone-marrow

Relying on the ideas of Dessauer's «X-ray bath», several test series were conducted between 1950 and 1970 to study the experimental and clinical possibilities of this method. FEREBEE (1958) tried for leukemia to eliminate the immunological resistance by intense irradiation and to implant bone-marrow. FEREBEE was moreover the first to use human hematopoetic tissue of feti 16–28 weeks old. The use of xenogenous fetal cells of liver and bone-marrow was the subject of a first publication by NIEHANS (1952). SCOTT, MATHIAS and others (1961) obtained by intravenous injections of fetal hematopoetic cells different results in 14 cases of anemia. These intravenous injections of suspensions of fetal cells were tolerated without complication, also if they were repeated. Used was freshly taken and immediately transmitted tissue of liver, and a permanent remission was obtained in two cases of chronic pancytemia. The expectations set in implantations of bone-marrow after irradiation in treatments of human leukemia (THOMAS 1957, FEREBEE 1958, KURNIK 1958, MATHE 1959) were not answered, though impressive temporary remissions were reached. WITTE (1961) took a similar way in acute leukemia by using first high doses of cytostatics and treating the resulting immuno-depression by subsequent transfusions of bone-marrow. According to his reports, 4 of 18 cases had a complete remission for up to 21 months, 4 cases of partial remission for 5–12 weeks. This experience corresponds to 4 cases of infantile leukosis treated by the author, which after intra-peritoneal injection of fetal liver and spleen showed remissions for up to 2 months. FLEISCHHACKER and STACHER (1960) saw also in leukosis treated cyto-statically with granulocytosis and thrombocytopenia complete remissions after transmitting bone-marrow of the same group.

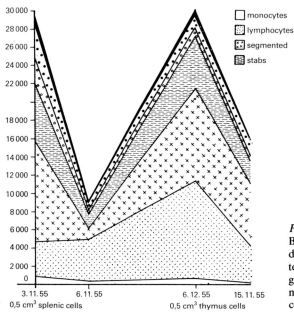

Legend:
□ monocytes ▦ juvenile forms
▦ lymphocytes ▦ myeloblasts
▦ segmented ■ mitosis
▦ stabs

3.11.55   6.11.55   6.12.55   15.11.55
0,5 cm³ splenic cells   0,5 cm³ thymus cells

Fig. 317:
Blood-counts (numbers of cells and differential blood-count) changed after injection of freeze-dried heterologous tissues. Decrease of cells, normalization of differential blood-count.

376

Relying on observations of transplantations of marrow after reactor-accidents, encouraged by experiments on animals in the 1960s, 203 transplantations on man were conducted by 1977 according to a statement by H. J. KOLB, but only 3 had a positive outcome. The insufficient immunosuppressive preliminary treatment was regarded as an essential reason for the failure of the transplants. The following methods were recommended: preliminary treatment of the recipient with 1000 rd complete irradiation and cytostatic chemotherapy in leukemia, and with 200 mg per kg of cyclophosphamide in bone-marrow aplasia. To avoid the secondary disease: methotrexate ($10 mg/m^2$ day on the 1st, 3rd, 6th and 11th days, then weekly till the 102 nd day), cyclophosphamide; the secondary treatment proper i. e. the settlement between the cells of the donor and recipient, should be effected with antithymocyte serum (7 mg per kg of IgG every 2nd day for 20 days). In bone-marrow aplasia, the mortality comes in this series to 70–90 %. A HLA-identical MLC-negative brother or sister must be available, the significance of bone-marrow aplasia must be established histologically.

G. F. WÜNDISCH (1977) reported on the successful transplantation of bone-marrow in a boy of 8 years with serious panmyelopathy, who had survived 22 months by the time of publication.

The present state of the questions connected with implantations of bone-marrow is described in two publications by NIETHAMMER, BIENZLE, KLEIHAUER (1977) and BHADURI et al. (1980).

After the first attempts to influence immunodefects by transplantations of bone-marrow between 1950 and 1970, this indication has meanwhile been extended to include aplastic anemia (panmyelopathia). Bone-marrow is taken from the crest of ilium of the anaesthetized donor by 100 and more aspirations, and treated with heparin to keep it from clotting. To dilute the bone-marrow it is filtered through sieves of various sizes, then the cell suspension is infused intravenously. Needed are about 1,5 times 10^8 nucleated cells per kg of body-weight of the recipient. In immunodefects this number is by 1–2 tenth powers lower than in aplastic anaemia. The risk of narcosis and a potential osteomyelitis are believed to be the only dangers to the donor. The risks to the recipient is microembolism, proceeding in part with dyspnoea, fever and chills. The main problems for the recipient are thought to be the following risks:

1. The toxicity of the high doses of cytostatics or irradiation during the conditioning.
2. Extreme predisposition to infection after the beginning of conditioning and in the first three months after the transplantation. The prevailing causes of death are interstitial pneumonia and pneumonia through Pneumocytis carinii on cytomegaly viruses as well as sepsis provoked by bacteria or candida.

Owing to this risk of infection, the patients must be isolated. The following is a list of indications for transplantations of bone-marrow:

1. *Combined immunodefects* (fig. 205);
2. *Aplastic anaemia* (fig. 309);
3. *Innate abnormalities of haemoglobin* with bad prognosis (fig. 318);
4. *Serious granulocyte defects* (e. g. infantile chronic granulomatosis);
5. *Leukemia* resistant to every therapy with cystostatics. BHADURI et al (1980) think transplantations of bone-marrow in serious aplastic anaemia the therapy of choice and

Suite see page 382

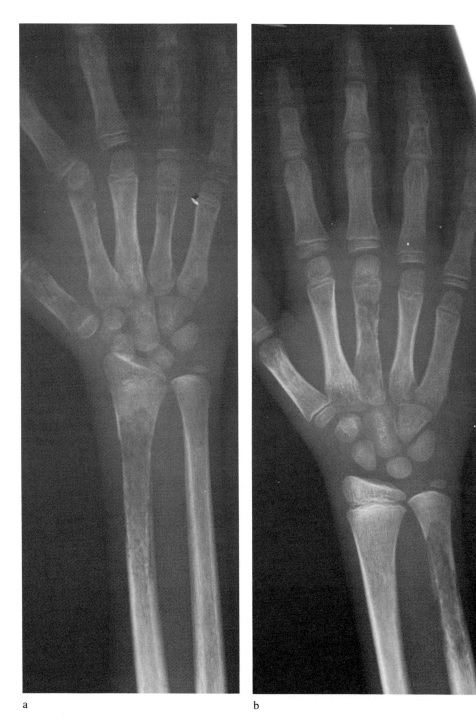

a   b

Fig. 318:
Sickle-cell anaemia; generalized osteomyelitis

378

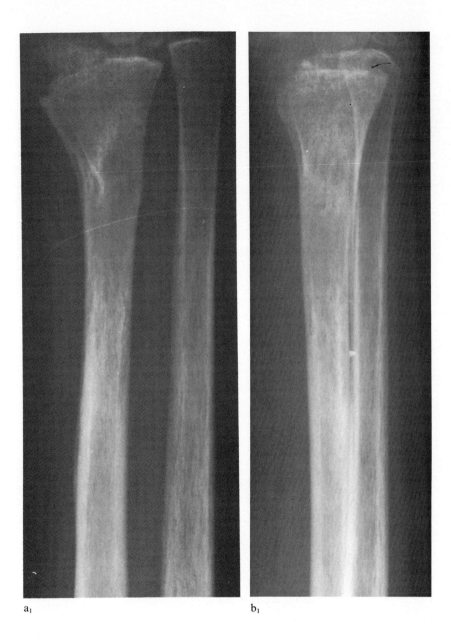

a₁   b₁

The 10-year-old Turkish boy had already been at several hospitals when he was admitted seriously ill in a cachectical condition; septic temperature, general icterus, many osteomyelitic fistulous wounds on all extremities. No normal adult haemoglobin.

HBS 89.5 %, the rest for HbF and HB A₂.

HBS in father 29.8 %, in mother 29.4 %.

Serious anaemia: Hb 4.8 (29 %), Ery 1.76 mill; reticulocytes 114 %. The suppurative fistulae had been

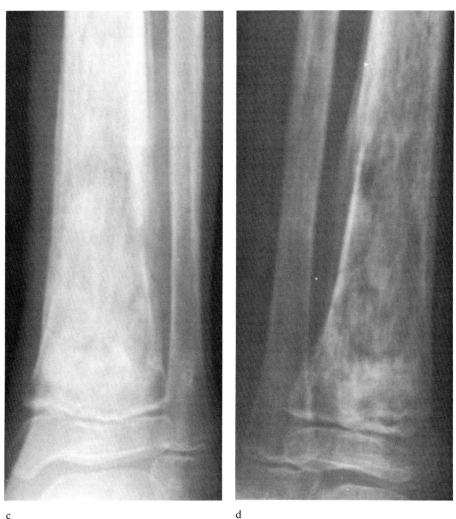

c   d

caused by extensive osteomyelitic focuses in the long hollow bones (a, b, c, d). Antiphlogistics, antibiotics and blood-transfusions had no influence on the septic temperatures. After two weeks of treatment as described, implantations of xenogenous tissues, fet. spleen (75 mg) and bone-marrow (100 mg). The fever declines within 3 days and the osteomyelitic focuses persisting for months heal gradually (a 1, b 1, c 1, d 1). Spleen and bone-marrow were implanted 3 × in all at intervalls of 4 weeks; additional treatment with vitamin-trace element-combinations.

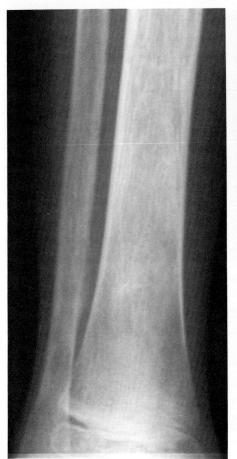

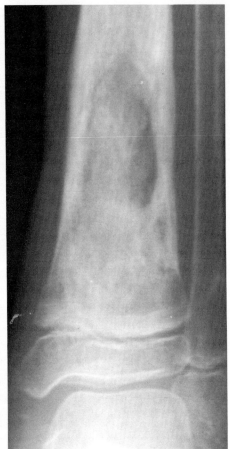

c₁

d₁

Tab. 52: **Results of bone-marrow transplantation in panmyelopathia**
(after Bhaduri et al.)

centre	number of patients	number of survivors	death by discharge	GVHR	infection	other cause
Seattle	110	50	27	22	10	1
Internat. Aplast. An. Study Group ACS/NIH	47	27	12	–	–	–
Marrow Transplant Reg.	38	18	13	3	4	
UCLA	20	7				
Leiden	19	9	3	3	3	2
Baltimore	22	7	10	2	3	1
Paris	25	9	13	3	0	0

Tab. 53: **Results of bone-marrow transplantation in acute leukaemia**

centre	number of patients	number of survivors	death by discharge	GVHR	infection	other cause
Seattle	120	16	1	44	19 (34 recurrences)	6
UCLA	33	5	0	1	22 (3 recurrences)	2
Results of bone-marrow transplantation in the remission						
Seattle	42	50–60%				
Duarte	15	ca. 70%				

saw longer times of survival than in patients treated with «customary methods». Transplantations of bone-marrow, however, should not be considered as a last alternative because a sensitization of the body by many preceding blood transfusions must be avoided. According to this statement, the results of bone-marrow transplantation in acute leukemia are better if the transplantation is effected during the remissions. The results obtained so far in the trans-plantation centres of the world have been compiled by Bhaduri et al. The figures and rates of survival in panmyelopathia and acute leukemia appear from Tab. 52, 53.

6. Panmyelopathy (fig. 308, 309).

The practical and clinical experience with the use of lyophilised xenogenous tissues are not extensive as only individual cases were published or reported verbally. Informative observations are represented in fig. 213, 308, 309, 318.

Tumour therapy

The collective name *«cancer»* comprehends the formations of new tissue threatening with autonomous growth the functions and existence of the organism in which they develop. These new formations are found in all living species including the plants (fig. 319, 320) but seem to be most frequent of all in long-lived and highly differentiated multicellular creatures. This may be the reason why cancer is the most frequent disease in man and the second most frequent cause of death behind the cardiac and circulatory diseases.

Biologically intact associations of cells integrate into an association of tissue or an organ by self-guidance and self-control of their growth i. e. they arrest their growth where they meet with neighbouring structures. The cancerous tissue has lost this self-control, does not stop its growth at areas of contact, continues expanding and infiltrating and thus forms a complex of tissue i. e. a tumour outside the functional laws of the organism. The concept of *«tumour»* is largely used as a synonym for *«cancer»* even though is does not strictly correspond. The *«malignity»* results from the parasitical character (consumption and withdrawal of foodstuffs at the expense of the economic requirements of the host),

Tab. 54:

Frequency of cancer with separation of the organs expressed as percentages in men and women, according to the US American Cancer Society:

Affections

Men		Women
23%	skin	13%
3%	oral space	2%
	breast	23%
19%	lungs	5%
11%	colon	13%
9%	other digestive organs	7%
11%	prostate	
	uterus	14%
6%	urinary organs	3%
7%	leukaemia and lymphoma . .	6%
11%	all others	14%

Table 55:

Frequency of cancer with separation of the organs expressed as percentages in men and women, according to the US American Cancer Society:

Causes of death

Men		Women
2%	skin	1%
3%	oral space	1%
	breast	21%
30%	lungs	9%
12%	colon	15%
15%	other digestive organs	13%
9%	prostate	
	uterus	7%
6%	urinary organs	3%
10%	leukaemia and lymphoma . .	10%
13%	all others	20%

on the one hand, and from the stubbornness of the growth against sound neighbouring tissues, on the other hand.

Frequency

The increase of life-expectancy and the changes of the human biological environment have for consequence that in the highly mechanized, densely populated industrial countries every 6th–8th individual nowadays suffers from cancer. The frequency of the cases (tab. 52, 53) differs from the pattern of the causes of death by cancer, according to the percentages worked out in the USA (MAUGH, Th. N. and MARX, J. L., 1979).

Forms

From the more than 100 diagnostically differentiated kinds of cancer, actually 3 main groups can be abstracted namely the mesenchymal, epithelial and mixed tumours. With the mesenchymal tumours subdivided by the degree of maturity and by clinical viewpoints, the following grouping results:

1. Mesenchymal tumours
   a) sarcoma
   b) lymphoma
   c) leukemia
2. Epithelial tumours
3. Mixed tumours

Sarcomata originate from derivatives of the mesoderm (bones, cartilage, connective tissue, vessels, muscles), form solid, rapidly growing and, therefore, very malign tumours; they occur frequently in young persons. The rate of their frequency among cancerous diseases comes to somewhat below 2%.

Malign lymphomata originate from the thymo-lymphatic tissue. Undifferentiated lymphocytes of the thymus, spleen and peripheral lymph-nodes proliferate locally into complexes; an increased volume of the affected organs and an impaired function characterize the clinical symptoms. *Lymphogranulomatosis (Hodgkin's disease)* is the most important of the subgroups. Malign lymphomata make 5% to 6% in general cancer statistics.

In *leukemia*, unripe white bloodcells from the bone-marrow are washed out. The total quantity in the peripheral blood can, but need not, be increased. The ripening can be arrested in the phase of the mother cells or myeloblasts as in leukosis of childhood with an increase of the mononuclear prophases (leukemia of the mother cells, myeloblasts, micromyeloblasts) or in the prophases of the myeloic-granulocytary series with proliferation of the promyelocytes, my-

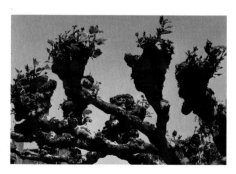 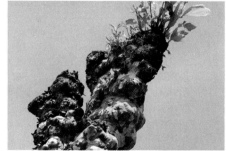

Fig. 319, 320:
Tumorous degenerations of trees (plane-trees); their biological development is prevented by continuous trimming.

384

elocytes and metamyelocytes. The unchecked proliferation of the unripe prophases of the one system suppresses the other systems.

Of the 655 000 cases of neoplasm diagnosed on an average every year in the USA (MAUGH and MARX, 1979), 3%–4% come under leukemia. Among the tumours of childhood, leukemia makes with 25% the largest group, followed by the tumours of the central nervous system.

Carcinoma (cancer in strictly sense) develops from epithelial tissue of the outer and inner limiting surfaces of the body. Starting points are the skin, mucosae of the respiratory, intestinal and urogenital tracts incl. their glands. Tumours of the central nervous system belong to this group as far as of ektodermal origin. About 85% of the human tumours are carcinoma, and the higher age-groups are more affected than the young.

Mixed tumours make a group of about 4% of the total. *Embryonic mixed tumours*, tumours of ovaries and testicles belong to them.

Principle of pathogenicity

Malign tumours have 4 common properties:

1. *Disproportion between the nucleus and cytoplasm;*
2. *Unchecked and uncontrolled growth;*
3. *Disdifferentiation in the sense of a formal arrest in prophases of cell maturation*
4. *Formation of metastasis.*

The disproportion between the nucleus and cellular body probably constitues the decisive fundamental principle of the cancer cells. The flow of energy and biochemical regulations depend on a harmonic coordination between the nucleus and cytoplasma organelles.

With the *«genetic space» (nucleus)* growing in proportion to the *«economic space»* of the cell (space between the cytoplasma membrane and nuclear membrane including the organelles) the ecologic harmony of the cell is lost. This misguidance is probably double-countertracked: the nucleus conveys its information wrongly coded (fig. 321) or not at all via the nucleolus to the centrioles and ribosomes. The centrioles lose the mechanism controlling the cell-division, the ribosomes can no longer form specific proteins integrable into the body. As all cell organelles depend on the information of the nucleus, the economic space of the cell can no longer exert its function of providing the cell with the substances and products of synthesis necessary for the correction of the false development. The accumulation of genetic material (DNA), which cannot be converted reasonably into structures (RNA-proteins), compels the centrioles to follow a dividing strategy as the comparatively small space of cytoplasm threatens the existence of the nucleus because the latter is inadequately supplied. The unchecked growth of formations that cannot be integrated into the systemic ecology is the fundamental principle of the malignity of the cell. The malignity of the boundless growth, which, unintegrable, does not stop before the physiological structures, is due to this mechanism.

The unchecked, uncontrolled in the sense of the systemic function, growth is accounted for by the loss of the ability to arrest the growth when getting into touch with neighbouring cells. On principle, primitive embryonic properties are redeveloped. The mesenchyme (from Greek «enchein» – to fill in) fills by rapid growth during the embryonic period the spaces between the endoderm and ektoderm, thus achieving virtually the form of a mammal organism. But whereas here the interplay between the mesenchymal dynamics and the ektodermal control works, this control mechanism no longer exists beyond the embryonic period.

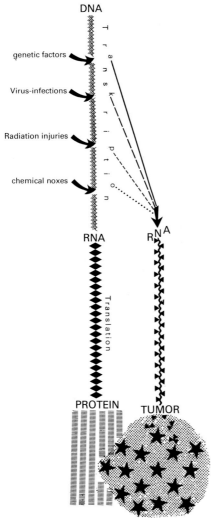

Fig. 321:
Theory of tumour genesis. Various noxae can change the transcription of the DNA so that with an abnormally coded RNA necessarily a protein differing from the autogenous structural law i. e. not integrable protein will develop. The ripening of the affected tissular formations may come to rest at any phase of development (= unripe tissues).

The term *«disdifferentiation»* is derived from the fundamental idea of a regression into embryonic prophases. For the pathobiological and therapeutic problems of malign tumours it would probably be more expedient to suppose a disturbance of ripening rather than a regression.

A further consequence of the uncontrolled growth is the formation of metastasis i. e. the property of malign tissues to form colonies in other regions of the body not immediately connected with the tumour.

Etiology

Without entering into particulars of etiological problems, it should be stated that 4 groups of causes are discussed for the origin of cancer because narrow connections between these noxae and cancer can be taken for granted.

1. *Genetic causes,* due to the accumulation of tumours and special kinds of tumour over generations of a family.

2. *Radiation genesis,* proved by the radiation cancer in the X-ray pioneers, the accumulation of leukemia after explosions of atomic bombs, the increased disposition to cutaneous cancer as a result of excessive exposure to natural radiation (cutaneous cancer of farmers) or radioactivity in the mining industry («Schneeberger's lung-cancer»).

3. *Chemical carcinogenesis.* Of the nearly 1000 compounds capable of producing cancer both in vitro or in man, some are of special importance as part of the natural environments. They provoke chiefly carcinoma of the outer (skin), still more of the inner contact (lung, nasal cavity) or excretory (bladder) surfaces. The most important substances belonging here are (MILLER, E. C., 1972):

386

soot, smoke of cigarettes, tars, mineral oils; 2-naphtylamin, 4-aminodiphenyl, benzidine, N-N-Bis (2-chlorethyl)-2-naphtylamin, Bis (2-chlorethyl) sulphide compounds of nickel and chrome, asbestoses.

The carcinogenetic substance used most frequently in experiments on animals is benzpyren.

4. *Viral carcinogenesis.* Two arguments have prevented any serious discussion of virus genesis for decades. Viruses normally lead to a specific immunity, not to a tumour; on the other hand, tumours are not infectious, as one should expect from a viral genesis.

Of the DNA viruses, adeno-, papova, SV40-, polyama viruses can provoke tumours in experimental animals and transform cells in the culture. But a connection with human cancer has been proved so far neither here nor for the herpes viruses (RAPP, F., 1974; TODARO, G. J., and HUEBNER, R. J., HUEBNER, R. J., 1972). The strongest indications are those for the *Epstein-Barr-virus,* which is said to account for the existence of the *Burkitt lymphoma.* Of the oncogenous RNA viruses (oncorna viruses, RNA tumour viruses), especially the C-RNA viruses classified in group C provoke mesenchymal tumours (sarcoma, lymphoma, leukemia). B-RNA viruses are associated with malignomata of the mammary glands, A-RNA viruses are not oncogenic.

The theoretical possibility with virus infections is there, as shown in a model by SHANNON, W. H. Everything depends on whether or not the DNA modified by viruses can be integrated into cellular DNA. Non-integration means proliferation of viruses and, possibly, subsequent immunity

whereas integration effects a chimerism between the systemic DNA and viral DNA, with failure of the transcription and translation, which leads to a transformation of the cells (fig. 321).

From the safe proofs of all 4 etiological groups appears the absence of a common cause though the initial point of the malign transformation of the cell seems to be largely uniform. The structural change of the DNA may be traced out genetically in the one group; in the chemical and radiation groups, chemical changes especially formations of epoxyde, and in the viral genesis, foreign nucleic acids will cause aberration of the DNA architecture and incorrect codes.

Tumour immunology

The disappointing results of the conventional therapies have much contributed to a renascence of the tumour immunology during the last years. H. HOEPKE (together with HEMPFING) mentioned already late in the twentieths and early in the thirtieths years of this century the importance of the «body-own defense», of the thymus and of the lymphocytes. In the fiftieths, HOEPKE resumed the tumour research with thymus and spleen implantations in animals, with different but not satisfying, after all, results. At the beginning of this century already, tests were conducted to take a

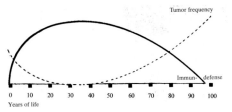

Fig. 322:
Reciprocity between the power of immunoresistance and frequency of tumour in the life profile.

therapeutic initiative with tumour transplantations.

There is probably a connection between the formation of a tumour and immunizing processes because the life profile of the immunocapacity practically constitutes a reciprocal to the frequency of tumours (fig. 322). During the last few years, the interest has been concentrating chiefly on the so-called «onco-fetal antigens». According to this theory, supported by many especially by REN-NER(H. RENNER, 1977), the tumour cells have on their membranes antigens differing immunologically from surface antigens of body cells. These membrane-associated tumour antigens provoke an immunoresponse of the body after the injection of fetal tissues (fig. 341). The «theory of immunesupervision» says that tumour cells are produced during the entire life but are destroyed by the immune-defense till this mechanism fails to work. This most probable of all theories is based on several facts:

a) the accumulation of tumours in the marginal periods of life of the not yet ripened (1st-5th years of life: leukemia, CNS tumours) and exhausted immune-defence (increasing frequency of carcinoma in old age, see fig. 322).
b) 10% of the patients with genetic syndromes of deficient immunocapacity suffers of tumours (GOOD, R., 1974; WALDMANN, T. A., et al., 1972).
c) Patients treated immunosuppressively suffer more frequently from cancer than comparative groups. According to PENN, I. (cit. MAUGH and MARX, 1979), patients with kidney transplantations and immunosuppression with the factor 100 will more frequently get sick of cancer than the equal agegroups.

There is no answer to the question whether the failure of the tumour-defense is caused finally by «blocking antibodies« (HELLSTRÖM, K. E. and HELLSTRÖM, I., 1974) or by «eliminating the immune-defense» with an excessive supply of antigens or by reducing the potential of immunocompetent cells. A correct estimation is difficult as immuno-stimulations accelerate rather than inhibit the growth of tumours under certain condition («enhancement phenomenon»).

Therapy

Though the fundamental research is chiefly preoccupied with the elementary processes of cellular transformation, the therapy has so far been following virtually other ways. «Steel and radiation» i. e. operation and X-ray therapy have limited possibilities on primary tumours. Chemotherapy has been successful in several systematized tumours such as leukemia and lymphoma, but seems to provide disadvantages rather than advantages in the most frequent kinds of cancer.

P. NIEHANS maintained early already (between 1950 and 1960) that cell therapy had a cancer-preventing effect; unfortunately his catamnestic reports in this respect on more than 1000 cell-treated patients have never been evaluated.

Starting from the basic process of cell transformation i. e. the prevention of the transfer of genetic information into corresponding structures, the RNA is no doubt very important. If the development of structures in plants is prevented by artificial interventions e. g. continuous trimming (fig. 319, 320), tumorous formations will originate. This circumstance was the primary starting point for the use of fetal connective tissue in cancer research, a trend from which later the product «fetal mesenchyme of the umbilical cord» (denoted as «Resistocell®») developed.

Comprehensive experimental and clinical experience on the effect of this fetal mesenchyme is available, namely systems of cell cultures (LANGENDORFF, v. L., 1977, 1979), morphological studies (HOEPKE, H.; LANDSBERGER, A., 1977–1980), immunological studies (RENNER, H., 1977, 1979, RENNER, H. et al. 1980); (FUENTE DE PERUCCHIO et al., FUENTE CHAOS, della A., GIANOLI, A. C. and PEREZ-QUADRADO, S., 1979) and clinical studies (LANDSBERGER, HOEPKE,

HAGMAIER, RENNER, 1979; ENDERLE, E., 1979; SCHNITZLER, A., 1978; HAGER, D. 1981; RENNER, K. H. et al. 1982).

The differentiation of the cell-culture systems has allowed to test fetal mesenchyme in 2 kinds of tumour in the tissue culture (LANGENDORFF, v. L. W., 1977, 1979). Arrangements of tests and results with a *Hodgkin-like lymphoma* will be given hereafter in the original, the results with a Wilms' tumour tissue as a summary.

The influence of fetal mesenchyme cells on a Hodgkin-like lymphoma cell strain
(L. v. LANGENDORFF)

Lymphoma cells modified in a culture containing, «siccacell mesenchyme» not only lose the capability of producing tumours but also exert a protective effect against subsequent inoculations of viable tumours from the cell culture or fresh tumours from SJL/J mice bearing tumours. It has turned out that the «immunity» lasts at least 4 months and resists even repeated inoculations of the same tumour.

Spontaneous course

The effect of fetal mesenchyme cells from sheep (siccacell) on Hodgkin-like lymphoma has been tested. This tumour develops spontaneously after nine months (but not earlier) in mice of an inbreeding strain. This model was chosen because it corresponds much to human cancer and, unlike other tumours in animals, does not involve virous or chemical induction. The tumour is easy to transplant, without impairment by histocompatibility barriers, and grows rapidly in a foreseeable way. It was reproduced over several generations in three to six weeks old female SJL/J mice and leads to death within two to three weeks in 80% of the animals.

Fig. 323 shows a tumour-bearing SJL/J mouse and fig. 324 the excised tumour.

Cultivation in the tissue culture

The tumour grows also in the tissue culture where its cultivation can be continued. The fig. 325–327 show the mixed culture, which was obtained from the tumour shown in fig. 324, after one, two and three weeks in RPMI 1640 culture medium. A uniform population of individual cells was cultivated from this mixed culture. Fig. 328 shows the cell strain after the lapse of one month. Fig. 329 and 330 demonstrate the increased density of the same strain after one- and two-week growth in the RPMI medium; the beginning formation of a lump appears from fig. 330. Fig. 331 shows the cell lump after another two weeks. Although the tumour in situ consists of a population of multiple cell types, its cultivation can be continued in the culture beyond this individual cell strain; it can stand an unlimited number of divisions and retain its full potency as a tumour-producing agent after each cell division. Injecting the cultivated cells intraperitoneally or subcutaneously into

389

the axilla of three to six weeks old SJL/J mice will produce tumours not differing from the original tumour as shown in fig. 332 and 333. But the tumours originating from the cultivated cells develop more rapidly and cause the deaths of 100% of the test animals within one to two weeks.

Modification by adding fetal mesenchyme cells

This culture of cultivated malign cells was modified by the addition of siccacell-mesenchyme to the nutritive substratum i. e. 15 mg/100 ml. Such a modified culture as appearing one month after the transplantation is seen in fig. 336. During that time it was supplied twice a week with fresh medium, which contained siccacell. The change of the form

is evident. Two weeks later, as seen in fig. 335, most of the cells have undergone necrosis, and the surviving cells are oblong in contrast to those of the original strain of cells. Whereas the cells grown in the standard medium RPMI 1640 retained their full tumour-producing effect even after 3 months and 15 transplantations, 70% of the cells cultivated in parallel cultures in the presence of siccacell had undergone necrosis after an equal time. The surviving 30% showed morphological changes. They were longer, became pyknic and the dendrite-like appendages were smaller.

Fig. 336 shows the modified culture in this stage. The cultivation of the surviving cells was continued, and while they propagated themselves, cell counts were used to adjust the quantities of the cells

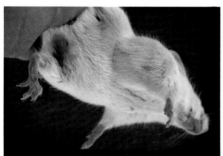

Fig. 323:
A tumour-bearing SJL/J mouse.

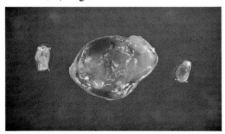

Fig. 324:
The excised tumour.

Fig. 325–327:
Mixed culture of tumour in fig. 324.

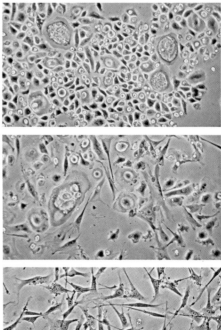

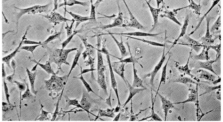

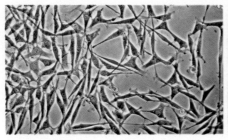

Fig. 328:
Cellular strain after 1 month.

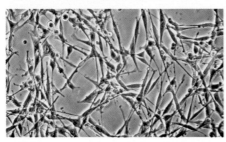

Fig. 329:
Cellular strain (fig. 328) after another week of growth.

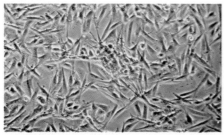

Fig. 330:
Cellular strain (fig. 328) after another 2 weeks of growth.

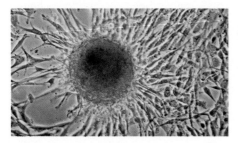

Fig. 331:
Cellular strain tumour tissue after 2 months.

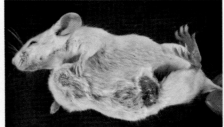

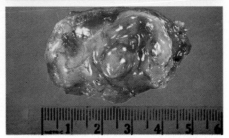

Fig. 332, 333:
Implantation tumour in SJL/J mice 3–6 weeks of age.

to be injected to the numbers of cells of the untreated cell strains, which were injected into the mice of control groups. Fig. 337 shows such a culture. After a month in a siccacell-containing medium, the cells were no longer capable of producing tumours. All mice that got injections of these pretreated cells were free from tumours after 3 months. A typical animal of this group is shown in fig. 338.

Protective effect

Further, the mice that had got modified cells, were protected from the effect of more inoculations of transplants of the original tumour or of the original cell strain of the tumour of the culture. No tumours developed if the mice were inoculated 4, 6, 8, 10 weeks after they had got an injection of cells cultivated in a nutritive medium containing siccacell. This appears from the diagram in fig. 340. On the left, once more the essential items of the test without siccacell-mesenchyme are shown: the tumour-

391

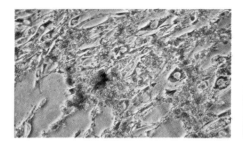

Fig. 334:
Addition of fetal mesenchyme cells to the nutritive medium, after 1 month.

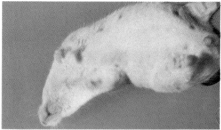

Fig. 338:
All mice that got injections of cells pretreated with mesenchyme are free from tumours after 3 months.

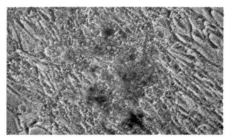

Fig. 335:
Culture 2 weeks later (2 × per week addition of siccacell).

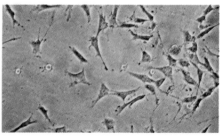

Fig. 336:
Death of tumour cells in the culture modified by addition of mesenchyme.

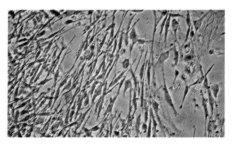

Fig. 337:
Modified culture in continued cultivation.

bearing mouse; the cell strain from the tumour culture and the rapid development of a fatal tumour after the injection of the cell strain. The upper line represents the changed morphology and the reduced number of cells, which results from the addition of siccacell mesenchyme to the nutritive medium, as well as the subsequent increase of the density growing to correspond to that of the unmodified cell strain. If these modified cells are injected into SJL/J mice, no tumour will develop. As seen on the right, the mice are free from tumours even after 10 weeks. If these mice get new injections 2–10 weeks after the implantation with siccacell-modified cells (either tumour-producing culture cell-strains / second line / or excised tumour from a tumour-bearing mouse /third line /), no tumours will develop. All pretreated animals remain free from tumours whereas all control animals succumbed to the tumour. Consequently, cells modified in a siccacell-mesenchyme-containing culture not only lose the capacity of producing tumours but also exert a protective effect against subsequent inoculations with viable tumours from the cell-culture or fresh tumours from tumour-bearing SJL/J mice. So far it has turned out that the «immunity» continues at least 4 months and resists even repeated inoculations of the same tumour.

LANGENDORFF, v. W. L. and his co-workers conducted similar tests to find out the influence of fetal lyophilised mesenchyme cells on the morphology and function of *Wilms-tumour tissue* cultures. The Columbia-Fürth-Wilms-tumour of the rat is a model corresponding much to the Wilms-tumour in children; it spreads in the same way and responds just so to therapeutic measures like the Wilms-tumour in man. This tumour is transplantable and can be transplanted over generations of Fürth-Wistar rats, which are predisposed to it. After the transplantation, a massive tumour develops within a week; it consists of hardly differentiated polygonal and fusiform cells, which are connected with each other in a loose texture. The tumour cell has a large central nucleus, which is surrounded by a small quantity of cytoplasm. The latter contains an endoplasmatic reticulum with much flocculent material, which indicates an active protein synthesis.

If lyophilisate of fetal mesenchyme from the umbilical cord is added to a growing tissue-culture of a Wilms-tumour tissue, part of the tumour-cells will die. The surviving cells show remarkable morphological changes. In comparison with the cells of the original culture, they become larger and flatter. The capacity of forming clusters of cells is lost. The re-transplantation into an original nutritive medium did not provoke a tumour, which suggested that after the addition of mesenchyme the transformation into a not tumour-forming kind of the cells is final (LANGENDORFF, v. W. L., 1979).

Tests of many years have proved beyound doubt the effect of fetal mesenchyme on various tumours. The prophylactic and protective action i.e. the prevention of metastases seems to be more important than the reduction of tumours. The explanation of this sequel is far more complicated than the experimental facts of the outcome. RENNER, H., supposes a cross immunity between the onco-fetal antigens and the fetal antigens of the mesenchyme. An immunostimulation against fetal antigens causes, thanks to the affinity to the tumour antigens, an immunization, which covers also the tumour cells. This explanations is substantiated by results obtained in the lymphocyte transformation test (fig. 341).

FUENTE PERUCCHIO et al. (1979) have drawn from the most extensive immunological tests ever conducted in this field the following conclusions: The influences of fetal mesenchyme (resistocell) on the lymphoblastic transformation by means of laboratory cultures of leukocytes from peripheral blood of 22 patients with swellings of the gastrointestinal tract and a carcinomatous mammal affection in certain phases of development showed clearly immunological effects. Ten patients (7 with cancer of the colon and 3 with gastric cancer) were given a dose of Resistocell® 30 days after the excision of the tumour, 5 got the second dose 160 days later. Phytohaemagglutinin (PHA) as a non-specific mitogen was added in 4 experimental models used for 4 in-vitro leukocyte cultures, one of them received moreover 0,5 ml of Resistocell. In the comparative study of the models with and without Resistocell, the results showed a positive effect of the fetal mesenchyme on the blastic transformation of the lymphocytes in the laboratory during the entire course of studies. The differences were statistically significant 55 days after the operation. As however the tests were not sufficient to draw valid conclusions on the therapeutic efficiency of the fetal mesenchyme, these statements are restricted to the immunimodu-

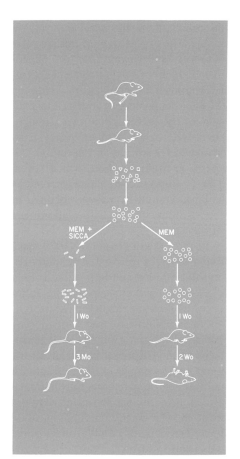

Fig. 339

Fig. 339:
is a diagram of these observations. An SJL/J mouse got an axillary injection of the Hodgkin-like lymphoma from another animal and develops the typical tumour. The tumour is excised and cultivated, a cellular strain is taken from the mixed culture. On the right, the processes after cultivation of the cellular strain in standard MEM or RPMI 1640 are represented. A week after the injection, a tumour has formed, and the animals are dead after another two weeks. The left side of the diagram shows, in contrast thereto, the outcome resulting from the addition of siccacell mesenchyme to the standard nutritive medium. Only few cells survive and have been changed morphologically. Their cultivation is continud till their density equals that of the tumour-producing controls, then they are injected into SJL/J mice. No tumour develops, the animals remain safe and sound for 3 months and longer. These mice remain permanently free from tumours.

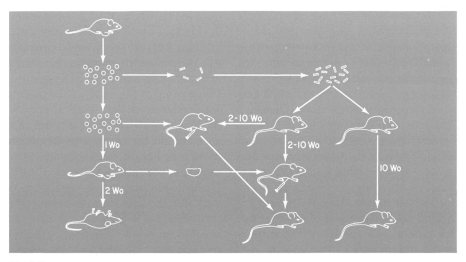

Fig. 340

394

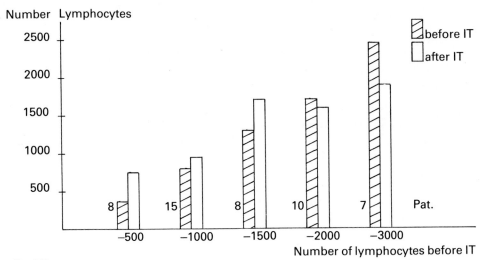

Tumor-Immunotherapy with fetal cells

Influence on the lymphocytes-number in tumor-patients

Fig. 341:
Tumour-immunotherapy with fetal cells. Influence on number of lymphocytes in tumour patients
(after H. RENNER).

lation using fetal mesenchyme in the cancer therapy.

Not until these last three years (1979–1982), methodical studies by A. LANDSBERGER et al., HAGER, D. 1981, WACKER 1982, provided another very essential point of view.

Fetal mesenchyme in the form of the Resistocell from the umbilical cord may be capable of increasing the *interferon* level to an extent impossible so far with other methods. As interferon is an essential component of the tumour defence, this component of the resistocell effect seems to be of considerable importance.

For all, partly interesting partly convincing, experimental and clinical detailed findings, the clinical reality of cancer prevention and cancer therapy is un-satisfactory. New ideas and reconsideration seem necessary to open promising ways. Moreover, the basic conception of « malignity» will have to be abandoned. As a rule, malignities result in biology from inhibitions of structures and functions. Consequently, it would be more expedient for the therapy to promote the ripening in order to eliminate the inhibition of ripening characteristic for all tumours. This basic conception ought to supersede the present conventional view that tumorous tissue, as a matter of principle, must be removed or destroyed. The deviations of cellular metabolism will become more important and the cell therapy will have to be put on a broader basis than hitherto.

The author's own patients

Relying on the experimentations on the passive transfer of tuberculin allergy by cells (1947–1951), the author's own work till 1967 centred on tests on animals in the cytochemical and immunological fields. Up to that year, about 60 children were treated in hospital or outdoor for maldevelopment, for which also cell-therapeutic measures were used.

A commission from the «Scientific Advisory Board to the Federal Chamber of Physicians»in 1969 prescribed to include a prospective study on 200 disabled children into the tests and long-term treatments so as to judge objectively of the effect of cell therapy on non-selected patients.

The use of cell therapy in addition to the customary therapeutic methods augmented rapidly the inquiries and requests for treatments beyond expectation. The prospective study was finished as soon as in 1972.

By April 1st, 1975, the recorded patients included:

976 cases of mongolism syndrome;
2271 cases of cerebral maldevelopment, among them in succession of their frequency:
 – infantile cerebral paresis (dyskinetic forms, hypertonic, spastic, mixed forms, cerebellar and cerebrospinal ataxia, hypotonic forms)
 – microcephalia;
 – postencephalic aspects;
 – impaired learning capacity and weakened concentration on an organic base;
 – degenerative diseases of the central nervous system.
140 cases of innate dysplasia;
 – mucopolysaccharidoses;
 – muscular dystrophia, innate defects of metabolism;
 – osteogenesis imperfecta;
 – posttraumatic conditions of the central nervous system;
 – appalic syndromes;
 – progeria;
 – sickle-cell anaemia, etc.

Since 1970, 1200–1800 babies and children with hereditary physical impairments and cerebral paresis have been cared for per year; implantations by injection were applied in 70–80% of the cases. A survey by groups of diseases for 1978 and the first 7 months of 1980, the latter also detailed in a geographical breakdown, is given in tab. 56, 57, 58 the number and geographical provenience of 7 month in 1982 in tab. 59. Since 1975, the numbers of requests for treatments from foreign countries in Europe and overseas have been growing so that patients of more than 54 countries have been treated so far. The diagnosis and the multidimensional therapy needs time and team-organization so that the capacity is limited. As most of the impairments require treatments of years, the possibility of admitting new treatments has been restricted during the last years, for the capacity was more than exhausted.

By the middle of 1980 (July 31st, 1980), the number of patients recorded since 1969 came to 4219 cases. The total number of documentated cases on July 31th 1982 was 4509. With an average of 7 series of implantations per patient and

Tab. 56:
Mental and multiple disabilities
Patients in 1978

	cases
1978	1422
Down's syndrome	944
cerebral paresis	294

hypertonous	64
hypotonous	16
dyskinetic	72
atactic	11
mixed forms	131

	cases
partial disabilities	43
cerebral defects + fits	34
fits	12
heredodegenerative diseases	23
apallic syndrome	9
deafness	4
syndromes	41
skeletal dysplasia	18

Achondroplasia	8
Osteogenesis imp.	3
Arthromyodysplasia	4
Enchondral Dysplasia	3

Tab. 57: **Diseases**
treated in the first 7 months in 1980, arranged by Diagnosis-groups

	cases
Down's syndrome	591
Infantile Cerebralparesis	
disturbed tonics	106
dyskinetic forms	54
cerebral attacks	11
metabolic disorders	21
skeletal dysplasia	20
syndromes and individual cases . .	48
	851

Tab. 58:
849 cases of mental and multiple disabilities
in the first 7 months of 1980, arranged by geographic origin.

Germany

postal code number	cases
1	11
2	16
3	25
4	92
5	89
6	185
7	59
8	131
total	608

foreign countries	cases
Switzerland	8
Austria	6
France	1
Luxembourg	2
Belgium	4
England	1
Norway	1
Holland	3
Spain	3
Portugal	2
Italy	7
Greece	4
Israel	4
Iran	2
India	2
Australia	46
USA	25
Canada	52
Mexico	60
Venezuela	1
Brazil	4
South-Africa	2
Jugoslavia	1
	241

Tab. 59: **Geographical origin of 1.700 in 1982 treated handicapped children and adults**

America	322	EUROPE	1.153
Canada	117	Finnia	10
USA	176	Sweden	1
Hawai	2	Norge	1
Mexico	14	Netherland	2
Venezuela	3	Belgia	18
Guatemala	1	Luxembourg	11
Brazil	2	France	2
Chile	6	Spain	11
Peru	1	Great Britain	13
		Ireland	5
		Austria	20
ASIA	**46**	Switzerland	15
Hongkong	1	Italy	10
India	1	Greece	7
Israel	43	Yugoslawia	2
Turkey	1	Hungary	1

AFRICA	2	Germany, F. R.	1.024
South-Africa	2	Post-Code 1	18
		2	30
		3	48
AUSTRALIA	174	4	174
		5	125
		6	305
POLYNESIA	3	7	120
		8	204

2,2 implantations per series taken as a base, more than 70 000 injection implantations were performed in the last 13 years since methodical records of these cases were adopted. These clinical cases and the experimental work preceding the clinical use of the method constitute the fundament of this book.

Till the final correctures of this book (31. 1. 1983) the documented number of outpatients was 4.616, included 1.814 Down's syndromes. Additionally about 200 patients treated only by hospital care and 400 patients in their different homelands. More and more treatment requirements came from overseas-countries. Table 59 gives an impression on the geographical origin of the patient in 1982. Several thousands of letters with recommendations for treatment and care must be answered in the last years.

Cell-therapeutic synopsis

The following alphabetical survey is intended to outline the tissues to be used for the more important aspects, syndromes and symptoms. The classification of first and second choice must be regarded just as a general rule as the selection of tissues depends chiefly on the individual situation and on the symptoms. In using this survey compiled to inform the reader at a glance, it should be noticed that cell therapy is always part of a wholistic, multidimensional therapy. The outcome will be the better the more carefully the tissues are selected and the more this biological method is integrated into necessary further medicamentous, dietetic, physiotherapeutic and psycho-social measures.

Disease syndrome symptom	Tissue 1 st choice	Tissue 2 nd choice
achondroplasia	cartilage liver osteoblasts	placenta connective tissue
acne vulgaris-globata	adrenal- gland skin	liver placenta
cerebral sclerosis	placenta heart diencephalon cerebral hemisphere	specific: cerebral regions
adrenal insufficiency	adrenal gland	hypothalamus (gonads)
agammaglobulinaemia	thymus spleen adrenal cortex	fet. mesenchyme liver
aged (senile) skin	skin placenta connective tissue	fet. skin extract

Disease syndrome symptom	Tissue 1 st choice	Tissue 2 nd choice
alcoholism	liver stomach-intestine placenta	hypothalamus frontal lobe adrenals heart
alopecia	adrenal gland diencephalon local: fet. skin extract	skin placenta liver
thallasemia	frontal brain temporal brain thalamus hypothalamus	placenta artery
amyotonia, cong.	spinal medulla occipital brain intestine	mesencephalon liver pancreas
anaemia, hypoplastic	spleen liver	bone-marrow fet. mesenchyme
antibody-deficiency	thymus spleen adrenal gland	bone-marrow liver mesencephalon
appalic syndrome	spinal medulla cerebrum cerebral cortex thalamus cerebellum	placenta cerebral regions by symptoms
arteriosclerosis	artery placenta heart liver	connective tissue gonads
arthritis chron.	adrenal gland cartilage connective tissue placenta	osteoblasts liver
arthromyodysplasia	cartilage placenta connective tissue osteoblasts	

Disease syndrome symptom	Tissue 1st choice	Tissue 2nd choice
arthrosis	cartilage placenta connective tissue liver adrenal gland	muscle parathyreoid gland
aseptic necrosis	cartilage placenta	connective tissue liver
asthma bronchiale	lung adrenal gland diencephalon	heart connective tissue liver
ataxia heredogenerative	liver intestine (mucosa) placenta	pancreas adrenal LPPM-Lyophilisate orally
ataxia teleangiectaca (Louis-Bar-S.)	thymus cerebellum	liver mesencephalon
ataxia	cerebellum spinal medulla mesencephalon	occipital brain
athetosis	diencephalon temporal brain basal ganglia	cerebellum thalamus
autism	frontal brain placenta	cerebellum hypothalamus temporal brain
Autoimmun-disease	adrenal gland liver placenta hypothalamus	Be careful of symptoms and contra-indications!
β-hypolipoproteinaemia	liver placenta gastrointestinal mucosa	cerebellum
bronchitis, obstructive	lung placenta connective tissue	mucosa adrenal gland

Disease syndrome symptom	Tissue 1 st choice	Tissue 2 nd choice
burns	fet. skin extract local	placenta skin sonnective tissue
cardiac insufficiency (not decompensated!)	heart liver lung (placenta)	artery adrenals
cat's-cry syndrome	diencephalon cerebral hemisphere placenta	cerebral regions record. to symptoms
cancer	Resistocell (fet. mesenchyme) adrenal gland	organo-specific selection general revitalization
carcinoma	fet. mesenchyme	org.-spec. tissues and revitalization
cerebral paresis, hypertonic	cerebral cortex spinal medulla cerebral thalamus; hemisphere	placenta mesencephalon
cerebralparesis, hypotonous	mesencephalon occipital brain spinal medulla cerebellum	parietal brain
cerebral paresis	tissues accord. to symptoms	
cerebral paresis, atactic	cerebellum occipital brain spinal medulla mesencephalon	
cerebral paresis, dyskinetic	diencephalon basal ganglia temporal brain cerebral cortex	hypothalamus frontal brain
cerebral atrophy	frontal brain hypothalamus cerebrum placenta	general revitalization

Disease syndrome symptom	Tissue 1 st choice	Tissue 2 nd choice
circulation disorder, peripherous	placenta artery heart	revitalization accord. to organ
colitis ulcerosa	liver adrenal gland intest. mucosa	thymus fet. skin extract oral
collagenosis	adrenal gland liver placenta hypothalamus	be careful of symptoms and contraindications
cutaneous defects	skin extract local	placenta skin connective tissue
depression	hypothalamus frontal brain liver placenta	gonads adrenal gland
diabetes insipidus	diencephalon hypothalamus hypophysis	
diabetes mellitus	pancreas liver gastrointestinal mucosa	diencephalon adrenal gland
disturbed fertility female	ovary adrenal gland female hypothalamus	placenta liver
disturbed fertility male	testis adrenal gland (male) hypothalamus	placenta liver
Down's syndrome	see Tab. 27	
Fabry's disease	fet. mesenchyme placenta liver	
Friedreich's ataxia	liver intestine mucosa placenta cerebellum	pancreas adrenal LPPM-lyophilisate orally

Disease syndrome symptom	Tissue 1 st choice	Tissue 2 nd choice
frontal brain syndrome	thalamus frontal brain	placenta temporal lobe
gangliosidosis	liver placenta intestine	adrenal gland connective tissue (fet. mesenchyme)
granulocytopenia	spleen liver bone-marrow	fet. connective tissue
Grigler-Najar syndrome	liver placenta basal ganglia	cerebellum
healing of fracture, retarded	fet. mesenchyme osteoblasts cartilage	placenta
hepatitis, chron.	intest. mucosa liver placenta	adrenal gland mesenchyme
hydrocephalus	cerebral hemisphere cerebral cortex thalamus placenta	
hypothyreosis	thyreoidea hypothalamus frontal brain	hypophysis adrenal gland
hyperammonaemia	liver placenta	cerebellum cerebral hemisphere
hypercorticism	diencephalon hypothalamus adrenal gland	
hypogonadism	hypophysis male hypothalamus adrenal gland testis	
hypoparathyreoidism	parathyreoidea	thyreoidea adrenal gland hypophysis

Disease syndrome symptom	Tissue 1 st choice	Tissue 2 nd choice
ichthyosis congen.	fet. skin extract local	placenta skin liver
immune deficiency	thymus adrenal gland	spleen lung liver mucosae
injuries cosmetics	fet. skin extract local	placenta connective tissue general revitalization
insomnia	hypothalamus frontal brain temporal brain	adrenal gland
keloids	fet. skin extract local	connective tissue placenta
liver cirrhosis comp.	liver placenta	adrenal gland connective tissue spleen
leukaemia	spleen liver bone-marrow	fet. mesenchyme
leukodystrophy	liver intestine (mucosa) placenta	pancreas adrenal LPPM-lyophilisate orally
lung emphysema	lung placenta heart	liver fet. connective tissue
lymphoma	fet. mesenchyme thymus spleen	liver
Ménière's syndrome	auditory nerve mesencephalon parietal brain temporal brain cerebellum	placenta

Disease syndrome symptom	Tissue 1 st choice	Tissue 2 nd choice
meta-epiphyseal dysplasia	cartilage osteoblasts placenta liver	bone-marrow
microcephaly	cerebral hemisphere cerebral cortex thalamus diencephalon mesencephalon	cerebral regions by anatomy and symptoms cerebral hemisphere
migraine	placenta frontal-temporal brain	adrenal gland liver
mongolism	see Tab. 27	
mucopolysaccharidosis	liver cartilage placenta connective tissue	osteoblasts
multiple sclerosis	liver intestine (mucosa) placenta	pancreas adrenal LPPM-lyophilisate orally
muscular dystrophy spinal	placenta liver spinal medulla cerebellum	
muscular dystrophy, progr.	(sic) liver muscle extract oral cartilage-bone-extract orally	adrenal gland
myocardiac infarction (not fresh!)	placenta heart artery liver	adrenal gland
nanism	differentiated selection of organ accord. to cause	see Tab. 41

Disease syndrome symptom	Tissue 1 st choice	Tissue 2 nd choice
nanism, adreno-genital	adrenal gland ovary or testis	hypothalamus
nanism, hepatic	liver placenta intest. mucosa	pancreas adrenal gland
nanism, hypophyseal	diencephalon hypothalamus hypophysis	adrenal gland
nanism, ossary	cartilage placenta	according to involved regions
nephritis, chronic	kidney placenta connective tissue	adrenal gland
nephrosis	kidney placenta liver	adrenal gland
Noonan's syndrome	adrenal gland gonads	placenta hypothalamus
Osteogenesis imperfecta	cartilage placenta osteoblasts bone-marrow	liver
Osteomyelitis chron.	fet. mesenchym sic osteoblasts	thymus adrenal gland
osteomyelofibrosis	bone-marrow fet. mesenchyme cartilage placenta	adrenal gland liver
osteoporosis	fet. mesenchyme cartilage bone-marrow liver placenta	gonads specific to sex parathyreoidea

Disease syndrome symptom	Tissue 1 st choice	Tissue 2 nd choice
panmyelopathia	spleen liver bone-marrow cartilage fet. mesenchyme	placenta adrenal gland
Parkinson's syndrome	basal ganglia diencephalon cerebellum	placenta artery connective tissue
potency disorders	hypothalamus adrenal gland testis	revitalization accord. to organs
Prader-Willi's syndrome	hypothalamus adrenal gland testis	placenta frontal brain liver
progeria	placenta liver diencephalon	adrenal gland
prostatic adenoma	prostata fet. mesenchyme testis adrenal gland	revitalization
radiation syndrome	spleen liver bone-marrow intest. mucosa fet. mesenchyme	adrenal gland gonads
retinitis pigmentosa	placenta retina nervus opticus	liver adrenal
revitalization, male	hypothalamus frontal brain adrenal gland testis liver placenta	depends on symptoms see Tab. 40

Disease syndrome symptom	Tissue 1 st choice	Tissue 2 nd choice
revitalization, female	hypothalamus frontal brain adrenal gland ovary liver placenta	depends on symptoms see Tab. 40
Reynaud's syndrome	placenta artery heart	organic revitalization
scalds	fet. skin extract local	placenta skin connective tissue
Scleroderma	skin placenta connective tissue liver	adrenal gland
Sheehan's syndrome	hypophysis diencephalon	adrenal gland ovary
spongy degeneration (Canavan-disease)	liver intestine (mucosa) placenta	pancreas adrenal LPPM-lyophilisate orally
sickle-cell anaemia	spleen liver placenta	fet. mesenchyme
thalassaemia	spleen liver placenta	
thrombocytopenia	spleen liver bone-marrow	adrenal gland thymus placenta
tuberous cerebral sclerosis	placenta liver	adrenal gland connective tissue
tumours	fet. mesenchyme	depend. on kind and localization of tumor

Disease syndrome symptom	Tissue 1 st choice	Tissue 2 nd choice
Turner's syndrome	adrenal gland gonads	diencephalon hypothalamus
ulcerous complaints	gastro-intest. mucosa liver adrenal gland	pancreas hypothalamus
wound-healing, retarded	fet. mesenchyme skin placenta	

Bibliography

The literature-index would be to voluminous, if all papers on cell-research and cell-therapy would be registered. The representative selection contains historically important, or critically sources and informative surveys.

A

ACKERMANN, G.: Behandlungsversuch bei fortgeschrittenem metastasierendem Prostata-Ca mit Humanplazenta. Münch. med. Wschr., *100,* 494 f., 1959.

ACKERMANN, G. A.: Ultrastructure and Cytochemistry of the developing Neutrophil. Lab. Invest. *19,* 290 (1968).

ADAMIKER, D.: Gerontologische Untersuchungen an Rattenlebermitochondrien. Inaugural-Diss., Tierärztl. Hochschule Wien 1963.

AEHNELT, E.: Erfahrungen mit der Trockenzellbehandlung bei Funktionsstörungen der Keimdrüsen großer Haustiere. Vortrag anl. d. 8. Arbeitstagung der Dt. Ges. f. Zellulartherapie, Bad Homburg, 1960. Berliner Ärzteblatt 73. Jg., Heft 18.

ALLAN, P. C. und KABAT, E. A.: Persistence of circulating antibodies in human immunized with dextran, levan and blood group substances. J. Immunol. *80,* 495 (1958).

ALTERAUGE, W.: Über allergische Reaktionen, Abderhaldenschen Reaktion und Zellulartherapie von Niehans in ihren Beziehungen zueinander. Berlinger Münchener tierärztl. Wschr., *70,* 70–74, 1957.

ALTMANN, PH. L. und KATZ, D. D.: «Cell-Biology»; 1976 by Feder. of American. Soc. F. Exper. Biology Bethesda, Maryland.

AMELUNXEN, F. und SPIESS, E.: Untersuchungen zur Struktur der Ribosomen. Ein Beitrag zur Konformation der 80 S-Ribosomen von Pisum sativum. Cytobiologie *4,* 293 (1971).

ANDRES, G.: Embryonic transplantation by the vascular route. Science, *111,* 456, 1950.

— Experiments on the fate of dissociated embryonic cells (chick) disseminated by the vascular route. Part. II Terotomas. J. Exper. Zool., Philadelphia, *122,* 507–540, 1953.

— Wachstumsreaktionen der Urniere und der Leber des Hühnerembryos auf Injektion von Zellbrei in die Blutbahn. Verh. d. Schweiz. Naturforsch. Ges., Lugano, 99, 1953.

— Growth reactions of mesonephros and liver to intravascular injections of embryonic liver and kidney suspension in the chick embryo. J. Exper. Zool., Philadelphia, *130,* 221–250, 1955.

— Wirkungsspezifität von Zellinoculaten beim embryonalen und heranwachsenden Organismus. In F. Schmid und J. Stein: Zellforschung und Zellulartherapie, Verlag Huber, Bern 1963, S. 241–264.

— Specific Effectiveness of Cell Inocula in Embryonic and Growing Organism. In F. Schmid and J. Stein: Cell Research and Cellular Therapy. Ott Publishers Thoune, Switzerland, 1967, p. 247–269.

— Injektion embryonaler Zellen in die Blutbahn der Hühnerembryos. Vorträge beim II. Internationalen Kongreß f. Zell- und Histotherapie. Wiesbaden. I. 6–11, 1959.

— Wirkung von Gewebsinjektionen auf den embryonalen Organismus. Vortrag anl. d. III. Intern. Kongr. für Zellulartherapie, Paris, 1961.

AYRES, W. W.: Production of Charcot-Leyden Crystals from eosinophils with aerosol. Blood, *4*, 595 (1949).

B

BABILLOTTE, J.: Ist eine causale Therapie der Depression möglich? Cytobiol. Rev. *2*, 31–35 (1978),

BABILLOTTE, J.: Die Migräne – Indikation für eine Zelltherapie? Cytobiol. Rev. *3*, 117–121 (1979).

BACH, M. K.: Immediate Hypersensitivity. Marcel Dekker Inc. New York and Basel 1978.

BAKER, R. W. R. et al.: Fatty acids-composition of brain lecithins in multiple sclerosis lancet, i. 26–27 (1963).

BANKER, B. Q., ROBERT; J. T. and VICTOR, M.: Spongy degeneration of central nervous system in infancy. Neurology (Minneapolis) *14*, 981–1001 (1964).

BARBEAU, A.: Friedreichs Ataxia 1979: An Overview J. Can. Scienc. neurol. *1979*, 311–319.

BARGMANN, W. und KNOOP, A.: Über die Morphologie der Milchsekretion. Licht- und elektronenmikroskopische Studien an der Milchdrüse der Ratte. Z. Zellforschg. *49*, 344 (1959).

BARRETT, A. J.: In Dingle, J. T., ed. Lysosomes; A Laboratory Handbook. North-Holland, Amsterdam 1972. S. 46–135.

BARTH, G.: Experimentelle Grundlagen für die Knochenmarktransplantation nach Ganzkörperbestrahlung. Dtsch. med. Wschr. *86*, 1331–1333, 1961.

BAUER, K. F.: Methodik der Zell- und Gewebezüchtung. S. Hirzel Verlag, Stuttgart 1974.

BECKER, F. F. and LANE, B. P.: Regeneration of the mammalian liver. Amer. J. Path. *47*, 783 (1965).

BEHRENS, M.: Über die Lokalisation der Hefenucleinsäuren in pflanzlichen Zellen. Hoppe-Seylers. Z. Physiol. Chem. *253*, 185 (1938).

BELL, G. I., PERELSON, S. S., PIMBLEY, G. H. JR.: Theoretical Immunology. Marcel Dekker. Inc. New York and Basel 1978.

BENNHOLD, H. Gefahren der Frischzellentherapie. Dtsch. med. Wschr. *79*, 704–711, 1954.

BERG, G.: Histologische Labortechnik. J. F. Lehmanns Verlag, München 1972.

BERNHARD, P.: Decken sich die Wirkungsvorgänge bei der Zellulartherapie mit der Genese der Endometriose? Therapiekongreß, 9–11, 1956. Therap. Woche, Karlsruhe, *7*, 43–51, 1956.

BERNHARD, P.: Merkmale und Behandlung des vorzeitigen und biologischen Alterns. Med. Mschr., Stuttgart, *10*, 361–367, 1956.

BERNHARD, P.: Über den Einfluß der Frischzellen-Implantation von Endometrium auf den Kastratenuterus des Kaninchens. Ber. v. d. 5. Tagg. d. Forschungskreises für Zellulartherapie, 45–47, 1958.

– Über die Wirkung von Frischzellen- und Trockenzellen-Implantationen von Kaninchenendometrium auf den Uterus kastrierter Kaninchen. Vorträge beim II. Intern. Kongr. f. Zell- und Histotherapie, Wiesbaden, I, 11–21, 1959.

BERNHARD, P. und KRAMPITZ, W.: Über die Wirkung von Frischzellen- und Trockenzellen-Implantationen von Kaninchenendometrium auf den Uterus kastrierter Kaninchen. Zschr. Geburtsh., Stuttgart, *156*, 1–19, 1960.

BERNHARD, P. und KRAMPITZ, W.: The Organ-Specific Cellular Effect of Implanted Rabbit Endometrium upon the Uterus of Castrated Rabbits. In F. Schmid and J. Stein: Cell Research and Cellular Therapy. Ott Publishers Thoune, Switzerland, 1967, p. 302.

BERNHARD, W., BAUER, A., GUERIN, M. et OBERLING, CH.: Étude au microscope éléctronique de corpuscles d'aspect virusal dans des épitheliomas mammaires de la souris. Bull. Ass. franç. Cancer *32*, 163 (1955).

BERSIN, TH.: Biochemie der Mineral- und Spurenelemente. Akad. Verlagsges. Frankfurt 1963.

BESSIS, H.: Living Blood Cells and their Ultrastructure, Springer-Verlag, Berlin-Heidelberg-New York 1972.

BESSIS, M. et LOCQUIN, M.: Sur la présence de mouvements propres de l'aster et des vacuoles contractiles dans les granulocytes. C.

412

R. Soc. Biol. *144*, 483 (1950).

BEUTNER, R.: Physical Chemistry of Living Tissues. Williams & Wilkins, Baltimore *1933*.

BHADURI, S., KURRLE, E., ARNOLD, R., LOHRMANN, H. P., PFLIEGER, H., KUBANEK, B. und HEIMPEL, H.: Knochenmarktransplantation (KMT). Klinikarzt *9*, 105–112 (1980).

BINDER, G.: Untersuchungen über die Verteilung und den zeitlichen Verlauf der Aktivität von L-Lysin-4,5-Tritium in Organen der Ratte nach peroraler Verabreichung. Inaugural-Diss. Tierärztl. Hochschule Wien, 1969.

BIRCHER, F. E.: Insuffisance surrénalienne et alimentation. Supplemento della Recerca Scientifica, *XXVII*, 1955, 3ème Journée de Diétique, Rome, 22–24 sept. 1955.

BIRCHER, F. E.: Thérapie cellulaire des troubles circulatoires terminaux. Rapports du 3ème Congrès Français de Thérapeutique cellulaire, Paris. Edit. du Centre-Méd. d'Etudes et de Rech. Paris 65–67, 1959.

BITTAR, E. E.: Membranes and Ion Transport, Wiley-Interscience a division of John Wiley & Sons Ltd. Volume 1, London *1970*, Volume 2 London *1970*, Volume 3 London *1971*.

BLACK, D. B., KATO, J. G. und WALKER, G. W. R.: A study of improvement in mentally retarded children accuring from Siccacell Therapy. Am J. of mental Deficieny, Jan. 1966, Vol. 70. Nr. 4, S. 499.

BLASIUS, W.: Vom Wesen des Lebens. Cytobiol. Rev. *3*, 31–37 (1979).

BLOCK, S.: Erfahrungsbericht aus über 30jährigen Praxis mit Frischzellentherapie bei über 45 000 Patienten. Biol. Med. *11*, 261–266 (1982).

BLUMENBERG, F. W.: Erste klinische Erfahrungen über die Zusatztherapie mit einem Zellpräparat zur Strahlen- bzw. Cytostatika-Therapie. Ref. Blatt Die Zelltherapie, Nr. 36, 1969.

– Erste klinische Erfahrungen über die Zusatztherapie mit einem Zusatzpräparat zur Strahlen- bzw. Zytostatika-Therapie. Die Heilkunst. 84. Jh., Heft 10. Okt. 1971.

BOMS, P.: Inwieweit kann der Schlachthoftierarzt, der Material für die Frischzellen-therapie entnimmt, schuldhaft sein? Archiv f. Lebensmittelhygiene, *7*, 171– 174, 1956. Archiv. f. Lebensmittelhygiene, *7*, 276–277, 1956.

BORSOOK, H., DEASY, C. L., HAAGEN-SMIT, A. J., KEIGHLY, G. and LOWY, P. H.: Metabolism of C^{14}-labeled glycine, l-histidine, l-leucine and l-lysine. J. Biol. Chem. *187*, 519 (1950).

BÖSCH, J.: Zellulartherapie, ja oder nein? Wien, klin. Wschr., *70*, 76–80, 1958.

BOSSE, J.: Kann man der vorzeitigen Alterung wirksam begegnen? Landarzt, Stuttgart, *34*, 164–168, 1958.

BRACHET, J.: Recherches sur la synthèse de l'acide thymonucléique pendant le développement de l'œuf d'oursin. Arch. Biol. *44*, 519 (1933). – La détection histochimique des acides pentosenucléique. C. R. Soc. Biol. 133, 88 (1940).

BRAMMER, H.: Neue Wege in der Behandlung von Alkoholkranken. Cytobiol. Rev. 6, 73–75 (1982)

BRANDIS, H.: Einführung in die Immunologie. Gustav Fischer Verlag Stuttgart 1975.

BRANDNER, R.: Die Zellulartherapie bei degenerativen Erkrankungen. Fortschr. Med., *76*, 453 f., 1958.

BRAUN, P.: Speech-Development-Analysis. Cytobiol. Rev. *5*, 73–75 (1981)

BRUECKEL, K. W.: Grundzüge der Geriatrie. Urban und Schwarzenberg, München-Berlin-Wien (1975).

BRUNNER, P.: Die Lunge des alten Mannes: Altersveränderungen und Krankheiten im Alter (im Druck)

BURGER, H.: Gerontologische elektronenmikroskopische Untersuchungen an Herzmuskelmitochondrien der Ratte. Inaugural-Diss., Tierärztl. Hochschule Wien, 1965.

BURNET, F. M.: The Clonal Selection Theory of Acquired Immunity. Vanderbilt Univ. Press, Nashville/Tenn., 1959.

BUSCHA, J.: Zelltherapie bei Asthma bronchiale? Cytobiol. Rev. *5*, 174–178 (1981).

BUTLER, I. A. V.: Vom Haushalt der Zelle. F. Vieweg u. S. Braunschweig 1958.

BYERS, B.: Structure and function of ribosome crystals in hypothermic Chick embryo cells. J. Mol. Biol. *26*, 155 (1967).

C

CAMERER, W.: Behandlung der Infertilität des Mannes. Therapie-Woche, Karlsruhe, *7*, 13, 1956.
- Über die Behandlung von Fertilitätsstörungen. Bericht v. d. 4. Tagg. d. Forschunghsf. Zellulartherapie, 47–50, 1957.
- Behandlung klimakterischer Beschwerden. Bericht v. d. 4. Tagg. d. Forschungskreises f. Zellulartherapie. *42*, 1957.
- Gibt es eine erfolgreiche Behandlung männlicher Fertilitätsstörungen mit Siccacell? Münch. med. Wschr., *100*, 1897–1900, 1958.
CAMERER, W.: Ist die Zellulartherapie schädlich? Landarzt, Stuttgart, *37*, 251–254, 1961.
CAMERER, W.: Infertilität – Diagnostik und Therapie. Cytobiol. Rev. , 12–16 (1978).
CAMITTA, B. M., THOMAS, E. D., NATHAN, G. et al.: Severe aplastic anemia: a prospective study of the effect of early marrow transplantation on acute mortality. Blood *48*, 63–70 (1976).
CARO, L. G. and PALADE, G. E.: Protein synthesis, storage and discharge in the pancreatic exocrine cell. An autoradiographic study. J. Cell Biol. *20*, 473 (1964).
CASPERSSON, T.: The protein metabolism of the cell. Naturwissenschaften *29*, 33, (1941).
CASTENS, C. E.: Vermeidung von Gefahren bei der Zellulartherapie. Hippokrates, Stuttgart, *28*, 40–45, 1957.
- Sichere Indikationen und Kontraindikationen der Zellulartherapie. therapie-Woche, Karlsruhe, *8*, 34–36, 1957. Therapie-Kongr. 6–10, 1957.
CHAO, F. C.: Dissociation of macromolecular ribonucleoprotein of yeast. Arch. Biochem. Biophys. *70*, 426 (1957).
CHASE, M. W.: The cellular transfer of cutaneous hypersensitivity to tuberculin. Proc. Soc. exp. biol. (N. Y.) *59*, 134 (1945).
CHERKIN, A., FINCH, C. E., KHARASCH, N., TAKASHI, M., SCOTT, F. L., STREHLER, B. S.: Physiology and cell Biology of Aging. Raven Press, Basel 1979.
CLAUDE, A.: Particulate components of cytoplasm. Cold Spring Harbor Symp. Quant. Biol. *9*, 263 (1941).

COGGIN, J. H. a.o.: Tumor immunity in hamsters immunized with fetal tissues. J. Immun. (1971).
COHEN, S. and PORTER. R. R.: Structure and Biological Activity of Immunglobulins. In Dixon, F. J. and Humphrey, J. H.: Advances in Immunology: Vol. 4, Academic Press; New York/London, 1964.
CONGDON, C. C., UPHOFF, D. and LORENZ, E.: Modification of acute irradiation injury in mice and guinea pigs by injection of bone marrow. J. Nat. Cancer Inst., Wash., *13*, 73–93, 1952.
COTTIER, H., ODARTCHENKO, N. and CONGDON, C. C.: Germinal Centers in Immune Response. Springer, Heidelberg/Berlin/New York. 1967.
CUMINGS, J. N. et al.: Lipid studies in the blood and brain in multiple sclerosis and motor neurons disease. J. Clin. Path. *18*, 641 (1965).

D

DAHMEN, H.: Tierkrankheiten, die gegebenenfalls durch Frisch- bzw. Trockenzellen auf den Menschen übertragen werden können. Bericht v. d. 1. Tagg. d. Arbeitsgem. f. Zellulartherapie, Frankfurt, 31–52, 1953.
- Ärztliche Sorgfaltspflicht bei der Anwendung der Zellulartherapie. Medizin heute, 5, 59–62, 1956.
DALTON, A. J.: A study of the Golgi material of hepatic and intestinal epithelial cells with the electron microscope. Z. Zellforschg. *36*, 522 (1952), Golgi apparatus and secretion granules. In: The cell, Vol. 2 eds. Brachet and Mirsky. New York and London, Academic Press 1961.
DANIELLI, J. F. and DAVSON, H.: J. Cellular Comp. Physiol. *5*, 495, 1935.
DANIELLI, J. F.: in K. B. WARREN (Ed.), Formation and Fate of Cell Organelles, Academie press, London *1967*, 239.
DAVID, J. M. und DAVID, AURELIA E. A. DE: Tratamiento de oligofrenias de etiologia diversa con la implantacion de tejidos frescos (Terapeutica celular). Sem. méd., Buenos Aires, *117*, 289 u. 329, 1960.

DAVISON, P. F.: Intermediate Filaments: Intracellular Diversities and Interspecies Homologies. In: Internat. Cell Biol. 1980–1981, p. 286–292; ed. H. G. SCHWEIGER. Springer-Verl. Berlin – Heidelberg – New York 1981.

DEAN, R. T.: In Dingle, J. T. and Dean, R. T., ed. Lysosomes in Biology and Pathology. North-Holland, Amsterdam 1975, 349–382.

DE DUVE, C.: The Lyosome. Sci. Am. *208*. 64, 1963.

DE DUVE, CHR.: Peroxyomes and related particles in historical perspective Annals New York Acad. Sciences *386*, 1–4 (1982)

DEGENS, E. T.: Über die Bedeutung von Metallionen in der biologischen Zelle. Cytobiol. Rev. *5*, 107–113 (1981)

DELONS, P. E. et COUGOULE, J.: Excitabilité neuro-musculaire et thérapie cellulaire. Rapports du 3ème Congrès Français de Thérapeutique Cellulaire. Paris. Edit. du Centre Méd. d'Etudes et de Rech., Paris, 52–55, 1959.

DESTUNIS, G.: The treatment of mental deficiency and encephalopathies in childhood by means of fresh tissue and Siccacell. Zellulartherapie bei Debilität und Encephalopathie. Ber. v. d. 4. Tagg. d. Forschungskreises für Zellulartherapie. 57–60, 1957.

– L'implantation de diéncéphale comme thérapie de dévelopment contre la débilité et l'encéphalopathie des enfants et son importance prophylactique. Rapports du 2ème Congrès Français de Thérapeutique Cellulaire, Tours. Edit. Du Centre Méd. d'Etudes et de Rech., Paris. 44–48, 1958.

– Die ärztliche Behandlung der Debilität und Encephalopathien. Medizinische, Stuttgart, *24*, 980–984, 1958.

– Zellulartherapie (Zwischenhirnimplantation) bei kindlichen Entwicklungsstörungen und Encephalopathien. Jahreskongreß 1958 für ärztliche Fortbildung, 341–345, VEB Verlag Volk u. Gesundheit, Berlin, 1958.

– La Terapia cellulare nelle turbe dell'infanzia. Relazioni I. Congresso Scientifico, Milano. Centro Italiano Terapie Istobiologica, Milano, Viale Lunigiana 46, 57–65 (1959). Die Zell- und Histotherapie, *1516*, 12–18, 1959.

– Zwischenhirnimplantationen bei Encephalopathien. Rotterdamse gesprecken over celtherapie. Ned. Uitgeversmaatschappij N. V., Leiden, 49–53, 1960.

DESTUNIS, G. und SCHMIDT, E.: Zwischenhirnimplantationen bei kindlichen Encephalopathien und Debilität verschiedener Genese, Med.-Klin., *51*, 768–770, 1956. Therapiekongreß 11–12, 1956.

DITS, A. TH.: Wurzelspitzenresektion und Knochenwundfüllung mit Osteoblasten «Siccacell-Trockenzellen». Heilkunst, München, *70*, 12–13, 1957.

DITTMAR, F.: Der Einfluß von Zellpräparaten auf Wachstum und Körpergewicht im Tierversuch. In F. Schmid und J. Stein: Zellforschung und Zellulartherapie. Verlag Huber, Bern 1963, S. 397.

DITTMAR, F., GROSS, A. und THOMAS, W.: Über den Einfluß der sogenannten Frischzellen auf Wachstum und Körpergewicht im Tierversuch. Medizinische, Stuttgart, *47*, 1637–1939, 1955.

DIXON, F. J. and HUMPHREY, J. H.: Advances in Immunology. Vol. 4. Academ Press. New York/London. 1964.

DIXON, K. C.: Cellular Defects in Disease. Blackwell Scient. Publ. Cambridge 1981.

DOLER, H. J. und SCHMID, F.: Infantile Cerebralparese. Früherkennung und Frühbehandlung. 3. Auflage. Dr. Schwappach-Verl. Gauting 1974.

DÖDERLEIN, G.: Die Indikation zur Implatation von Kalbs- und Schweine-Hypophysen. Münch. med. Wschr. *95*, 969, 1953.

DÖDERLEIN, G., FANCONI, G. und NONNENBRUCH, W.: Wie sind Theorie und Leistung der Frischzellen-, Frischdrüsen-, beziehungsweise Serumtherapie nach Niehans, Zajicek und Bogomoletz zu beurteilen? Münch. med. Wschr., *97*, 710–712, 1955.

DOLCE, G.: Neurophysiologische Untersuchungen zur Wirkung von Pyrithioxin auf das zentrale Nervensystem der Katze. Pharmakopsychiatrie *3*, 355–370 (1970).

DOLCE, G.: Beeinflussung der akuten alkohol-bedingten Veränderung des EEG, der evoked potentials sowie des Verhaltens bei der Katze durch Pyrithioxin. Act nerv. sup. (Praha) *16*, 1 (1974).

DOMAGK, G. F.: Zur Biochemie des Lernens. In: G. NISSEN: Intelligenz, Lernen und

Lernstörungen. Springer-Verlag, Berlin-Heidelberg-New York 1977.

DORNBUSCH, S.: Die Beeinflussung der experimentellen Cholesterinsklerose durch Siccacell-Placenta. Zellulartherapie in Klinik und Praxis. Kuhn, W. Hippokrates-Verlag. Stuttgart, 134–140. 1956. Bericht v. d. 3. Tagg. d. Forschungsgemeinschaft f. Zellulartherapie, 19–20. 1956.

– Der Einfluß von Placenta-Zellinjektionen auf die experimentelle Cholesterin-Arteriosklerose bei Kaninchen. Medizinische. Stuttgart, 43, 1533–1535. 1956. Bericht v. d. 5. Tagg. d. Arbeitsgemeinschaft für Zellulartherapie, Bad Homburg, 1–2, 1956.

DORNBUSCH, S.: Die Beeinflussung der Angiopathien der experimentellen Gefäßsklerose durch Placenta-Zellen. In F. Schmid und J. Stein: Zellforschung und Zellulartherapie. Verlag Huber, Bern 1963, S. 378.

– Action of Placenta Cells in Experimentel Arteriosklerosis. In F. Schmid and J. Stein: Cell Research and Cellular Therapy. Ott Publishers Thoune, Switzerland, 1967, p. 380.

DREIER, H. K.: Aktivitätsverteilung in verschiedenen Organen der Ratte nach s.c. Verabreichung Tritium-markierter Organhomogenate. Inaugural-Diss. Tierärztl. Hochschule Wien, 1972.

DUBOIS, A. M. et GONET, A.: Régénération des îlots de Langerhans, au cours de la Correction du diabète expérimental du rat par bréphoplastie pancréatique. Zschr. Zellforsch., 53, 481–491, 1961.

DUMONDE, D. C.: The Role of Lymphocytes and Macrophages in the Immunological Response. Springer, Berlin/Heidelberg/New York, 1971.

DVORAK, ANN M.: Biology and Morphology of basophilic Leukocytes. In: BACH, M. K.: Immediate Hypersensitivity. Marcel Dekker Inc. New York and Basel 1978, S. 369–406.

E

Editorial: Die Abderhaldensche Reaktion. Cytobiol. Rev. 2, 44–45 (1978).
Editorial: Marrow Transplantation for Non-malignant Disorders. New Engl. J. Med. *298,* 963 (1978).

EHNI, L. und DUVE, G.: Zur Beurteilung und Therapie hypophysär-diencephaler Regulationsstörungen im Entwicklungsalter. Medizinische, Stuttgart, *38,* 1381–1384. 1957.

EHRLICH, P. und MORGENROTH, J.: Über Hämolysine, Berlin, Klin. Wschr. *36,* 1, 481, (1899); *37,* 453, 581 (1900).

EICKSCHEN, H.: Fetales Mesenchym (Resistocell) bei Osteomyelitis. Cytobiol. Rev. *2,* 39–40 (1978).

EMÖDI, G.: Die Beeinflussung des Immunsystems durch Interferon und klinische Behandlungsmöglichkeiten neoplastischer Erkrankungen. Cytobiol. Rev. *1,* 27–29 (1977).

ENDERLE, E.: Ergebnisse einer prophylaktischen und therapeutischen Anwendung von fetalem Mesenchym (Resistocell) bei DÄNA-induzierten Tumoren. 2/3, 7–9 (1979).

ERNST, W., KANZOW, U. und OETTGEN, H.: Untersuchungen zur Zellulartherapie. 3. Mitteilung: Über den Einfluß von Placenta-Zellinjektionen auf die Blutlipoide. Medizinische, *7,* 277–281, 1958.

F

FAGRAEUS, A.: The plasma cellular reaction and its relation to formation of antibodies in vitro. J. Immunol. *58,* 1 (1948).

– Antibody production in relation to the development of plasma cells. In vivo P., GIBSON, G. E., KARK, R.A.P. and CARREL, R. E.: Ketonic diet in the management of pyruvate dehydrogenase deficiency. Pediatrics *58,* 713–721 (1976).

FANTON, E.: La terapia cellulare nel Mongolismo. Relazioni I. Congresso Scientifico, Milano. Ediz. Centro Italiano Terapia Istobiologica, Milano. Viale Lunigiana *46,* 67–69, 1959.

FAWCETT, P. W.: Structural and functionell variations in the membranes of cytoplasm. In: Intracellular membraneous structure. Proc. first Int. Symp. Chemistry 1963, Okayama: Chugoku Press Ltd. 1965.

FEDERLIN u. Mitarb.: Inselzell-Transplantation – eine Chance für die Behandlung des Diabetes mellitus? Med. Welt *29, 535–543* (1978).

FELDMANN, H. S.: A propos du traitement médicamenteux des obligophrènes. Revue Suisse d'Utilité Publique, *98,* 1/2. 1959.

– Valeur de la thérapie cellulaire dans les retards du développement chez l'enfant. Vortrag anl. d. III. Intern. Kongresses für Zellulartherapie. Paris. 1961. Rev. méd. Suisse rom., LXXXI/11, 773–796, 1961.

FELDMANN, H. S.: The value of Cell therapy for cases of retarted development in children. In: IIIRD International Congress for cellular therapy, Hans Huber, ed. Bern, pp 89–116 (1961).

FELDMANN, H. S.: Present Drug Treatments for Mental Retardation. (A Comparative Longitudinal Study of 100 Cases). Cytobiol. Rev. *3,* 55–69 (1979).

FELDWEG, TH.: Die Zuckerkrankheit und ihre biologische Behandlung. Heinr. Schwab, Gelnhausen 1965.

FEULGEN, R., BEHRENS, M. und MAHDIHASSAN: Darstellung und Identifizierung der in den pflanzlichen Zellkernen vorkommenden Nucleinsäure. Hoppe-Seyler's Z. Physiol. Chem. *246,* 203 (1937).

FISCHER, K. J.: Niehans, Arzt des Papstes. Wilhelm Andermann Verlag, München-Wien 1957.

FISHMAN, M. and ADLER, F. L.: Antibody formation in vitro. Immunpathologie IIIrd Internat. Symposium. S. 79. Basel u. Stuttgart: Benno Schwabe & Co. 1963.

FREDERICKS, R. E. and MALANEY, W. C.: The basophilic granulocyte. Blood *14,* 571 (1959).

FUENTE CHAOS, DE LA A.: Filosofía de la terapia en el cáncer. Cytobiol. Rev. *2*/1, 10–12 (1978).

FUENTE-PERUCHO, DE LA A., FUENTE-CHAOS, DE LA A., PAYA-PARDO, J. M., GIANOLI, A. C., MORENO-KOCH, M. C. e PEREZ-CUADRADO: Terapia celular con Resistocell e immunidad en oncologia. Cytobiol. Rev. *3,* 83–104 (1979).

FUJIKI, Y., FOWLER, S. HUBBARD, A. L. a. LAZAROW, P. B.: Polypeptide and phospholipid composition of the membrane of rat liver peroxysomes. J. Cell. Biol. 1982

G

GARNIER, CH.: Contribution à l'étude de la structure et du fonctionement des cellules glandulaires séreuses. Du rôle de l'ergastoplasma dans la sécrétion. Thesis Nancy 1899.

GEIGER, H.: Krebskrankheit und Placenta-Substrate. Medizinische. *1958,* 1099–1103.

GERSTL, B. et al.: Alterations in myelin fatty acids and plasmalogens in multiple sclerosis. Ann. N. Y. Acad. Sci. *122,* 405–416 (1965).

GIANOLI, A. C.: Therapie des Morbus Parkinson. Fortschr. Med. *87,* Nr. 35/36 (1969).

GIANOLI, A. C.: Neuere Erfahrungen auf dem Gebiet der Zelltherapie. Die Zelltherapie *42,* 3–18 (1975).

GIANOLI, A. C.: Revitalisationstherapie in Klinik und Praxis. Z. praeklin. Geriatrie *5,* 186–192 (1975).

GIANOLI, A. C.: Der heutige Stand der Organtherapie in Klinik und Praxis. Cytobiologische Revue 1, 30–34 (1977).

GIANOLI, A. C.: Revitalization. Cytobiol. Rev. *4,* 70–74 (1980).

GIANOLI, A. C.: Où en est le traitement cellulaire du point de vue international? Cytobiol. Rev. *4,* 145–146 (1980)

GIANOLI, A. C.: Behandlung der Parkinsonschen Krankheit. Cytobiol. Rev. *6,* 184–188 (1982).

GIANOLI, A. C. a. PEREZ-CUADRATO, S.: Immunmodulation and Restoration with Resistocell. Cytobiol. Rev. *6,* 138–139 (1982)

GIESE, H.: Die Zellulartherapie homosexueller Männer. Nervenarzt,Berlin, *30,* 133 ff., 1959.

GILKA, L.: Schizophrenia: A Disorder of Tryptophan Metabolism. Acta psych. scand. Suppl. 258, 1975. Parkinson's Disease – A New Approach 10th Internat. Congr. Neurol. Barzelona 1973.

GILLHAM, N. W.: Organelle Heredity. Raven Press, Basel 1978

GLEICH, G. J., LOEGERING, D. A. and MALDONADO, J. E.: Identification of a major basic protein in guinea pig eosinophil granules. J. exp. Med. *137,* 1459 (1973).

GOLDSTEIN, H.: Siccacell Therapy in Children. Arch. Pediatr. N. Y., *73,* 234–249, 1956.

– La terapia «Siccacell» en los ninos afectados de lesiones cerebrales con trastornos de la evolution. Sintesis Medica IV, No. 26, Sept. 1959.

– Siccacell-Therapie bei hirngeschädigten, entwicklungsgestörten Kindern. Zellulartherapie nach Dr. P. Niehans in Wissenschaft und Praxis, Sonder-Nr. 1959.

– Siccacell Therapy for retarded children. General Practice, Jan. 1961.

GOLGI, C.: Sur la structure des cellules nerveuses. Arch. ital. Biol. *30,* 60, (1898).

GOOD, R. A.: Immunbiology, Cellular Engineering and Cancer. Pediatric Research Vol. 12, Nr. 4, Part. 2. Williams a. Wilkins Co. Baltimore 1978.

GOOD, R. A. and PAPERMASTER, B. W.: Autogeny and Phylogeny of Adaptive Immunity. In Dixon, F. J., Humphrey, J. H.: Advances in Immunology. Vol 4. Academic Press, New York/London. 1964.

GOOD, R. und BACH, F.: Clinical Immunbiology. Academic Press, New York 1974.

GOOD, R. A., MARTINEZ, C., DALMASSO, A. P., PAPERMASTER, B. W., and GABRIELSEN, A. E.: Studies on the role of the thymus in developmental biology, with a consideration of the assoziation of thymus abnormalities and clinical disease. Immunopathologie. IIIrd Internat. Symposium. Basel u. Stuttgart: Benno Schwabe & Co. 1963.

GORDONOFF, T.: Pharmakologische Unter suchungen einiger Siccacell-Präparate. Med. Welt, *44,* 2303–2307. 1960.

GOSLAR, H. G.: Recherches histophysiologiques sur la réalité de l'action de divers extraits d'organes lymphatiques. Rapports du 3ème Congrès Français de Thérapeutique Cellulaire, Paris. Edit. du Centre Med. d'Etudes et de Rech., Paris 29–33, 1959.

– Beiträge zur Korrelation von Thymus, Schilddrüse und Nebenniere. Vorträge beim II. Intern. Kongr. f. Zell- und Histother., Wiesbaden, I, 22–24, 1959.

– Morphologische Untersuchungen zur Objektivierung einer differenten Wirkung von Extrakten lymphatischer Organe. Rotterdamse gesprekken over celtherapie. Ned. Uitgeversmaatschappij N. V., Leiden 55–57, 1960.

GOWANS, I. L., and MCGREGOR, D. D.: The origin of antibody-forming cells. Immunpathologie. IIIrd Internat. Symposium. S. 89, Basel u. Stuttgart: Schwabe & Co. 1963.

GRAUPNER, H.: Die Niehanssche Zellulartherapie. J. F. Lehman's Verlag, München, 1955.

GRIFFEL, A.: The latest developments in Dry Cell Therapy (Siccacell). Arch. Pediatr., N. Y., *74,* 325–342, 1957.

GRÜBER, H.: Experimentelle Studien mit Trockenzellen bei der Salvarsan-Nephrose. Ber. v. d. 2. Tagg. d. Forschungsgem. f. Zellularth. 49 f., 1955.

– Die Wirkung tierischer Trockenzellen auf den Arsenobenzolschaden der Tiere. Frankf. Zschr. Path., *66,* 362–375, 1955.

– Experimentelle Untersuchungen zur Zellulartherapie. Vortrag auf der Herbsttagg. d. Nord- und Westdtsch. Pathologen in Bad Ems. Sept. 1954. Ref. Blatt «Die Zellulartherapie». Nr. 6, 7–8. 1955.

GRUMET, F. C., PAYNE, R. O., KONOSHI. J., KRISS, J. P.: HLA-antigens as markers for disease susceptibility and autoimmunity in Graves disease. J. Clin. Endocrinal. Metab. *39,* 1115 (1974).

GUTTMANN ; G.: Neurospychologie des Lernens. In Nissen G.: Intelligenz, Lernen und Lernstörungen. Springer-Verlag, Berlin – Heidelberg – New York 1977.

H

HAGER, D.: Kongreßbericht über den Kurs «Lyophilisationstechnologie». Cytobiol. Rev. *5,* 212–213 (1981).

HAGER, D.: Immunstimulation und Interferon-Induktion in der Tumortherapie. Cytobiol. Rev. *5,* 144–148 (1981).

HAGMAIER, W.: Zelltherapie in der postoperativen Phase. Ref. Blatt «Die Zelltherapie» Nr. 40. Aug. 1973.

HAGMAIER, W.: Erfolgreiche Behandlung von Weichteilverletzungen mit Nekrosen. Eiterungen, osteomyelitischen Veränderungen und unüberbrückbaren Hautdefekten durch lyophilisiertes Mesenchym (Resistocell). Cytobiol. Rev. *2,* 36–38 (1978).

HAGMAIER, W., HOEPKE, H., LANDSBERGER. A. und RENNER, H.: Erfolgreiche Behandlung Krebskranker durch Immuntherapie mit fetalem Mesenchym-Lyophilisat. Cytobiol. Rev. *3*, 10–14 (1979).

HAILER, B. Y. u. BRAUNE, J.: Die Blut-Hirnschranke Cytobiol. Rev. *5*, 166–170 (1981)

HALPERN, B. N., BENACERRAF, B. and DELAFRESNAYE. J. F.: Physiopathology of the reticuloendothelial system. Oxford: Blackwell, Paris: Masson & Cie. 1957.

HARBERS, E.: Tierexperimentelle Untersuchungen zur Beeinflussung künstlich gesetzter Leberschäden durch Frisch- und Trockenzellen. Bericht v. d. I. Tagg. d. Forschungsgemeinschaft für Zellulartherapie. 8–10, 1954.

HARBERS, E.: Tierexperimentelle Untersuchungen mit radioaktiv markiertem Trokkengewebe. Bericht v. d. 3. Tagg. d. Arbeitsgem. f. Zellulartherapie, Frankfurt, 13, 1954. Bericht v. d. 2. Tagg. d. Forschungsgemeinschaft f. Zellulartherapie. 31 f., 1955.

HARMS, A.: Zelltherapie – Endlich Licht in das Dunkel. Gesunde Medizin 1978/12. 54–58.

HARTMANN, G.: Quantitative elektronenmikroskopische Studien an Lebermitochondrien der Ratte nach Injektionen von Placenta- und Hodengewebe. Inaugural-diss. Tierärztl. Hochschule Wien, 1964.

HARVEN DE. E. and BERNHARD, W.: Etude au microscope électronique de l'ultrastructure du centriole chez les vertébrés. Z. Zellforsch. *45*, 378 (1956).

HASHIMOTO, T.: Individual peroxysomal β-oxidation enzymes. Annals of the New York academy of sciences, *386*, 5–12 (1982).

HASSELMANN, H.: Zum Problem einer Therapie der Keratosis palmaris et plantaris hereditaria. Hippokrates, Stuttgart, *30*, 184f., 1959.

HAUBOLD, H.: Bisherige Erfahrungen über kombinierte Vitamin- und Zellbehandlung bei endokrinen Störungen. Bericht v. d. 1. Tagg. d. Forschungsgemeinschaft für Zellulartherapie, 29–38, 1954.

HAUBOLD, H.: Neue therapeutische Möglichkeiten bei Mongolismus. Vorschlag einer Nachreifungsbehandlung. Ärztl. For-schung, München, IX, I/211-I/228. 1955. Neue therapeutische Möglichkeiten beim Mongolismus. Therapiekongreß, 12–15, 1954. Therapie-Woche, Karlsruhe, *5*, 275–282, 1955.

– Vergleich zwischen ärztlicher Nachreifungstherapie und heilpädagogischer Behandlung ohne ärztliche Hilfe bei mongoloiden und anderen entwicklungsgehemmten Kindern. Ber. a. d. 6. Tagg. d. Arbeitsgemeinschaft f. Zellulartherapie, Bad Homburg, 37–41, 1957.

HAUBOLD, H., LOEW, H. und HAEFFELE-NIEMANN, R.: Möglichkeiten und Grenzen einer Nachreifungsbehandlung entwicklungsgehemmter, insbesondere mongoloider Kinder. Landarzt, Stuttgart, *36*, 378–380, 1960.

HAUPT, E.: Das Verhalten von Milz und Thymus beim intraperitonealen Yoshida-Aszites-Tumor von Ratten. Medizinische, Stuttgart, *4*, 157–160, 1958.

HAUROWITZ, F.: Immunochemistry and the Biosynthesis of Antibodies. New York, 1968.

HAUSWIRTH, A.: Die Stellung der Zellulartherapie in der inneren Medizin. Prakt. Arzt, Wien, XII, 352–361, 1958.

HAYFLICK, L.: Die celluläre Basis des biologischen Alterns. Verh. Dtsch. Ges. Path. *59*, 52–66 (1975).

HEIDELBERGER, M.: Lectures in Immunochemistry. Acad. Press. Publ., New York, 1956.

HEINSTEIN, G. u. ENDERLE, E.: Versuch der Prävention DÄNA-induzierter Karzinome durch immunologische Antezedenz. Cytobiol. Rev. *5*, 135–143 (1981)

HEINTZ, R.: Die Zellulartherapie bei der chronisch differenzierten Glomerulonephritis, Therapie-Woche, Karlsruhe, *5*, 282–284, 1954/55.

HELLSTRÖM, K. E. and HELLSTRÖM, I.: The role of cell-mediated immunity in control and growth of tumors. In Good and Bach: Clinical Immunbiology, Bd. II. Academic Press 1974.

HENNING, N. und WITTE, S.: Erfahrungen mit Knochemarktransfusionen bei akuten Leukämien. Vortrag anl. d. 66. Tagg. d. Dt. Ges. f. inn. Medizin. Medizinische, Stuttgart, *21*, 1172, 1960.

419

HERRSCHAFT, H.: Die Wirkung von Pyritinol auf die Gehirndurchblutung des Menschen. Münch. Med. Wschr. 1978.

HERS, H. G. and HOOF, VAN F.: Lysosoms and Storage Diseases. Academic Press, New York 1973.

HETTICH, U.: Das Verhalten von Milz und Thymus bei Aszites-Tumor-Ratten nach Impfung mit Thymus-Placenta- und Milz-Trockenzellen nach Niehans. Medizinische, Stuttgart, 48, 1785–1789, 1957.

HEUBNER, W.: Zum Thema: Einfluß der Zellen auf das Endokrinum, Therapie-Woche, Karlsruhe, 7, 52 f., 1957.

HIERONYMI, G.: Veränderungen der Lungenstruktur in verschiedenen Lebensaltern. Verh. Dtsch. Ges. Path. 44, 129–130 (1969).

HIRSCH, G. C.: Mikrosomen: Handb. d. allgem. Pathol. Bd. II/I. Springer-Verlag Berlin-Göttingen-Heidelberg 1955, S. 116.

HIRSCH, G. C.: Form- und Stoffwechsel der Golgi-Körper. Protoplasmamonographie 18, Berlin 1939.

HIRSCH, J. G.: Cinematographic observations on granúle lysis in polymorpho-nuclear leucocytes during phagocytosis. J. exp. Med. 116, 827 (1962).

HÖHLER, H.: Changes in Facial expression as a result of plastic surgery in mongoloid children. Aesth. Plast. Surg. 1, 245–250 (1977).

HOEPKE, H.: Über Grundlagen einer Geschwulst-Bekämpfung bei Ratten. Medizinische, Stuttgart, 36, 1205–1207. 1954.

– Milz- und Thymuszelltherapie bei Geschwülsten. Zellulartherapie in Klinik und Praxis, Kuhn, W. Hippokrates-Verlag, Stuttgart, 70–70, 1956.

– Über die Wirkung von Zellinjektionen bei Ratten-Tumoren. Therapiekongreß bei Ratten-Tumoren. Therapiekongreß, 32–37, 1955.

– Cellular therapy in experimental animal tumors. Symposium on Cellular therapy, Cairo, 1960.

– Zellulartherapie an Tiergeschwülsten. Ein Überblick. Med. Welt, 35, 1758–1762, 1960.

– Zellulartherapie bei Geschwülsten. In F. Schmid und J. Stein: Zellforschung und Zellulartherapie. Verlag Huber, Bern

1963, S. 485.

– Behandlung von Benzpyren-Tumoren der Ratte mit Nabelschnur-Trockenzellen vom Schaf. Der Landarzt, 41, 1421–1424 (1965).

– Cellular Therapy in Tumors. In F. Schmid and J. Stein: Cell Research and Cellular Therapy. Ott Publishers Thoune. Switzerland, 1967, p. 481.

– Immunsuppression, Krebsgeschehen, Zellulartherapie. Fortschr. Med. 86, 1102–1107, 1968.

HOEPKE, H.: Zur Lage der Zelltherapie. Ref. Blatt Die Zelltherapie Nr. 35, 1968.

– Die wissenschaftlichen Grundlagen der Zelltherapie. Aus: Zur Wirkungsweise unspezifischer Heilverfahren. Hippokrates-Verlag, Stuttgart, 1972.

– Gibt es etwas Neues in der Frischzellentherapie? Fragen aus der Praxis. Selecta Nr. 44, 1972.

HOEPKE, H. und FLUHR, F.: Zellulartherapeutische Beobachtungen an experimentellen Ratten-Tumoren. Therapiekongreß, 15–17, 1954. Therapie-Woche, Karlsruhe, 5, 377–282, 1954/55.

HOFECKER, G.: Untersuchungen über die Verteilung und den zeitlichen Verlauf der Aktivität von Tritium-markiertem L-Histidin in Organen der Ratte nach peroraler Verabreichung. Inaugural-Diss. Tierärztl. Hochschule Wien, 1969.

HOFECKER, G., KMENT, A., SKALICKY. M. und NIEDERMÜLLER, H.: Messungen des biologischen Alters. Cytobiol. Rev. 3, 49–54 (1979).

HOFF, F.: Über Therapieschäden. Medizinische, Stuttgart, 17, 587–596. 1957.

HOFFMANN, P.: Die Zellulartherapie und verwandte Methoden. Objektivierung und therapeutische Anwendung (Bericht v. Therapiekongreß 1960). Ärztl. Sammelbl. Stuttgart, 49, 383f, 1960.

HOFFMAN, P. N. a. LASEK, R. J.: J. Cell Biol. 66, 351–366 (1975).

HOLMER ; A. J. M.: Implantation von embryonalen Eierstocksgewebe in Fällen von gonadaler Agenesie. Geburtsh. u. Frauenhk., Stuttgart, 18, 621–626, 1958.

HÖTZL, H. A.: Die Behandlung chronischer Leberentzündungen und Leberzirrhosen mit Leber-Mitochondrien-Suspensionen.

420

Münch. med. Wschr., *102*, 1670–1674, 1960.
– Die Behandlung chronischer Leberentzündungen und Leberzirrhosen mit Leber-Mitochondrien-Suspensionen. Therapie-Woche, Karlsruhe, *11,* 506–509, 1961.
– Therapie mit Mitochondrien. Reine Leberzellmitochondrien als neues, biologisch-therapeutisch hochwirksames Prinzip. Ärztl. Wschr., *11,* 634–641, 1956.
HOTOVY, R., ENENKEL, H. J., GILLISEN, J. u. a.: Zur Pharmakologie des Vitamin B_6 und seiner Derivate. Arzneimittel-Forschung, *14,* 26–29 (1964).
HOYER, S.: Zur Wirkung von Centrophenoxin auf Durchblutung und oxydativen Stoffwechsel des Gehirns bei organischem Psychosyndrom. In KUGLER, J.: Hirnstoffwechsel und Hirndurchblutung, Schnetztor-Verlag 1976, S. 98.
HOYER, S., OESTERREICH, K. and STOLL, K. D.: Effects of Pyritinol-HCl on Blood D.: Effects of Pyritinol-HCl on Blood Flow and Oxidative Metabolism of the Brain in Patients with Dementia. Arzneimit.-Forsch. *27,* 671–674 (1977).
HÜLSMANN, H.: Die Gefahren der Zellulartherapie aus der Perspektive des Tierarztes. Bericht v. d. 5. Tagg. d. Arbeitsgem. f. Zellulartherapie, Bad Homburg, 13, 1956.
HUMPHREY, J. H., WHITE, R. G.: Kurzes Lehrbuch der Immunologie. Thieme, Stuttgart, 1971.
HUPFELD, D. P. und WENZEL, U.: Landry-Guillain-Barré-Syndrom nach Frischzellentherapie. Mat. med. *32,* 104–110 (1980).

I

IVERSEN, G.: Zellulartherapie bei altersbedingten Abnutzungserscheinungen und Krankheiten. Landarzt. Stuttgart, *33,* 956–962, 1957.
IVERSEN, G.: Gedanken über die bisherige Kritik der Zellulartherapie nach Niehans. Landarzt, Stuttgart, *32,* 537–539
IVERSEN, G.: Bericht über die 2. Tagg. d. Arbeitsgem. f. Zellulartherapie in Frankfurt. Med. Klin. *49,* 421–423, 1954.
– Bericht über die 3. Tagg. d. Arbeitsgem. f.

Zellulartherapie in Frankfurt. Med. Klin., *35,* 1414–1417, 1954.
– Bericht über die 4. Tagg. d. Arbeitsgem. f. Zellulartherapie in Bad Homburg. Med. Klin., *50,* 1497–1499, 1955.
– Fragen aus Theorie und Praxis der Zellulartherapie. Therap. Gegenw., München, 94/6, 1955.
– Die Niehanssche Zellulartherapie im Gewirr der Meinungen, Schlesw.-Holstein. Ärzteblatt, II, 1955.
– Placebo-Versuche – Placebo-Komplexe? Ärztl. Mitt., Köln, *41,* 1021–1025, 1956.
– Bericht über die 6. Tagg. d. Arbeitsgem. f. Zellulartherapie in Bad Homburg. Med. Klin., *52,* 2013–2015, 1957. Landarzt, Stuttgart, *33,* 903–906, 1957.
– Zur bisherigen Kritik der Zellulartherapie und zur Bedeutung des Zweifels an den sogenannten Außenseiter-Methoden in der Medizin. Vortrag anl. d. I. Intern. Symp. f. Zell- und Histotherapie, Bad Ischl. Die Zell- und Histotherapie, 1, 5/6, 6–11, 1959.

J

JANSON, PH.: Probleme des männlichen Klimakteriums und der Sexualität des alternden Mannes. Hippokrates, Stuttgart, *23,* 539, 1952.
– Zur Therapie der Dystrophia adiposogenitalis, des Klimakteriums virile und des Eunuchoidismus. Ärztl. Praxis, München, *VII/23,* 1955.
JANSON, PH.: Moderne Auffassungen über die Ätiologie der Rosacea und moderne Rosacea-Therapie. J. med. Kosmet., Berlin, *53/12,* 1953.
– Behandlung der Acne vulgaris . J. med. Kosmet., Berlin, *53/5,* 1953.
– Frischzellentherapie in der Dermatologie. Bericht v. d. 3. Tagg. d. Arbeitsgem. f. Zellulartherapie, Frankfurt, 26–29, 1954.
– Dermatosen und Störungen der Leberfunktion. Ärztl. Praxis, München, VII/44, 1955.
– Seborrhoische Dermatose. Ärztl. Praxis München, VII/51, 11, 1955.
– Behandlung der Lichen chron. simplex. Ärztl. Praxis, München, VII/51, 1955.

- Therapie der Sklerodermie, Ärztl. Praxis, München, VII/3, 1955, Med. Klin., *51*, 2152, 1956.
- Hautorgan und Frischzellentherapie. Dtsch. Drogistenzeitung, 17, 596, 1955.
- Zellulartherapie in der Dermatologie Sammelmanuskript d. Referate d. I. Fortbildungskurses f. Zellulartherapie in Österreich, I, 25–29, 1957.

JANSON, PH.: Der derzeitige Stand der Therapie und Prophylaxe des Mongolismus. Hippokrates, Stuttgart, *27,* 623–625, 1956. Eigene Ergebnisse der Nachreifungstherapie des Mongolismus nach Haubold. Hippokrates, Stuttgart, *28,* 310–312, 1957.

JAKOBS, R.: Über die Behandlung schwachsinniger anstaltsgebundener Kinder, Materia med. Nordmark, *XII/9,* 387–395, 1960.

JELENIK, C.: Beitrag zur kinematographischen Registrierungsmethode der Aktivität von Ratten im Rahmen der Revitalisierungsforschung. Inaugural-Diss., Tierärztl. Hochschule Wien, 1971.

JELLINGER, K. und SEITELBERGER, F.: Akute tödliche Entmarkungs-Encephalitis nach wiederholten Hirntrockenzellen-Injektionen. Klin. Wschr. *36,* 437–441, 1958.

JORES, A.: Kritisches zur Zellulartherapie nach Niehans und zu den «Außenseitermethoden» in der Medizin. Hippokrates, Stuttgart, *26,* 206–209, 1955.

JUSSEK, E. G.: Cellular Therapy: Allergic problem, Effectiveness and mode of action. Vortrag anl. d. 35th Congress of the Pan American Medical Association in Mexico City, 1960.
- Critical Review of Contemporary Cellulartherapy (Celltherapy). J. of Gerontology, 1970, Vol. 25, no. 2, 119–125.

K

KABAT, E. A.: Einführung in die Immunchemie und Immunologie. Springer, Berlin/Heidelberg/New York, 1971.

KALB, H.: Experimentelle Untersuchungen über die stoffwechselsteigernde Wirkung von Zellen und Organextrakten. Vorträge beim II. Intern. Kongr. f. Zell- und Histotherapie, Wiesbaden, I. 36–40, 1959.

- Über die spezifisch stoffwechselsteigernde Wirkung von Organextrakten in vitro. Inaugural-Dissertation. München 1959.

KALK, H.: Zellulartherapie der Leberkrankheiten. Problematik und Klinik der Zellulartherapie. Rietschel, H. G. Verlag Urban & Schwarzenberg, München/Berlin, 118–124, 1957.

KANIG, K., TENCHEVA, Z. S., NITSCHKI, J. und DINGLER, W. J.: Der Einfluß von Centrophenoxin auf den ^{32}P-Einbau in Nucleinsäuren und Adenosinphosphate des Rattengehirns. In Kugler, J.: Hirnstoffwechsel und Hirndurchblutung, Schnetztor-Verlag. Konstanz 1976, S. 40.

KANOWSKI, S.: Zum Wirkungsnachweis der enzephalotropen Substanzen (Pyrithioxin und Pirazetam). Z. Gerontol. *8,* 333–338 (1975).

KANZOW, U.: Untersuchungen zur Zellulartherapie – 5. Mitteilung: Weitere klinische Ergebnisse. Medizinische, Stuttgart, 10, 400–404, 1958.
- Zellulartherapie, Bericht über den 9. Kongreß für ärztliche Fortbildung 1960 in Berlin, Naturwiss. Rundschau, *14,* 147 f., 1961.

KANZOW, U.: Kritisches zur Zellulartherapie. Dtsch. med. J., 11, 524–528, 1960.

KANZOW, U. und KINDLER, M.: Untersuchungen zur Zellulartherapie – 4. Mitteilung: Die Antikörperbildung nach Zellinjektionen. Medizinische, Stuttgart, *8,* 312–316, 1958.

KANZOW, U. und SCHULTEN, H.: Untersuchungen zur Zellulartherapie – I. Mitteilung: Über den Wert der Abderhaldenschen Abwehrferment-Reaktion für die Praxis. Medizinische, Stuttgart, *13,* 447–450, 1957.

KANZOW, U. und WALLOSECK, R.: Untersuchungen zur Zellulartherapie – 2. Mitteilung: Die Behandlungsergebnisse bei primär-chronischem Gelenkrheumatismus und Arthrosen. Medizinische, Stuttgart, *37,* 1335–1338. 1957.

KARK, R. A. P, RODRIGUEZ-BUDELLI, M., PERLMAN, S., GULLEY, W. F. a. TOROK, K.: Preclinical diagnosis and carrier detection in ataxia associated with abnormalities of lipoamide dehydrogenase. Neurology *30,* 502–508 (1980)

KENT, S.: Can cellular therapy rejuvenate the aged? New Frontiera of Research Geriatrics *1977,* 92–99.

KERP, L. und STEINHAEUSER, G.: Klin. Wschr. *39,* 762 (1961).

KETTY, S. S.: The biological substrates of mental illness. Pediatric Research Vol. 12, Nr. 4 Part. 2, Williams a. Wilkins Co., Baltimore 1978.

KIBLER, M.: Schulmedizin und Außenseitermethoden. Hippokrates, Stuttgart, *26,* 210–214, 1955.

KIHN, B.: Über systematische Zellulartherapie. Therapie-Woche, Karlsruhe *11,* 509–521, 1961.

KIHN, B.: Über die Epilepsie-Behandlung der Gegenwart. Ärztl. Sammelbl., Stuttgart, *47,* 403–406, 1958.

KIMBALL, I. W.: Biologie der Zelle. G. Fischer-Verlag Stuttgart 1972.

KINDL, H. and LAZAROW, P. B.: Peroxysomes and Glyoxysomes. Annals of the New York Academy of Sciences Vol. *386* (1982).

KLEINMAIER, H.: Experimentelle Untersuchungen zur Schockbereitschaft durch Trockenzellen. Zschr. Immunit. Forschung, Stuttgart, *112,* 382–392, 1955.

KLEINSORGE, H.: Erfahrungen bei der Behandlung von Myodegeneratio cordis mit der Zellulartherapie. Bericht v. d. I. Tagg. d. Forschungsgemeinschaft für Zellulartherapie, 38–42, 1954.

– Klinische Ergebnisse nach Placenta-Injektionen bei peripheren Durchblutungsstörungen. Therapiekongreß. 26 f., 1956. Bericht v. d. 5. Tagg. d. Arb. Gem. f. Zellularth. Bad Homburg, 2–3, 1956.

KLEINSORGE, H.: Der Einfluß von Placenta-Zellinjektionen auf die tier-experimentelle Arteriosklerose. Bericht von d. 5. Tagg. d. Forschungskreises f. ZT. 11–14. 1958.

KLEMKE, R. E.: Zur Fehlsteuerung der Gen-Expression in den Zellkernen maligner Tumorzellen. K. F. Haug-Verl., Heidelberg 1981.

KLIMA, J.: Zytologie, G. Fischer, Stuttgart *1967.*

KLIMA, J.: Einführung in die Cytologie, Stuttgart, G. Fischer-Verlag, 1970.

KLUDAS, M.: Histologische Organschnitte von Meerschweinchen nach Injektion mit lyophilisierten Placenta-Zellen. Bericht v. d. 1. Tagg. d. Forschungsgem. f. ZT. 3–8. 1954.

KLUDAS, M. und RIESENBERG, J.: Über die Wirkungsdynamik der Zellulartherapie. Die Zellulartherapie, Niehans, P. Verlag Urban & Schwarzenberg, München/Berlin, 457–464. 1954.

KLUDAS, M.: Pharmakologische Wirkungen von Organpräparaten im Tierversuch. Bericht v. d. 5. Tagg. d. Forschungskreises f. ZT 59–64, 1958. Medizinische, Stuttgart, *41,* 1624–1629, 1958.

KMENT, A.: Der Revitalisierungsbegriff und seine tierexperimentelle Objektivierung. Gerontol. Symposium Lugano (1975).

KMENT, A.: Altern und Geriatica aus der Sicht der experimentellen Gerontologie Act. Gerontol. 8, 241–252 (1978).

KMENT, A.: Zur Physiologie des Hypothalamus. Die Zellther. *35,* 1–17 (1968).

KMENT, A.: Untersuchungen der Meerschweinchenschilddrüsen-Aktivität mit Radioisotopen (J 131) nach Siccacell-Präparaten. Bericht v. d. 5. Tagg. d. Forschungskreises f. ZT 33–40, 1958.

– Untersuchungen an Ratten über den Revitalisierungseffekt von Herzmuskelzellen, Herzmuskelkernen und Herzmuskelmitochondrien. 18. Kongreß f. ZT, 29./9. 73, Referatenblatt Die Zelltherapie Nr. 41, 1974.

– Scheidenepithelstudien an der Maus unter lyophilisiertem Organmaterial. Med. Klin., *53,* 645–647, 1958.

– Allgemeines über Zellstrukturen und ihre Funktionen. In F. Schmid und J. Stein: Zellforschung und Zellulartherapie, Verlag Huber, Bern 1963, S. 25–51.

– Die tierexperimentelle Objektivierung des Revitalisierungseffektes nach Zellinjektionen. In F. Schmid und J. Stein: Zellforschung und Zellulartherapie. Verlag Huber, Bern 1963, S. 407–479.

– Quantitative elektronenmikroskopische Studien an Herzmitochondrien der Ratte nach Injektionen von Placenta- oder Testis-Gewebe. Zschr. f. Tierphysiologie, Tierernährung und Futtermittelkunde Bd. 21, Heft 4, S. 206–210.

– the Objective Demonstration of the Revitalization Effect after Cell injections. In F.

Schmid and J. Stein: Cell Researche and Cellular Therapy. Ott Publishers Thoune. Switzerland, 1967. p. 401–476.

– General Aspects of Cell-Structures and their Functions. In F. Schmid and J. Stein: Cell Research and Cellular Therapy. Ott Publishers Thoune. Switzerland. 1967, p. 29–55.

KMENT, A.: Experimentell-gerontologische Untersuchungen der Revitalisierung. Cytobiol. Rev. 1, 4–9. (1977).

KMENT, A.: Aktivitätsstudien an Ratten unter Verwendung lyophilisierter Organpräparate. Therapiekongreß 12–16. 1956.

– Objective demonstration of revitalization by cell-injections in animals. Symposium on Cellular Therapy. Cairo, 1960.

KMENT, A.: Altern und Revitalisierung aus wissenschaftstheoretischer Sicht. Cytobiol. Rev. 7, 10–14 (1983).

KMENT, A. und HOFECKER, G.: Aktuelle Probleme der experimentellen Gerontologie. Wien. Tierärztl. Monatsschr. 64, 109–116 (1977).

KMENT, A., HOFECKER, G., NIEDERMÜLLER, H., und SKALICKY, M.: Neue Ergebnisse der Revitalisierungsforschung. Cytobiol. Rev. 3, 44–48 (1979).

KMENT, A., HOFECKER, G., NIEDERMÜLLER, H.u. SKALICKY, M.: Altern und Revitalisierung. Cytobiol. Rev. 6, 125–133 (1982)

KMENT, A., LEIBETSEDER, J. und STEININGER, K.: Versuche zur tierexperimentellen Objektivierung des Revitalisierungseffektes nach Zellinjektionen. Therap. Woche Karlsruhe, 11, 489–495, 1961.

KMENT, A., HOFECKER, G. und NIEDERMÜLLER, H.: Die Verteilung tritiummarkierter Herz-, Leber- und Nierenzellen bei alten Ratten. Inaugural-Diss. Tierärztl. Hochschule Wien. 1972.

KMENT, A. und NIEDERMÜLLER, H.: Untersuchungen über die Auswirkung der Revitalisierung bei Ratten auf die Resorption. Verteilung und Ausscheidung von Penizillin V. 17. Kongreß f. ZT. 24./25. 9. 72. Ref. Blatt «Die Zelltherapie» Nr. 40. August 1973.

KNÜCHEL, F.: Einige Untersuchungsmethoden zur Objektivierung und zur Erkennung des Schweregrades arteriosklerotischer Veränderungen. Bericht v. d. 5. Tagg.

d. Forschungskreises f. Zellulartherapie, 14f., 1958.

KNÜCHEL, F.: Encephalitis nach Frischzelleninjektion? Medizinische. Stuttgart, 8, 1956.

KNÜCHEL, F.: Harnsteroidausscheidung beim Menschen nach Injektion getrockneter Zellen tierischer innersekretorischer Drüsen. Bericht v. d. 2. Tagg. d. Forschungsgemeinschaft f. Zellulartherapie, 5–10, 1955.

– Untersuchungen über den Einfluß der Zellulartherapie auf die Funktion innersekretorischer Drüsen. Therapiekongreß, 2–5, 1955, Therapie-Woche, Karlsruhe, 6, 123–128, 1955.

– Über den Einfluß von Zellen des Endokrinium. Therapiekongreß, 6–9, 1956. Therapie-Woche, Karlsruhe, 7, 41–43, 1956.

KNÜCHEL, F.: Antikörperbildung nach parenteraler Zufuhr fetaler tierischer Organe. Verhandlg. d. dt. Ges. f. innere Med., 60. Kongreß. Verlag J. F. Bermann, München, 273–276, 1954.

KNÜCHEL, F. und KUHN, W.: Therapeutisch-experimentelle Ergebnisse nach Siccacell-Behandlung. Medizinische, Stuttgart, 16, 587–593, 1955.

KOCH, G. L. E.: The Anchorage Cell Surface Receptors to the Cytoskeleton. In: Internat. Cell Biol., p. 321–330; ed. H. G. SCHWEIGER, Springer-Verl. Berlin – Heidelberg – New York 1981.

KOLB, H. J.: Knochenmarktransplantationen bei Knochenmarkaplasie und akuter Leukämie – Voraussetzungen, Erfolge. Indikationen. Klin. Pädiatrie 189, 60–67 (1977).

KÖNIG, W.: Struktur und Funktion des eosinophilen Leukozyten. Immunität und Infektion 6, 97–105 (1978).

KOPFF, R.: Gerichtsärztliche Beurteilung von Todesfällen nach Frischzellenbehandlung. Jahrbuch d. Akademie f. Staatsmedizin. Düsseldorf, 102–109. 1959.

KORTING, G. W.: Die Zellulartherapie bei Hauterkrankungen. Bericht v. d. 4. Tagg. d. Forschungskreises f. Zellulartherapie. 12–16. 1957.

KÖSTERS, W.: Rückbildung diabetischer Glomerulusveränderungen nach Inselzell-Transplantationen. Fortschr. Med. 97, 825

(1979).

KOTSOVSKY, D.: Therapie von Alterserscheinungen mit embryonalen Wirkstoffen. Ärztl. Praxis. München, *V/40*, 1953.

KROKOWSI, E. und TIBURTIUS, H.: Möglichkeiten des biochemischen Strahlenschutzes für die Augenlinse. Strahlentherapie. Band 119, Heft 2. 1962.

KRSTIĆ, R. V.: Ultrastruktur der Säugetierzelle. Springer-Verlag, Berlin-Heidelberg-New York 1976.

KRÜPE, M.: Immunreaktionen. In: Handb. d. Biologie, Bd. II, S. 265. Konstanz, Akadem. Verlagsges. Athenaion, 1962.

KUGLER, J.: Hirnstoffwechsel und Hirndurchblutung, Schnetztor Verlag, Konstanz 1976.

KUHN, W.: Klinische Erfahrungen und statistische Erhebungen zur Zellulartherapie. Therapiekongreß, 5–11, 1955. Therapie-Woche, Karlsruhe, 6, 117–123, 1955.

– Zellulartherapie in Klinik und Praxis. Hippokrates-Verlag, Stuttgart, 1956.

KUHN, W. und KNÜCHEL, F.: Allgemeinbiologische und immunologische Untersuchungen zur Klärung der Wirkung von tierischen Organtrockenpräparaten. Die Zellulartherapie, Niehans, P. Verlag Urban & Schwarzenberg, München/Berlin, 414–456, 1954.

KUHN, W. und KNÜCHEL, F.: Zur Wirkung von Placenta-Trockengewebe auf arteriosklerotische Veränderungen. Med. Klin., *48*, 1363–1366, 1954.

KURLAND, C. G.: Functional Organization of the 30-S Ribosomal Subunit. In Nomura. Tissieres and Lengyel: Ribosomes. Cold Spring Harbor Laboratory 1974, S. 309–332.

KURTZAHN, H. und HÜBENER, H.: Schilddrüsenüberpflanzung durch Injektion. Zbl. Chir., 27. 1666–1696, 1927.

KÜTTNER, H.: Sitzungsbericht der Breslauer Chirurgischen Gesellschaft vom 22. 1. 1912. Zbl. Chir., 392, 1912.

KÜTTNER, H.: Die Injektionstransplantation endokriner Drüsen. Brun's Beitr. klin. Chir., Berlin. *145,* 721–723, 1929.

KWAPINSKI, J. B. G.: Methodology of Immunochemical and Immunological Research. Wiley-Interscience. New York/London/Sydney/Toronto, 1972.

L

LACY, D.: The morphology of the Golgi apparatus in neurons and epithelial cells of the common limpet patella vulgata. Proc. Europ. Conf. Electron Microscop. Stockholm 1956.

LAKE, J. A., SABATINI, D. D. and NOMURA, Y.: Ribosome Structure as studied by Electron Microscopy. In Nomura, Tissieres and Lengyel: Ribosomes. Cold Spring Harbor Laboratory 1974, S. 543–558.

LAMBERT, G.: Niehans ou la vieillesse vaincue. Libraire Artheme Fayard, Paris 1958.

LANDSBERGER, A.: Die Wirkung von Mastzellensubstanzen auf das Tumorwachstum. In F. Schmid und J. Stein: Zellforschung und Zellulartherapie. Verlag Huber, Bern 1963, S. 495.

– Results of Animal Experiment on Malignant Cells with Special Consideration of the Body's Own Tumor Defense. In F. Schmid and J. Stein: Cell Research und Cellular Therapy. Ott Publishers Thoune, Switzerland, 1967, p. 492.

– Morphologische Untersuchungen über die Wirkung der Zelltherapie mit Semi-Dünnschnitt-Technik und Elektronik-Mikroskopie. 17. Kongreß f. ZT, 23./24. 9. 72, Ref. Blatt «Die Zelltherapie» Nr. 40, August 1973.

– Licht- und elektronenmikroskopische Untersuchungen zur Zelltherapie. 18. Kongreß f. ZT. 29./30. 9. 1973. Referatenblatt Die Zelltherapie Nr. 41, Dezember 1974.

LANDSBERGER, A.: Aktivierung der körpereigenen Abwehr durch Zelltherapie. Die Heilkunst. 84. Jg. Heft 10. Okt 1971.

LANDSBERGER, A.: Zur Frage der Hirnregeneration durch Zelltherapie. Die Zelltherapie 42.. 19–21 (1975).

LANDSBERGER. A.: Tumortherapie durch Implantation fetaler xenogener Gewebe. Cytobiol. Rev. *2*, 7–9 (1978).

LANDSBERGER, A.: Krebstherapie – zugleich Immuntherapie. Cytobiol. Rev. *3,* 15–17 (1979).

LANDSBERGER, A.: Regeneration, Immunstimulation und Interferon-Induktion Cytobiol. Rev. *4*, 133–136 (1980).

LANDSBERGER, A.: Cancer Immunotherapy. Cytobiol. Rev. *4*, 76–79 (1980)

425

LANE, N. J. and NOVIKOFF, A. B.: Effects of arginine deprivation, ultraviolett radiation and X-radiation on cultured KB cells. A cytochemical and ultrastructural study. J. Cell Biolog. *27*, 603 (1965).

LANGENDORFF. W. LANGER VON: Die Bedeutung enzymatischer Aktivitäten der Placenta in ihrer Beziehung zur Zelltherapie. 5. Internat. Kongreß f. Zelltherapie (14. Arb. Tagg. dt. Ges.) 5./6. 77. 69 Referatenblatt Die Zelltherapie Nr. 36. Dez. 1969.

LANGENDORFF, W. LANGER VON: Vergleichende Versuche zur Revitalisierung von Zellen in vitro. 16. Kongreß f. ZT. 9./10. 10. 1971. Ref. Blatt Die Zelltherapie Nr. 39, August 1972.

LANGENDORFF, W. LANGER VON: Schutzwirkung der Zelltherapie gegen emphysembedingte Lungendegeneration. Re-Blatt Die Zelltherapie Nr. 41, 1974.

LANGENDORFF, W. LANGER VON: The Effect of Fetal Mesenchymal Cells on a Hodgkins-like Lymphoma Culture. Cytobiol. Rev. *2/* 1, 3–6 (1978).

LANGENDORFF, W. LANGER VON: The Effect of Fetal Mesenchyme Cells on the Morphology Growth Characteristics and Function of an Experimental Wilm's Tumor Culture. Cytobiol. Rev. *4*, 131/134 (1979).

LAUBE, H.: Inselzell-Autotransplantation. Ref.: Praxis-Kurier *21*, 4 (1979): 85. Tagung der Deutschen Gesellschaft für Innere Medizin, Wiesbaden, April 1979.

LAUDAHN, G.: Grundlagen und tierexperimentelle Untersuchungen zur Frage einer therapeutischen Anwendbarkeit isolierter Mitochondrien. Ärztl. Forschung. München, *10*, I/513–I/524, 1956.

LAUDAHN, G. und LÜDERS, C. J.: Die Wirkung isolierter Leberzellmitochondrien auf die akute Schädigung der Rattenleben durch Tetrachlorkohlenstoff. Arzneimittel Forsch., Aulendorf. *10*, 978–985. 1960.

LAWRENCE, H. S.: The cellular transfer of cutaneous hypersensitivity to tuberculin in man. Proc. Soc. exp. Biol. (N. Y.) *71*, 516 (1949).

LECHNER, E.: Quantitative elektronenmikroskopische Studien an Herzmitochondrien der Ratte nach Injektionen von Placenta- oder Hodengewebe. Inaugural-Diss., Tierärztl. Hochschule Wien. 1965.

LEHNINGER, A. L.: The Mitochondrion, W. A. Benjamin, New York *1964*.

LEIBIG, A.: Über die Behandlung von Arthrosen und Arthritiden mit Placenta. Medizinische, Stuttgart, *51*, 1823–1825, 1956.

LENDRUM, R., WALKER, G., CUDWORTH, A. G., THEOPHANIDES, C., PYKE, D. A., BLOOM, A. and GAMBLE, D. R.: Islet cell antibodies in diabetes mellitus. Lancet 11. 1273 (1976).

LEPOW, I. H., NAFF, G. B., TODD, E. W., PENSKY, J. and HINZ jr. C. F.: Chromatographic resolution of the first component into three activities. J. exp. Med. *177*, 983 (1963).

LETTRÉ, R.: Gewebekulturversuche mit Frisch- und Trockenzellen. Ber. v. d. 1. Tagg. der Forschungsgem. f. ZT, 1, 1954.
– Zellkonfrontation in der Gewebekultur. Bericht v. d. 2. Tagg. d. Forschungsgem. f. ZT. Frankfurt, 28–30, 1955.

LETTRÉ, H.: Versuche zur Klärung der Wirksamkeit der Zellulartherapie nach Niehans. Umschau in der Wissenschaft u. Technik, 23, 708 ff., 1954.
– Untersuchungen an Frisch- und Trockenzellen. Bericht v. d. 1. Tagg. d. Forschungsgemeinschaft Zellulartherapie, 2–3, 1954.

LETTRÉ, H.: Prüfung der organspezifischen Wirkung von Zellinjektionen. Therapiekongreß, 17–19, 1954. Therap. Woche, Karlsruhe, 5, 152–156. 1955.
– Experimentelle Studien über die Wirkung von Zellfragmenten. Bericht v. d. 2. Tagg. d. Forschungsgem. f. ZT. 30 f., 1955.

LINDER, G.: Untersuchung der Zellatmung von Herz, Niere und Leber bei Hühnern in Beziehung zum Lebensalter. Inaugural-Diss. Tierärztl. Hochschule Wien. 1961.

LINDMARK, D. G. a. MÜLLER, M.: Hydrogenosome, a cytoplasmic organelle of anaerobic flagellate Trichomonas foetus and its role in pyruvate metabolism. J. Biol. Chem. *248*, 7724–7728 (1973).

LINTZ, R. M.: Implantation of Placental Tissue in Patients with Rheumatoid Arthritis. Ann. Rheumat. Dis., London, *13*, 63–66, 1954.

LITTLEFIELD, J. W. and KELLER, E. B.: Incorporation of C^{14} amino acids into ribonucleoprotein particles from the Ehrlich mouse ascites tumor. J. Biol. Chem. *224*,

13 (1957).

LORENZ, E., UPHOFF, D., REID, T. R. and SHELTON, H.: Modification of irridiation injury in mice and guineapigs by bone marrow injections. J. of NCl *12*, 197 (1951).

LORENZ, E. and CONGDON, C. C.: Modification of Letal Irradiation Injury in Mice by Injection of Homologous or Heterologous Bone. J. Nat. Cancer Inst. Wash., *14*, 955–961, 1954.

M

MACKENZIE, C. D., RAMALHO-PINTO, F. J., MCLAREN, D. J. and SMITHERS, S. R.: Antibody-mediated adherence of rat eosinophils to shistosomula of shistoma mansoni in vitro. Clin. exp. Immunol. *30*, 97 (1977).

MARCOLONGE, R. and DI PAOLA, N.: Fetal Thymic Transplant in Patients with Hodgkins Disease. Blood *41*, 625 (1973).

MARGRAF, O.: Minder- und Zwergwuchs, Cytobiol. Rev. *3*, 122–123 (1979).

MARQUARDT, P. und FRANZ, G.: Zur Wirkung von Trockenzellpräparaten bei intravenöser Injektion. Arzneimittel-Forschung. Aulendorf,*11*, 544 f., 1961.

MARSHAK, A. und WALKER, A. C.: Effect of Liver Fractions on Mitosis in Regenerating Liver. Amer. J. Physiol., *149*, 226–234, 1946.

MAUGH, TH. H. und MARX, J. L.: Zerstörendes Wachstum, G. Thieme Verlag, Stuttgart 1979.

MCLAREN, D. J., MACKENZIE, C. D. and RAMALHO-PINTO, F. J.: Ultrastructural observations on the in vitro interaction between rat eosinophils and parasitic helminths. Clin. exp. Immun. *30*, 105 (1977).

MEDAWAR, P. B.: Immunological tolerance: Nobel lecture. Nature *189*, 14 (1961).

MEHNERT, H.: Stoffwechselkrankheiten. Thieme-Verlag, Stuttgart 1975.

MEISS, L., RONIEN, CL. und SERON, B.: Immuntherapie des Krebses. Dtsch. med. Wschr. *98* 1, 1179 (1973).

MERTELMANN, R., KOCH, G., SCHUMPELICK, V. und TACHEZY, H.: Implantation von fetalem Thymusgewebe bei Patienten mit progredienten bösartigen Geschwulstkrankheiten. Münch. med. Wschr. *166*, 2063–2066 (1974).

METCHNIKOFF, E.: Lectures on the Comparative Pathology of Inflammation. London 1893.

METSCHNIKOFF, E.: L'inflammation. Paris 1892. – Immunität bei Infektionskrankheiten. Jena: Gustav Fischer 1902.

MEYER, W.: Experimentelle Pankreastransplantation. Fortschr. Med. *97*, 1280–1284 (1979).

MIEHLKE, K.: Hypophysen-Implantation bei chronischer Polyarthritis. Ärztl. Praxis, München, *V/37*, 1953. Ber. v. d. I. Tagg. d. Arb. Gem. f. Zellulartherapie, Frankfurt, 9–12, 1953.

– Zur Behandlung der Arthrosis. Ber. v. d. 4. Tagg. d. Arbeitsgem. f. Zellulartherapie, Bad Homburg, 22–24, 1955.

MILLER, E. C. and MILLER, A.: Approaches to the mechanisms and control of chemical carcinogenesis. In: Environment and Cancer. Williams and Wilkins, Baltimore 1972.

MILLER, J. F. A. P.: Immunological function of the thymus: Lancet 1961 II: 748.

MILLER, I. F. A. P. und DUKOR, P.: Die Biologie des Thymus nach dem Stand der heutigen Forschung. Frankfurt: Akad. Verlagges. 1964.

MILLER, F.: Acid phosphatase localisation in renal protein absorption droplets. Proc. Intern. Congr. Electron. Microscopy. 5th Philadelphia Academic. Press. Inc. New York 1962.

MOENCH, A.: Der Einfluß heterologer Gewebetrockenzellen auf die experimentelle Nephritis des Kaninchens. Bericht v. d. 2. Tagg. d. Forschungsgem. f. ZT. 49, 1955.

MOENCH, A. und BURCKHARD: Über die Wirkung von Siccacell und Kaninchentrokkenserum auf die experimentelle Neosalvarsan-Nephrose der weißen Ratte. Bericht v. d. 4. Tagg. d. Forschungskreises f. ZT, 6–8, 1957.

MÖLBERT, E.: Die Orthologie und Pathologie der Zelle. Handb. allgem. Pathol. Band II/5. 238–466. Springer-Verlag, Berlin-Heidelberg-New York 1968.

MÖLBERT, F.: Das endoplasmatische Reticulum. In H. W. Altmann u. a., Handb. allgem. Pathol. II/5. Die Zelle, S. 336–403. Springer-Verlag, Berlin-Heidelberg-New York 1968.

MÖSE, J. R.: Serologische Untersuchungen bei Behandlung mit lyophilisierten Organzellen oder Organextrakten. Vorträge beim II. Intern. Kongreß f. Zell- und Histotherapie, Wiesbaden. I. 54–62, 1959.

– Beeinflußbarkeit von Heterohämolysinen und Normal-Bakterien-Agglutininen durch Behandlung mit lyophilisierten Organzellen. Vortrag anl. d. III. Intern. Kongr. f. ZT, Paris, 1961.

MÖSE, J. R., WENNIG, F. und STEIN, O.: Änderung des Heterohämagglutinationstiters nach Injektion lyophilisierter Organzellen. Medizinische, Stuttgart, 31/32, 1200–1202, 1958.

MOMMSEN, H.: Über die Behandlung des Mongolismus mit Frischzellen. Ber. v. d. 4.Tagg. der Arbeitsgem. f. Zellulartherapie, Bad Homburg, 25–27, 1955.

– Hippokrates, Stuttgart, 27, 619–623. 1956.

– Zellulartherapie bei entwicklungsgestörten Kindern. Ber. v. d. 4. Tagg. d. Forschungskreises f. Zellulartherapie, 61 f., 1957.

– Die Zellulartherapie des Mongolismus. Ärztl. Praxis, München, XIII/II, 646 f., 1961.

MOORE, F. D.: Transplantation. Springer, Berlin/Heidelberg/New York. 1970.

MORGAN, W. T. J. and WATKINS, W. M.: Biochemistry of human bloodgroup substances. Brit. med. Bull. 1959, 112.

MOUNT, H. T. R.: Multiple Sclerosis and other demyelinating diseases. Canadian Med. Ass. J. 108, 1356–1358 (1973).

MÜLLER, O.: Antikörper- und Autoantikörperbildung nach intraperitonealer Injektion von heterologen lyophilisierten Zellen. Inaug.-Diss. a. d. Albert-Ludwigs-Univ., Freiburg, 1956.

MÜLLER, E. A.: Die Anwendung der Frischzellentherapie nach Dr. Niehans bei Endangiitis obliterans. Med. Klin., 48, 1294 f., 1953.

MÜLLER, I.: Selbstversuch mit Resistocell. Cytobiol. Rev. 2/2, 30 (1978).

MÜLLER, L. FELIX: Therapieversuche mit Lebermitochondrien beim experimentellen Tetrachlorkohlenstoff-Schaden des Hundes. Berliner Münchener tierärztl. Wschr. 74, 130–132, 1961.

MÜLLER-EBERHARD, H. J.: Chemical aspects of human complement components IInd Internat. Symp. Immunopath. p. 23. Basel u. Stuttgart, Benno Schwabe & Co. 1962.

N

NEUBERT, H.: Frischzellentherapie beim Diabetes mellitus. V. Wissen. Kongreß München 1978, Kongreßbericht S. 25–48.

NEUBERT, H.: Wissenswertes über langjährige Erfahrungen stationärer Frischzellentherapie. Biolog. Medizin 8, 436–447 (1979).

NEUBERT, H.: Einsatz der Zelltherapie bei Diabetes mellitus. Cytobiol. Rev. 6, 22–27 (1982)

NEUMANN, K. H.: Versuche zur therapeutischen Wirksamkeit von Frisch- und Trockenzellen, getestet an ovariektomierten Mäusen. Ber. v. d. 1. Tagg. d. Forschungsgem. f. ZT, 10 f., 1954.

– Konservierungsverfahren, Herstellung und Eigenschaften von Trockengewebe. In F. Schmid und J. Stein: Zellforschung und Zellulartherapie Verlag Huber, Bern 1963, S. 72–99.

– Pharmakologische Grunduntersuchungen zur Zellulartherapie. In F. Schmid und J. Stein: Zellforschung und Zellulartherapie. Verlag Huber, Bern 1963, S. 101–124.

– Methods of Conservation and Preparation of Desiccated Tissues and their Properties. In F. Schmid and J. Stein: Cell Research and Cellular Therapy. Ott Publishers Thoune. Switzerland, 1967, p. 83–108.

– Basic Pharmacological Studies concerning Cellular Therapy. In F. Schmid and J. Stein: Cell Research and Cellular Therapy. Ott Publishers Thoune, Switzerland. 1967, p. 110–132.

NEUMANN, K. H.: Gefriertrocknung und ihre Leistungen für die Konservierung von Organpräparaten. Zellulartherapie in Klinik u. Praxis, Kuhn, W. Hippokrates-Verlag, Stuttgart, 39–69, 1956.

– Untersuchungen über die therapeutische Wirksamkeit von Injektionen von Nierengewebe bei experimentell erzeugter Nephrose. Ber. v. d. 6. Tagg. d. Arbeitsgem. f. ZT, Bad Homburg, 1–3, 1957.

– Über die Wirkung von Trockenzelleninjek-

tionen auf Gewicht und Bau einzelner Organe der Maus. Bericht von der 5. Tagg. d. Forschungskreises f. ZT, 54–59, 1958.
- Induktion des Organwachstums durch Implantation von homologen Geweben. Vorträge beim II. Intern. Kongreß f. Zell- und Histotherapie, Wiesbaden, I. 62–68, 1959.
- Induktion des Organwachstums durch Implantation von homologen Geweben. In F. Schmid und J. Stein: Zellforschung und Zellulartherapie. Verlag Huber, Bern 1963, 328–335.
- Beeinflussung experimenteller Leberschädigung durch Gewebeinjektionen. In F. Schmid und J. Stein: Zellforschung und Zellulartherapie, Verlag Huber, Bern 1963, S. 366–376.
- Induction of Growth in Organs by the Implantation of Homologous Tissues. In F. Schmid und J. Stein: Cell Research and Cellular Therapy. Ott Publishers Thoune, Switzerland, 1967, p. 331–337.
- The Influence of Tissue Injections on Experimental Liver Damage. In F. Schmid and J. Stein: Cell Research and Cellular Therapy. Ott Publishers, Thoune, Switzerland, 1967, p. 368–377.
NIEDERMÜLLER, H.: Untersuchungen an der Ratte über die Resorption, Verteilung und Ausscheidung von Penicillin V in Abhängigkeit vom Lebensalter und nach Revitalisierung. Inaugural-Diss. Tierärztl. Hochschule, Wien 1972.
NIEHANS, P.: Die endokrinen Drüsen und die Methoden der Verjüngung. Vortrag am XV. Schweiz. Chirurgen-Kongreß. Verlag Benno Schwabe, Basel, 1928.
- Les glandes endocrines et les méthodes de rajeunissement. Verlag Benno Schwabe, Basel 1930.
- Krebs und endokrine Drüsen. Benno Schwabe, Basel 1933.
- Das Alter, seine Beschwerden und die Verjüngung. Hans Huber, Bern 1936.
- Die endokrinen Drüsen des Gehirns. Hans Huber, Bern 1938.
- Krebs-Krankheit. Hans Huber, Bern 1945.
- Biologische Behandlung kranker Organe bei Menschen und Tieren. Hans Huber, Bern 1948.
- Biologische Behandlung kranker Organe durch Einspritzen lebender Zellen. Verlag

A. Schmid & Co, Bern 1949.
- Die Zellulartherapie (Lehrbuch). Verlag Urban & Schwarzenberg, München 1954.
- Einführung in die Zellulartherapie. Hans Huber, Bern 1957.
- Introduction to Cellular Therapy. Coopers Square Publ., New York 1960.
NIETHAMMER, D., BIENZLE, U., KLEIHAUER, E.: Knochenmarktransplantation. Erg. Pädiatr. Onkologie 1, 70–73 (1977).
NIETHAMMER, D.: Behandlung mit immunologisch kompetenten Zellen und Zellextrakten. Monatsschr. Kinderheilk. 127, 381–388 (1979).
NIKOLOWSKI, W.: Behandlung männlicher Potenzstörungen. Therapie-Woche, Karlsruhe, Kongreßausgabe, 604–608, 1956.
NOMURA, M., TISSIÈRES, A. and LENGYEL, P.: Ribosomes. Cold Spring Harbor Laboratory 1974.
NOMURA, M. and HELD, W. A.: Reconstitution of Ribosomes: Studies of Ribosome Structure, Function and Assembly. In Nomura, Tissières and Lengyel: Ribosomes. Cold Spring Harbor Laboratory 1974, S. 193–224.
NOSSAL, G. I. V. and MITCHELL, JUDITH: The nature of RNA synthesis in immune induction. Immunpathologie. IIIrd Internat. Symposium. S. 113. Basel u. Stuttgart, Benno Schwabe & Co. 1963.

O

OBERLING, CH.: The structure of cytoplasm. Int. Rev. Cytol. 8, 1 (1959).
OETZMANN, H. J.: La thérapeutique cellulaire dans les maladies hépatiques. Rapports du 2ème Congrès Français de Thérapeutique Cellulaire, Tours. Edit. de Centre Méd. d'Etudes et de Rech., Paris 49–53, 1958.
- Kritisches zur Zellulartherapie chronischer Leberererkrankungen. Vorträge beim II. Intern. Kongreß f. Zell- und Histotherapie, Wiesbaden I, 69–73, 1959.
OHNISHI, T.: Gann 49, 233 (1958). Peroxidbildung im Gewebe, zit. Bersin.
OLBRISCH, R. R.: Plastische Chirurgie bei mongoloiden Kindern. Fortschr. Med. 97, 1475–1477 (1979).
OPITZ, H. und SCHMID, F.: Handbuch der

Kinderheilkunde, Bd. IV, Springer-Verlag, Berlin-Heidelberg-New York 1965.

OPPERDOES, F. R. a. BORST, P.: Localization of nine glycolytic enzymes in microbody-like organelle in Trypanosoma brucei The glycosome. FEBS Lett. *80*, 360–364 (1977)

ORTIZ, R. F.: Evaluacion de la Citoterapia en los Retrasos del Desarrollo físico e intelectual del niño. Mexico 1973.

– Sinopsis de terapeutica celular. Mexico 1971.

– Citaterapia en las Enfermedades reumáticas. Mexico 1974: Cytobiol. Revue 4, H. 3 (1980).

P

PALADE, G. E.: A small particulate component of the cytoplasm. J. Biophys. Biochem. Cytol. *1*, 59 (1955).

PALADE, G. E.: A study of fixation for electron microscopy. J. exp. Med. *95*, 285 (1952).

PALADE, G. E.: Studies on the endoplasmatic reticulum. II. Simple dispositions in cells in situ. J. biophys. biochem. Cytol. *1*, 567 (1955).

PALADE, G. E.: Relations between the endoplasmatic reticulum and the plasma membrane in macrophages. Anat. Rec. *121*, 445 (1955).

PAPPENHEIMER, A. M.: The Golgi apparatus: personal observations and a review of the literature. Anat. Rec. *11*, 107 (1916).

PARADE, G. W.: Somatophysische Wirkungen der Epithelkörperchenüberpflanzung. Beiträge zur Zellulartherapie. Festschrift zum 70. Geburtstag von P. Niehans. Verlag Urban & Schwarzenberg, München/Berlin, 34–43, 1952.

PARAT, M.: Appareil de Golgi, vacoume, colorations vitales pH intracellulaire, Arch. exp. Zellforschg. *6*, 109 (1928).

PARKMANN, R., RAPPOPORT, J., CASSADY, R., LEVEY, R., NATHAN, D. G. and ROSEN, R. S.: Correction of the Wiskott-Aldrich-Syndrome by Bone-Marrow-Transplantation. New Engl. J. Med. *298*, 921–927 (1978).

PEDRERO, A. e SCHMID, F.: Down-Syndrom (span) Cytobiol. Rev. *5*, 197–211 (1981).

PETERMANN, M. L., HAMILTON, M. G. and MIZEN, N. A.: Elektrophoretic analysis of the macromolecular nucleoprotein particles of mammalian cytoplasm. Cancer Res. *14*, 360 (1954).

PFEIFFER, I.: Die lebende Zelle, Time-Life, International (Nederland) 1965.

PICOURET, A.: La thérapeutique cellulaire dans les artérites des membres inférieurs. Rapports du 2ème Congrès Français de Thérapeutique Cellulaire, Tours. Edit. du Centre Méd. d'Etudes et de Rech., Paris, 36–43, 1958.

– La thérapeutique cellulaire dans les affections vasculaires des membres inférieurs. Rapports du 3ème Congrès Français de Théapeutique Cellulaire, Paris. Edit. du Centre Méd. d'Etudes et de Rech., Paris, 41–51, 1959.

PISCHINGER, A.: Schicksal und Wirkung körperfremden Gewebes im Organismus. Stuttgart, *23*, 767–771, 1953.

PISCHINGER, A.: Frischzellentherapie. Zur Kritik der Theorie und zum Wesen der Frischzellentherapie nach Niehans. Wien, med. Wschr., *105*, 952–957, 1955.

PLICARD, A. et BESSIS, M.: Etude sur l'élément vivant en pathologie cellulaire l'emploi de la microcinématographie en contraste de phase. Rev. Hémat. *8*, 57 (1953).

POLICARD, A., BESSIS, M., BRETON-GONUS, J. et THIERY, J. P.: Polarité de la centrosphère et des corps de Golgi dans Exp. Cell Res. *14*, 221 (1958).

POLLISTER, A. W. and POLLISTER, P. F.: The structure of the Golgi apparatus. Int. Rev. Cytol. *6*, (1957).

PORTER, K. R.: The fine structure of cells. Fed. Proc. *14*, 673 (1955).

PORTER, K. R.: Current views of the cytoskeleton. Pediatric Research Vol. 12, Nr. 4, Part 2. Williams & Wilkins Co, Baltimore 1978.

PORTER, K. R. und BONNEVILLE, M. A.: Einführung in die Feinstruktur von Zellen und Geweben, Springer-Verlag, Berlin-Heidelberg-New York 1965.

PREHN, R.: Immunological surveillance: pro and contra. In: GOOD and BACH. Clinical Immunbiology, Bd. II, Academic Press, New York 1974.

Q

QUADBECK, G., LANDMANN, H. R., SACHSSE, W. und SCHMIDT, J.: Der Einfluß von Pyrithioxin auf die Bluthirnschranke. Medicina experim. *7*, 144–154 (1962).

R

RANSWEILER, V.: Tierexperimentelle Untersuchungen über die therapeutische Wirksamkeit von Trockenzellen. Inaugural-Dissertation, Med. Fakultät der Universität Heidelberg, 1960.
RAPP, F.: Herpesvirus and cancer. Advanc. Cancer Res. *19*, 265 (1974).
RAPPOLD: Erfordern die Gefahren der Zellulartherapie im Lande NRW gesetzliche Schutzvorschriften? Österr. Zschr. Kinderheilk., *19*, 204–206, 1957.
READING, CH. M., MCLEAY, A. and NOBILE, S.: Down's Syndrome and Thiamine Deficiency. Journ. Orthomol. Psych. *8*, 4–12 (1979).
REITZ, W. und SCHOOP, W.: Ein tödlich verlaufener anaphylaktischer Schock nach Trockenzellinjektion. Medizinische Stuttgart *13*, 416f., 1957.
RENNER, H.: Onko-fetale antigene und Tumor-Immuntherapie. Fortschr. Med. *92*, Nr. 5 (1974).
RENNER, H.: Immunologische Wirkung fetaler Zellen. Cytobiol. Rev. *1*, 24–26 (1977).
RENNER, H.: Klinische Aspekte einer Tumor-Immuntherapie mit lyophilisierten fetalen Zellen. Cytobiol. Rev. *3*, 3–6 (1979).
RENNER, K. H., RUNGE, T. u. ZEINZ, M.: Erfahrungen mit Resistocell als Zusatztherapie beim metastasierenden Mamma-Carcinom. Cytobiol. Rev. *4*, 109–114 (1980).
REVEL, J. P. and HAY, E. D.: An autographic and electron microscopic study of collagen synthesis in differentiating cartilage. Z. Zellforschg. *61*, 110 (1963).
REZEPECKI, R. M., LUKASIEWICZ, M., ALEKSANDROWICZ, J., SNAGIEL, Z., SKOTNICKI, A. and LISIEWICZ, J.: Thymus Transplantation in Leukemia and malignant Lymphogranulomatosis. Lancet 1973/I, 508.
RIEKKINEN, P. J. and CLAUSEN, J.: Proteinase Activity of Myelin. Brain Research *15*, 413–430 (1969).
RIES, W. et al.: Methodische Probleme bei der Ermittlung des biologischen Alters. Innere Medizin *4*, 109 (1976).
RIESEN, W. F. und BARANDUN, S.: Struktur und Funktion von Antikörpern. Allergologie *2*, 153–159 (1979).
RIETSCHEL, H. G.: Problematik und Klinik der Zelltherapie, Verlag Urban und Schwarzenberg, München-Berlin (1957).
RIETSCHEL, H. G.: Frischzellentherapie und ihre Gefahren. Wien, med. Wschr. *105/46*, 1955.
– Nutzen und Gefahren der Frischzellentherapie. Therapiekongreß. 9–12, 1954. Therapie-Woche, Karlsruhe, *5*, 161–170, 1955.
– Ein Zwischenfall bei der Zellulartherapie. Erfahrungsheilkunde, *5*, 177–180, 1956.
ROBERTS, A. N. and HAUROWITZ, F.: Intracellular localization and quantitation of tritated antigens in reticuloendothelial tissues of mice during secondary and hyperimmune responses. J. exp. Med. *116*, 4 (1962).
ROBERTS, R. B.: Microsomal particles and protein synthesis. Pergamon Press. New York 1958.
ROBINSON, D.: Enzyme *18*, 114–134 (1974)
ROCHELS, R.: Anthropometrische Untersuchungen zum Down-Syndrom, Cytobiol. Rev. *5*, 65–74, 129–134, 179–183 (1981)
RODEMANN, H. P. und BAYREUTHER, Ks.: Die Zellteilungskapazität von menschlichen diploiden Fibroblasten und Gliazellen in quantitativen Gewebekultursystemen unter dem Einfluß von Centrophenoxin. In Kugler, J.: Hirnstoffwechsel und Hirndurchblutung. Schnetztor-Verlag. Konstanz 1976, S. 32.
ROEDER, F.: Über die maximale Behandlung des Parkinsonsyndroms. Wiss. Beiblatt zur Materia Medica Nordmark. Nr. 59, April 1967.
ROEDER, K. H.: Behandlung eines Falles von chronischer Nephritis mit hochgradiger Nephrose mit Trockenzellsubstanz nach Dr. P. Niehans, Med. Klin. *47*, 1572, 1962.
ROITT, I.: Immunologie, Dr. Dietrich Steinkopff, Darmstadt 1977.
ROMEIS, B.: Mikroskopische Technik. R. Oldenbourg Verlag, München 1978.

ROTHER, CL.: Experimentelle immunbiologische Studien nach der Verwendung von Niehans-Trockenzellen. Ber. v. d. 3. Tagg. d. Forschungsgemeinschaft f. ZT. 33–34, 1955.
– Sensibilisierungsvorgänge nach Niehans-Zellulartherapie. Bericht v. d. 3. Tagg. d. Forschungsgemeinschaft f. ZT. 3–5, 1956.
ROTHER, K.: Komplement. Dr. Dietrich Steinkopff Verlag, Darmstadt 1974.
ROTHER, K.: Schäden durch direkte Bindung von Antikörpern am Gewebe. Allergologie 2, 160–167 (1979).
RÜMELIN, K.: Zur Prophylaxe und Therapie allergisch-anaphylaktischer Reaktionen. 5. Intern. Kongr. f. Zelltherapie (14. Arb. Tagg. Dt. Ges.) 5./6. 7. 1969. Ref. Blatt Die Zelltherapie Nr. 37, 1969.
RUMPF, K. D.: Methoden zur Funktionskontrolle transplantierter Langerhansscher Inseln. Langenbecks Arch. Chir. 343, 293–305 (1977).
– Transplantation isolierter Langerhansscher Inseln zur Diabetes-Behandlung. Fortschr. Med. 96, 1227–1232 (1978).
RUPP, J.: Kritisches zur Frischzellentherapie, Ärztl. Praxis. München. VII/47, 1955. Ärztl. Mitt., Köln, 40/47, 1955.

Sch

SCHAFFER, J.: Über das Vorkommen eosinophiler Zellen im menschlichen Thymus. Zbl. Med. Wiss. 29, 401 (1891).
SCHEIB, D.: Properties and role of acid hydrolases of the Müllerian ducts during sexual differentiation in the male chickembryo in A. V. S. de Reuck and M. P. Cameron (eds.), Ciba Found, Symp. Lysosomes, J. and A. Churchill, Ltd. London 1963, p. 264.
SCHLANGE, H.: Die passive Übertragung der Tuberkulinempfindlichkeit durch Blutaustauschtransfusionen und die Übertragung der erworbenen Tuberkulinnegativität. Arch. Kinderheilk. 148, 2 (1954).
SCHMID, F.: Schicksal und Wirkung injizierter Fremdgewebe. Vorträge beim II. Intern. Kongreß f. Zell- und Histotherapie, Wiesbaden, I, 85–88, 1959.
– Haben injizierte Zellsuspensionen eine spezifische Wirkung? Rotterdamse gesprekken over celtherapie. Ned. Uitgeversmaatschappij N. V., Leiden, 97–194, 1960.
– Aufnahme und Verteilungsprinzipien injizierter Fremdgewebe. Vortrag anläßlich d. III. Intern. Kongr. f. ZT, Paris 1961.
– Nachweis biochemischer Substanzen in frischentnommenen und lyophilisierten fetalen Geweben. In F. Schmid und J. Stein: Zellforschung und Zellulartherapie, Verlag Huber, Bern 1963, S. 126.
– Demonstration of Biochemical Substances in Fresh and Lyophilized Tissues. In F. Schmid and J. Stein: Cell Research and Cellular Therapy. Ott Publishers Thoune. Switzerland, 1967, p. 134.
SCHMID, F.: Tierexperimentelle Untersuchungen über die Organspezifität von injizierten Zellsuspensionen. Bericht v. d. 5. Tagg. d. Forschungskreises f. ZT. 41–44. 1958.
– Les cellules fraîches et sèches ont-elles une action spécifique aux organes? Rapports du 3ème Congrès Français de Thérapeutique Cellulaire, Paris. Edit. du Centre Méd. d'Etudes et de Rech., Paris, 3–10, 1959.
– Wirkung und Wirkungsspezifität auf leukämische Blutbildverschiebungen. In F. Schmid und J. Stein: Zellforschung und Zellulartherapie. Verlag Huber, Bern 1963, S. 275.
– Aufnahme und Verteilungsprinzipien injizierter Fremdgewebe. In F. Schmid und J. Stein: Zellforschung und Zellulartherapie. Verlag Huber, Bern 1963, S. 135–145.
– Effect and Specific Effectiveness on the Change of the Blood Picture in Leukemia. In F. Schmid and J. Stein: Cell Research and Cellular Therapy. Ott Publishers Thoune, Switzerland, 1967, p. 280.
– Acceptance and Distribution-Patterns of Injected Foreign Tissues. In F. Schmid and J. Stein: Cell Research and Cellular Therapy. Ott Publishers Thoune, Switzerland, 1967, p. 143–152.
SCHMID, F.: Biologische Aspekte der Leukose-Behandlung. Kinderärztl. Praxis. Leipzig, 26, 485–493, 1958.
– Experimentelle Grundlagen der Therapie mit Geweben und Gewebsfraktionen. Die Therapiewoche 12, 11, 1962.
– Wachstumsimpulse heterologer Gewebe

in der Gewebekultur. In F. Schmid und J. Stein: Zellforschung und Zellulartherapie. Verlag Huber, Bern 1963, S. 386–396.
– Growth-Stimulation of Heterologous Tissues in Tissue Cultures. In F. Schmid and J. Stein: Cell Research and Cellular Therapy. Ott Publishers Thoune, Switzerland, 1967, p. 388–397.
Schmid, F.: Der immunologische Mechanismus der Zelle. In F. Schmid und J. Stein: Zellforschung und Zellulartherapie. Verlag Huber, Bern 1963, S. 219–231.
– The Immunological Mechanism of the Cell. In F. Schmid and J. Stein: Cell Research and Cellular Therapy. Ott Publishers Thoune, Switzerland, 1967, p. 226–235.
– Fundamental Immunological Principles. In F. Schmid and J. Stein: Cell Research and Cellular Therapy. Ott Publishers Thoune, Switzerland, 1967, p. 157–203.
Schmid, F.: Prof. Dr. Paul Niehans (Aktuelle Übersicht). Fortschr. Med. 86. J., Nr. 24, 1968.
– Zelltherapie: Analyse und Aspekte. Selecta Nr. 19 Jg. XIV v. 8. 5. 1972.
Schmid, F.: Das Mongolismus-Syndrom. Hansen u. Hansen, Münsterdorf 1976.
Schmid, F.: Das Mongolismus-Syndrom. Sammelsonderdruck aus Fortschr. d. Med., Jg. 87, 29: 1185, 1204; 30:1248, 1252, 31:1324, 1969.
– Mehrschichtige Therapie bei Mehrfachbehinderten. Ref. Blatt Die Zelltherapie Nr. 40, Aug. 1973 und Phys. Med. und Rehabilitation, 3. Jg., Juni 1972, Heft 6.
– Therapeutischer Nihilismus beim Mongolismus ist heute nicht mehr zu verantworten. Medical Tribune, Jg. 9, Nr. 10 vom 8. 3. 1974.
Schmid, F.: Das apallische Syndrom, Cytobiol. Rev. 1, 10–16 (1977).
Schmid, F.: Die Zelle als biologische Elementareinheit. Cytobiol. Rev. 1, 40–42 (1977).
Schmid, F.: Fetaler Hautextrakt – ein neues therapeutisches Prinzip. Cytobiol. Rev. 1, 35–39 (1977).
Schmid, F.: Down's Syndrome. Treatment and Management. Cytobiol. Rev. 2, 25–32 (1978).
Schmid, F.: Zelltherapie – Experimentelle

Grundlagen und Klinik. Cytobiol. Rev. 2, 3–11 (1978).
Schmid, F.: Cytomembranen. Cytobiol. Rev. 2, 20–23 (1978).
Schmid, F.: Mitochondrien. Cytobiol. Rev. 2, 17–19 (1978).
Schmid, F.: Ribosomen. Cytobiol. Rev. 2, 28–32 (1978).
Schmid, F.: Lysosomen. Cytobiol. Rev. 2, 23–30 (1978).
Schmid, F.: Der Golgi-Apparat, Cytobiol. Rev. 3, 70–74 (1979).
Schmid, F.: Centriolen, Cytobiol. Rev. 3, 105–107 (1979).
Schmid, F.: Geistige und Mehrfachbehinderungen: Konzept einer Behandlungs-Systematik. Cytobiol. Rev. 2, 3–22 (1978).
– Antigene. Fortschr. Med. 82, 475 (1964).
– Antigene Determinanten. Fortschr. Med. 82, 684–685 (1964).
– Antikörper. Fortschr. Med. 82, 644–645 (1964).
– Antigen-Antikörper-Beziehungen. Fortschr. Med. 82, 774–775 (1964).
– Das Immunsystem. In Mikroökologie und Therapie. Vol. 7, 1977, S. 20–31. Institut für Mikroökologie D-6348 Herborn.
– Die generalisierten Tuberkulosen, Literaturzusammenstellung «RES und Immunität». Stuttgart: Georg Thieme 1951.
– Klinische Aspekte des Mesenchymproblems. Med. Welt 1960, 1207.
– Immunobiologie. In Handbuch der Kinderheilkunde. Bd. V, S. 646. Berlin-Göttingen-Heidelberg: Springer 1963.
– Das «aktive Mesenchym», Fortschr. Med. 82, 446 (1964).
– Lebensprofil der Immunabwehr. Mkurse ärztl. Fortbild. 15, 76 (1965); – Selecta 1965.
Schmid, F.: Staffelung der immunologischen Abwehrvorgänge. Dtsch. Ärzteblatt, 63, 3009 (1966).
– Immunmangelzustände. Pädiatr. Praxis 14, 555 (1974).
– Cytobiologie der Immunocyten. Die gelben Hefte 12, 481 (1966).
Schmid, F.: Konstitutionsanomalien des Skelettes. Handb. Inn. Med. VI/1 B, 981–1055. Herausgeb. Kuhlencordt, F. und Bartelheimer, H. Springer Verlag Berlin-Heidelberg-New York 1980.

SCHMID, F.: Immunbiologische Synopsis. Cytobiol. Rev. *4*, 3–44 (1980)

SCHMID, F.: Cell Therapy-Experimental Basis and Clinics. Cytobiol. Rev. *4*, 63–69 (1980).

SCHMID, F.: Zelltherapie – die Medizin der Zukunft. Cytobiol. Rev. *4*, 141–143 (1980)

SCHMID, F.: Das Gehirn; Entwicklung, Morphogenese und Funktion. Cytobiol. Rev. *5*, 51–64 (1981)

SCHMID, F.: Elemente als Determinanten biologischer Strukturen. Cytobiol. Rev. *5*, 122–128 (1981)

SCHMID, F.: Down-Syndrom: Situationsanalyse (Situation analysis). Cytobiol. Rev. *5*, 184–196 (1981)

SCHMID, F.: Down-Syndrom: Behandlung und Betreuung – Treatment und Care (deutsch u. englisch); Cytobiol. Rev. *6*, 28–41 (1982)

SCHMID, F.: Down-Syndrom – Grundlagenforschung. Cytobiol. Rev. *6*, 140–152 (1982)

SCHMID, F.: Mineralien und Spurenelemente in lyophilisierten Geweben. Cytobiol. Rev. *6*, 89–95 (1982).

SCHMID, F.: Die degenerativen Krankheiten der weißen Gehirnsubstanz; The degenerative diseases of the white brain matter. Cytobiol. Rev. *6*, 189–197 (1982).

SCHMID, F. et al.: Beeinflussung der mongoloiden Dyszephalie durch Injektionsimplantationen fetaler, heterologer Gehirngewebe. Fortschr. Med., 1181–1186 (1972).

SCHMID, F. und HAGGE, W.: Beeinflussung unspezifischer Zellreaktionen durch die Tuberkulose-Allergie. Beitr. Klin. Tuberk. *109*, 139–142 (1953).

SCHMID, F., SCHUSTER, W. und KREBS, H.: Haben Frisch- und Trockenzellen eine organ-spezifische Wirkung? Med. Klin. *54*, 1202–1206, 1959.

SCHMID, F. und STEIN, J.: Zellforschung und Zelltherapie, Verlag H. Huber. Bern – Stuttgart 1963.

SCHMID, F. und STEIN, I.: Cell Research and Cellular Therapy; Ott Publishers Thoune, Switzerland 1967.

SCHMID, R. G.: Cytochemischer Vergleich fetaler und maternaler Gewebe. Cytobiol. Rev. *2*, 2–10 (1978).

SCHMID, R. G.: Stoffwechselstörungen. Cytobiol. Rev. *3*, 151–154 (1979).

SCHMID, R. G.: Diagnostisch-therapeutische Probleme in der Betreuung cerebraler Anfallsleiden. Cytobiol. Rev. *5*, 76–78 (1981).

SCHMIDT, H.: Die bei Zellulartherapie in Betracht kommenden immunologischen Reaktionen. In F. Schmid und J. Stein: Zellforschung und Zellulartherapie. Verlag Huber, Bern 1963, S. 199–206.

– The Immunological Reactions in Cellular Therapy. In F. Schmid and J. Stein: Cell Research and Cellular Therapy. Ott Publishers Thoune, Switzerland, 1967, p. 206.

SCHNEIDER, H.: Immunreaktion, I. Pathomechanismen. Cytobiol. Rev. *3*, 139–148 (1979) II. Klink. Cytobiol. Rev. *4*, 45–54 (1980).

SCHNEIDER, H.: Die Überlebenszeit lebenswichtiger Organe. Cytobiol. Rev. *2*, 19, (1978).

SCHNEPPENHEIM, P. und GRÜNBERG, H.: Experimentelle Untersuchungen über die Wirkung von Nebennierenrinden-Trokkenzellen. Zschr. exper. Med., Berlin, *126*, 319–333, 1955.

SCHNITZER, A.: Untersuchungen mit fetalen Zellen beim chemisch induzierten Hautcarcinom des Kaninchens. Vortr. anl. d. 13. Arb. Tagg. d. Dt. Ges. f. ZT. 15.9. 1968.

SCHNITZER, A.: Wirkungsmechanismen bei der Zelltherapie. Cytobiol. Rev. *2*, Heft 4, 33–37 (1978).

SCHOLZ, K.: Zur Therapie des Morbus-Down-Syndroms im ersten und zweiten Lebensjahr. Ref. Blatt: Die Zelltherapie Nr. 40. Aug. 1973.

– Erfahrungen mit der Zelltherapie beim Morbus-Down-Syndrom. Ref. Blatt: Die Zelltherapie Nr. 41, 1974.

SCHREIBER, A.: Einflüsse von Injektionsimplantationen auf cerebrale Anfallsleiden. Ref. Blatt: Die Zelltherapie Nr. 41, 1964.

SCHREIER, K.: Die angeborenen Stoffwechselanomalien. Thieme-Verlag, Stuttgart 1979.

SCHUBERT, E. v.: Zur Therapie des Mongolismus. Ber. v. d. 6. Tagg. d. Arbeitsgem. f. Zellulartherapie, Bad Homburg, 9–12, 1957, Medizinische, Stuttgart, *40*, 1452–1454, 1957.

SCHUCK, W.: Biologische Behandlung von

Verbrennungen und Verbrühungen im Kindesalter. Cytobiol. Rev. *6*, 10–14 (1982).

SCHULTEN, H.: Wissenschaft als Gewissen des Arztes, dargestellt am Beispiel der Zellulartherapie. Mts. Kurse f. d. ärztl. Fortbildung, 9. 378–385, 1957.

SCHULTZE, H. E.: Immunitätslehre. Klin. Gegenw. *IX,* 423 (1960).

SCHÜTZE, E.: Wesen, Wert und Gefahren der Zellulartherapie. Ärztl. Forschg. München, X, 1/431–I/441, 1956.

S

SCOTT, R. B. et al.: Hypoplastic Anaemia treated by Transfusion of Foetal Haemopoietic Cells. Brit. Med. J., *2,* 1385–1388, 1961. Referiert: Selecta, *IV/9,* 11, 1962.

SEIDL, W.: Zellulartherapie bei neurologischen psychiatrischen Erkrankungen. Sammelmanuskript d. Referate d. I. Fortbildungskurses f. Zellulartherapie in Österr. I, 30–32, 1957.

– Die Pathobiologie der Schizophrenie und die Zelltherapie. Vortrag anl. d. I. Intern. Symp. f. Zell- und Histotherapie. Bad Ischl. Die Zell- und Histotherapie, I, *5/6,* 21–26, 1959.

SHELDON, W. H. und CALDWELL, I. B. H.: Die mononucleare Zellphase in der Entzündungsreaktion des Neugeborenen. Bull. Johns Hopk. Hosp. *112,* 258 (1963).

SHELDON, H. and KIMBALL, F. B.: Studies on cartilage. III. The occurence of collagen within vacuoles of the golgi apparatus. J. Cell Biol. *12,* 599 (1962).

SIEGMUND, H. D.: Reticulo-Endothel und aktives Mesenchym. Beitr. klin. Med. *1927* I.

SJÖSTRAND, F. S. and HANZON, V.: Membrane structures of cytoplasma and Mitochondria in exocrine cells of mouse pancreas as revealed by high resolution electron microsopy. Exp. Cell Res. *2,* 393 (1954).

SPITZNAGEL., J. K.: In Cell Biology 1976, s. ALTMANN und KATZ.

SPRADO, K.: Die Gefahren der Zellulartherapie. Dtsch. med. Wschr. *80,* 1262–1264, 1955.

– Die Frischzellentherapie, der Prügelknabe unter den umstrittenen Heilmethoden. Landarzt, Stuttgart. *34,* 161–164, 1958.

SPRADO, K.: Kombinationsbehandlung peripherer Durchblutungsstörungen. Hess. Ärzteblatt, 1, 10–12, 1958. Landarzt, Stuttgart, *33,* 452–456, 1957.

St

STEIN, J.: Immunological Reactions after Cellular Therapy. Symposium on Cellular Therapie. Cairo, 1960.

– Spezielle immunbiologische Probleme der heterologen Gewebeimplantation. In F. Schmid und J. Stein; Zellforschung und Zellulartherapie. Verlag Huber, Bern 1963, S. 207–218.

– Special Immunological Problems in the Implantation of Heterologous Tissues. In F. Schmid and J. Stein: Cell Research and Cellular Therapy. Ott Publishers Thoune, Switzerland, 1967, p. 214.

STEIN, J.: Die Implantation hämatopoetischer Gewebe als Therapie der Strahlenschäden. In F. Schmid and J. Stein: Zellforschung und Zellulartherapie. Verlag Huber, Bern 1963, S. 505.

– Grundlagen und Technik der Zelltherapie. Die Heilkunst, 84. Jg., Heft 10, Okt. 1971.

– Grundlagen und Entwicklung der Zelltherapie. Der Dt. Apotheker, 23. Jg., Heft 6, Juni 1971.

– Erfahrungen mit Zelltherapie. Ein Kongreßbericht – Haut-Verlag 1971. – Technik der Zelltherapie. Ref. Blatt: Die Zelltherapie Nr. 38, 1971.

– Gibt es etwas Neues in der Frischzellentherapie? Fragen aus der Praxis. Selecta Nr. 44, 1972. – Zelltherapie. Annabelle-Enzyklopädie. Nr. 38, Okt. 1972.

– Der Mensch und Arzt Paul Niehans. Bayrischer Rundfunk, Abt. Kirchenfunk, Titel: Besuch am Krankenbett, Febr. 1973.

STEIN, J.: Specific Effect of Implanted Endocrine Tissues. In F. Schmid and J. Stein: Cell Research and Cellular Therapy. Ott Publishers Thoune, Switzerland, 1967, p. 340.

STEIN, J.: Die Objektivierung organspezifischer Wirkung zellulärer Präparate. F. Schmid und J. Stein: Zellforschung und Zellulartherapie. Verlag Hubert, Bern 1963, S. 289.

STEIN, J.: Vitalität, Vitalitätseinbuße und Re-

435

vitalisierungstherapie. Die Heilkunst, Heft 11, Nov. 1972, 85. J.

STEIN, J.: Vitalität-Charakterisierung eines biologischen Phänomens. Cytobiol. Revue 3, 38–43 (1979).

STEIN, J.: Zellimplantationen bei Diabetes mellitus. Cytobiol. Rev. 6, 15–21 (1982)

STEIN, J.: Die Zelltherapie endokriner Dysfunktionen. Cytobiol. Rev. 6, 134–137 (1982).

STEINERT, P. M., IDLER, W. W. a. WANTZ, M. L.: Biochem. J. 187, 913–916 (1980).

STEININGER, U. und THEILE, H.: Funktionsdiagnostik im Kindesalter. Thieme-Verlag Stuttgart 1974.

STEPANTSCHITZ, G. und SCHREINER, B.: Erfahrungen mit der Siccacell-Therapie bei Gefäßerkrankungen. Therap. Umschau 10, 1956.

STEPANTSCHITZ, G. und SCHREINER, B.: Erfahrungen mit der Schilddrüsenimplantation bei Gelenkerkrankungen. Wien. Klin. Wschr., 981, 1952, Ref. Blatt Die Zelltherapie, 6, 10–11, 1955.

STICKL, H. und SCHMID, F.: Impfprobleme Problem-Impfungen. Dtsch. Ärzteverlag, Köln, 1975.

STOBB, R., THOMAS, E. D., BUCKNER, D. et al.: Marrow transplantation in untransfused patients with severe aplastic anemia. Blood 50: Suppl. 1, 316 (1977).

STÖWER, P.: Untersuchungen über die Einwirkung von Niehans-Trockenzellen auf regenerierendes Leber-Gewebe. Inaugural-Dissertation. Justus-Liebig-Hochschule, Gießen, Pharmakologisches Institut der Akademie für medizinische Forschung und Fortbildung 1956.

STÜHLINGER, H.: Erfahrungsbericht über 30 Jahre Zelltherapie. Cytobiol. Rev. 5, 171–173 (1981).

STUBBLEFIELD, E. and BRINKLEY, B. R.: Architecture and function of the mammalian centriole. In Warren, K. B. ed.: Formation and fate of cell organelles. Symp. internat. Soc. Cell Biol. 6, 175 (1967), Acad. Press, New York.

STURM, A.: Einfluß von Thyreoidea-Siccacellen auf den Jodstoffwechsel der Schilddrüse. Medizinische, Stuttgart, 47. 1634–1637, 1955.

SULMAN, F. G.: Objektivierung des Erfolges der Zelltherapie durch Neurohormon-Analyse vor und nach der Behandlung. Die Zelltherapie 43, 3–11 (1976).

SULMAN, F. G.: Neue Methoden zur Behandlung der Migräne. Cytobiol. Rev. 3, 108–116 (1979).

SUZUKI, K. et al.: Myelin and Multiple Sclerosis. Arch. Neurol. 28, 293–297 (1973).

T

TEIR, H. and RAVANTI, K.: Mitotic Activity and Growth Factors in the Liver of the white Rat. Exper. Cell. Res., 5, 500–507, 1953.

TIBURTIUS, H. und EHLING, U.: Ein Beitrag zur experimentellen Prüfung der Zellulartherapie bei einer erblichen Katarakt des Kaninchens. Klin. Mbl. für Augenheilkunde. Stuttgart, 134, 687–692, 1959.

TIBURTIUS, H. und KROKOWSKI, E.: Über Versuche, die Entstehung der Röntgenkatarakt des Kaninchens auf zellulartherapeutischem Wege zu beeinflussen. Graefes Arch. f. Ophth., 163, 572–546, 1961.

TISSIÈRES, A.: Ribosome Research: Historical Background. In Nomura, Tissières and Lengyel: Ribosomes. Cold Spring Harbor Laboratory 1974.

TODARO, G.J. and HUEBNER, R. J.: The viral oncogene hypothesis. Proc. nat. Acad. Sci. (Wash.) 69, 1009 (1972).

TOURAINE, J. L., MALIK, M. C., PERROT, H., MAIRE, I., REVILLARD, J. P., GROSSHANS, E. and TRAEGER, J.: Maladie de Fabry: deux malades améliorés par la greffe de cellules de foie foetal. Nouv. Presse Méd. 8, 1499–1503 (1979).

TRINCHER, K.: Das Krebsproblem in struktur-thermodynamischer Sicht. Cytobiol. Rev. 5, 114–121 (1981).

U

UHLENBRUCK, P.: Die Stoffwechseltherapie des Herzens. Münch. med. Wschr., 102, 859–864, 1960.

UHLENBRUCK, P.: Introduction. In F. Schmid and J. Stein: Cell Research and Cellular Therapy. Ott Publishers Thoune, Switzerland, 1967, p. 19.

ULLRICH, K.: Diabetes insipidus beim Hund. Deutsches Tierärzteblatt, *6/5,* 78, 1958.

UHRICH; K.: Bekämpfung des Alterns mit Injektionen von Aufschwemmungen tierischer Embryonen. Ärztl. Praxis, München, XI/43, 1529–1532, 1959.

V

VALLS CONFORTO, A.: The Dependency of Immunological Reactions on the Blood Content of Implants. In F. Schmid and J. Stein: Cell Research and Cellular Therapy. Ott Publishers Thoune, Switzerland, 1967, p. 239.

VAN HOLDE, K. D. and HILL, W. E.: General Physical Properties of Ribosomes, In: NOMURA, TISSIÈRES and LENGYEL: Ribosomes. Cold Spring Harbor Laboratory 1974, S. 53–92.

VELLEY, G. C.: Effects des injections de suspensions cellulaires et endocellulaires sur les organes greffés dans la chambre antérieure de l'œil. Bericht v. d. 5. Tagg. d. Forschungskreises f. ZT, 52–54, 1958.

VIDAL SAPRIZA, C. und GAYOSO, M.: Resultado de la implantacion de placenta en las arteriopatias obstructivas de los miembros inferiores. Biol. Soc. cir Uruguay, XXVII/6, 1956.

VORSTER, R.: Zur Siccacell-Behandlung von Amenorrhoe und Sterilität. Hippokrates, Stuttgart, *29,* 565 f., 1958.

VORLÄNDER, K. O.: Gefahren der Zellulartherapie. Fortschr. d. Med., *76,* 239–241, 1958.

VORLÄNDER, K. O., FITTING, W. und GIERLICH, G.: Der Einfluß heterologer Gewebszellen (Nierentrockenzellen nach Niehans) auf die Masugi-Nephritis der Ratte. Klin. Wschr., *32,* 1065–1073, 1954.

VOYNOW, P. and KURLAND, C. G.: Stoichiometry of the 30 S ribosomal proteins of Escherichia coli. Biochemistry *10,* 517, (1971).

W

WACKER, A.: Interferon-Induktion durch xenogenes Gewebe (Resistocell) Cytobiol. Rev. *6,* 182–183 (1982).

WAKSMAN, B. H., ARNASON B. G. and JANKOVIC, B. D.: Role of the thymus in immune reactions in rats. III. Changes in the lympoid organs of thymectomized rats J. exp. Med. *116,* 187 (1962).

WALDMANN, T. A., STROBER, W. and BLAESE, R. M.: Immundeficiency disease and malignancy. Ann. intern. Med. 77, 605 (1972).

WALLNÖFER, E.: Das Verhalten der Spontanaktivität und des Kollagens von Ratten nach s. c. Injektionen von Herzmuskelzellkernen oder Herzmitochondrien. Inaugural-Diss. Tierärztl. Hochschule Wien, 1973.

WARNATZ, H.: Immunsystem. In: Siegenthaler, Klinische Pathophysiologie. G. Thieme-Verlag, Stuttgart 1979.

WARNER, N. L., SZENBERG, A.: The Thymus in Immunbiology. Eds: R. A. Good, A. E. Gabrielson, Harper & Row, New York 1964.

WEISS, P. and TAYLOR, A. C.: Reconstitution of complete organs from single-cell suspensions of chick embryos in advanced stages of differentiation. Proceedings of the National Academy of Siences, Sciences, *46,* 1177–1185, 1960.

WESTPHAL, O.: Immunchemie. Springer, Berlin/Heidelberg/New York, 1965.

WIETEK, H. F. und TAUPITZ, E.: Der Einfluß lyophilisierter Placenta auf die experimentelle Arteriosklerose von Ratten. Arzneimitt.-Forsch., Aulendorf, *7,* 479–485, 1957.

– Der Einfluß von Siccacell-Placenta auf die experimentelle Arteriosklerose von Ratten. Bericht v. d. 4. Tagg. d. Forschungskreises f. Zellulartherapie 26–30, 1957.

WILHELM, J.: Das Verhalten von Hydroxyprolin, Succinodehydrogenase und Lipofuscin in verschiedenen Organen der Ratte nach s. c. Injektion von Herzmuskelzellkernen und Herzmitochondrien. Inaugural-Diss. Tierärztl. Hochschule Wien, 1973.

WITTE, S.: Klinische Erfahrungen mit der Knochenmarktransfusion. Dtsch. med. Wschr. *86,* 1334–1337, 1961.

– Die Behandlung der zytostatisch bedingten hämatologischen Nebenwirkungen durch Knochenmarktransfusion. Münch. med. Wschr. *102,* 1251–1253, 1960.

437

WOLF-JURGENSEN, P.: The basophilic leuko-cyte. Series haemat. I. Nr. *4*, (1968).

WOLF, N.: Zellulartherapie bei hirnatrophi-schen Prozessen des mittleren und reifen Lebensalters. Psychiatria et Neurologica, Basel. 152. 230–245, 1966. Möglichkeiten und Erfolge der Zelltherapie bei hirnatro-phischen Prozessen. Fortschr. Med. *87*, H. 15 (1969).

– Zelltherapie bei cerebralen Krankheitspro-zessen. Die Heilkunst, 84. Jg., Nr. 10. Ok-tober 1971.

WOLF, N.: Klinische Ergebnisse der Zellthe-rapie bei hirnatrophischen Prozessen des mittleren und reifen Lebensalters. Aktuelle Gerontol. *6*, 635–639 (1976).

WOLF, N.: Klinische Ergebnisse der Zellthe-rapie bei hirnatrophischen Prozessen des mittleren und reiferen Lebensalters. Cyto-biol. Rev. *1*, 21–23 (1977).

WOLF, N.: Der Begriff Vitalität aus psychia-trischer Sicht. Cytobiol. Rev. *2*, 13–16 (1978).

WOLF, N.: Bestätigung und Reproduzierbar-keit therapeutischer Ergebnisse. Cytobiol. Rev. *3*, 18–20 (1979).

WOLF, N.: Behandlungsergebnisse der Zell-therapie bei Patienten mit fortgeschritte-nen cerebralen Abbauerscheinungen. Cy-tobiol. Rev. *4*, 128–132 (1980).

WOLF, N. und HENNING, W.: Heterologe In-jektionsimplantationen bei hirnatrophi-schen Prozessen des mittleren und reifen Lebensalters. Verlaufsbeobachtungen aus psychologischer Sicht. Ref. Blatt Die Zell-therapie Nr. 36, 1969.

WORTMANN, F.: Serologische Untersuchun-gen bei einem Fall von Serumkrankheit nach Frischzell-Implantation. Dermatolo-gica. Basel. *117*, 428–432, 1958.

WRBA, H.: Die Wirkung von Organextrakten und -seren auf den Stoffwechsel von Or-gankulturen. Vortrag anl. d. Xème Con-grès International de Biologie Cellulaire. Pathologie-Biologie. 2. 581–583. 1961.

– Wachstumsfördernde Stoffe und Hemm-faktoren in Warmblütlergeweben (uniden-tifizierte humorale Regulationsstoffe). Na-turwissenschaften. *49,*97–101. 1962.

WRBA, H. und KALB. H. W.: Vergleich des Phosphatumsatzes embryonaler und adul-ter Organe in vitro. Naturwissenschaften, *46,* 405, 1959.

WÜNDISCH, g. F.: Behandlung der Panmyelo-pathie im Kindesalter durch Knochemark-transplantationen, Klin. Pädiatrie *189,* 50–59 (1977).

Y

YOKE, M. S. and SAINTE-MARIE, G.: Granu-locytopoiesis in the Rat Thymus. Brit. J. Haemat. *11,* 613 (1965).

YOUNG, Gordon: Doctors without Drugs. Frederick Muller Lim. London 1962.

– Conquest of Age. The extraordinary story of Dr. Paul Niehans. Rinehart u. Comp. New-York-Toronto 1959.

Z

ZABAKAS, G.: Vergleichende Untersuchun-gen über die Verteilung der spezifischen Aktivität in Organen der Ratte nach per-oraler Verabreichung von L.-Histidin-2,5-Tritium bzw. L-Lysin-4,5-Tritium. In-augural-Diss. Tierärztl. Hochschule Wien, 1968.

Zeitgeschichte: Down-Syndrom; Stellung-nahme der Deutschen Gesellschaft für Zelltherapie zu den Fragen zur Anhörung des Petitionsausschusses des Deutschen Bundestages am 7. 12. 1977. Cytobiol. Rev. *2,* 35–39 (1977).

ZELANDER, T.: Ultrastructure of articular car-tilage. Z. Zellforschg. *49,* 720 (1959).

ZELLER, W.: Entwicklungsdiagnostik und Entwicklungstherapie. Ber. v. d. 4. Tagg. d. Forschungskreises f. Zellulartherapie, 54–57, 1957.

ZUCKER-FRANKLIN, D.: The Properties of Eo-sinophils. In: BACH, M. K.: Immediate Hypersensitivity. Marcel Dekker Inc., New York and Basel 1978.

Index

VIP 299, 315
viral carcinogenesis 387
Virus infections 124
Vision, disturbances 294
Vitafestal 215, 302
Vitality 280
vital-stored, cells 94
Vitamins 235
Vitamin B1 213
Vitamin B6 213
Vitamins, Down-S. 214
Vitamin metabolism 253
Vitiligo 337
«Vitium cerebri» 257

W

Waldeyer's lymphatic glands 127
weak resistance 219
WILM's Tumour 106
WILM's-tumour tissue 393
WILSON's disease 253, 297

WISKOTT-ALDRICH-syndrome 168
Wobe-Mugos 216
Wobenzyme 216, 275, 302
WOLF-HIRSCHHORN-syndrome 208
WOLMAN, Morbus 184
Wound-healing 410
Wounds 346
Writing-disorders 260

X

xenogenic 91
xenogenous 113

Z

Zinc 86, 138, 146, 214, 235
Zn, in lyophil. tissues 85
Zone of migration 102
Zoonosis 204